Social Accountability of Medical Schools

Mohamed Elhassan Abdalla
Mohamed Hassan Taha • Charles Boelen
Editors

Social Accountability of Medical Schools

Empowering the Future of Medical Education and Healthcare Systems

Springer

Editors
Mohamed Elhassan Abdalla
School of Medicine University of Limerick
Limerick, Ireland

Charles Boelen
SCIEZ, France

Mohamed Hassan Taha
College of Medicine and Medical Education Center
University of Sharjah
Sharjah, UAE

ISBN 978-3-031-94434-5 ISBN 978-3-031-94435-2 (eBook)
https://doi.org/10.1007/978-3-031-94435-2

This Springer imprint is published by the registered company Springer Nature Switzerland AG
The registered company address is: Gewerbestrasse 11, 6330 Cham, Switzerland

Foreword

People's Needs, Health System Changes, and Medical Schools

The rich collection of experiences related to this book reflects some of the numerous endeavors around the world to steer health professional education towards improving health service delivery to every citizen in society. The gap between education and actual health service delivery is large. It may remain large unless educational institutions are led by a strategic commitment to create partnerships with other key stakeholders in the health system to optimize their combined impact on people's health. The "partnership pentagram" illustrates the concept of social accountability as an expectation of synergy to better serve people's health needs, through a common engagement to serve values such as quality of person-centered care, social justice, relevance to social determinants, and efficient use of resources.

Today and for some time in the future, health systems will face challenges in properly responding to the increased health needs and expectations from citizens and societies due to important demographic, political, socioeconomic, cultural, and environmental evolutions. We learned from history that the ambitious goal of universal health coverage can only be attained if each key health stakeholder is prepared to make important internal transformations and collaborate in joint operations with other external complementary forces.

This observation is explicitly confirmed by the last 2023 progress report of the United Nations "Sustainable Development Goals" strategy covering the period 2015–2030, comprising 17 goals, 4 of which being health specific and others with indirect influence on health. The report warns explicitly that goals would be attained **only** if measures are taken "… *to improve accountability of governments and other stakeholders*." In 1992, a paper published in *Academic Medicine* defined medical education as "*the science and art of preparing future physicians to function* *properly in society, which should imply responsibility for influencing circumstances and conditions under which they practice. To ensure durable impact of educational reforms, educational institutions must accept social accountability for their products.*"

As health practitioners and health professional educators, we are aware that changing a health system is a huge political undertaking due to inherent resistance to renewal along the long sequence of steps for relevant production of graduates, proper deployment of workforce, innovative practice models, interdisciplinary teamwork, and collaborative patterns with social and economic jurisdictions.

While acknowledging the complexity of the context, important thresholds have been crossed since the 1995 WHO definition of social accountability of medical schools as "an *obligation to direct their education, research, and service activities toward addressing the priority health concerns of the community, the region, or nation they have a mandate to serve. The priority health concerns are to be identified jointly by governments, healthcare organizations, health professionals and the public.*" The Global Consensus for Social Accountability of Medical Schools in 2010 brought a clearer vision of how to implement the concept by suggesting ten strategic directions.

Medical Education as a Gearwheel Toward Better Health

By becoming socially accountable institutions, medical schools will serve as models to other health professional schools, to academic institutions in general, and eventually to other stakeholders in the health system. Today, more than ever, medical education must be regarded not only as an instructional design but also as a strategy conveying a political vision by projecting which aptitudes the future physician should possess to meet society's needs, which mechanism to install for a better share of duties with other health and health-related professionals, and which innovative practice models to experiment within the healthcare delivery system to ensure newly acquired aptitudes of graduates are fully rewarded.

Along with such prospects, medical schools should establish collaborative links with health actors outside of their walls to assess in real life whether and how their investments do meet expectations, eventually by striving to attain specific priority health objectives within a defined territory. Subsequently, it is likely that such explicit engagement to improve people's well-being in the field may somehow lead to question the fundamental notion of "excellence" of any academic institution. Indicators of excellence used for accreditation purposes should not only explore the number of papers published in peer-reviewed journals or rewards for outstanding specialty achievements but also for innovative measures leading to sustainable impact on people's health status.

As one begins to realize that everyone and every institution must contribute to preserve our planet and people's well-being, and therefore accept some important cultural, social, economic, and political adjustments, principles of social accountability have gathered impetus worldwide. Readers will find inspiration from ideas and experiences proposed in this comprehensive book on ways to translate the concept of social accountability into meaningful institutional transformations and practical interventions and will therefore be encouraged to continue the wonderful voyage of discoveries for better mankind.

International consultant, Charles Boelen
Former coordinator of the WHO program
of human resources for health
SCIEZ, France

Preface

The global health landscape is evolving rapidly. Health inequities, shifting demographics, and rising public expectations call for medical schools to move beyond traditional education models. Social accountability offers a powerful framework for aligning medical education with the priority health needs of the communities we serve.

Social Accountability of Medical Schools: Empowering the Future of Medical Education and Healthcare Systems presents a comprehensive and practical guide for embedding social accountability into institutional structures, curricula, and partnerships. This book brings together global thought leaders, educators, and practitioners who have pioneered and implemented socially accountable practices in diverse settings. Their collective insights offer direction, tools, and evidence for action.

Developed with the involvement of more than 61 scholars from across the world, this book reflects deep expertise and wide-ranging perspectives in social accountability and health professions education. Contributors include medical educators, researchers, policy leaders, and institutional innovators who have led change in their own systems and collaborated globally to advance this agenda.

The book is organized into five structured parts, each focusing on a critical dimension of social accountability:

Part I—*Social Accountability: Concepts, Principles, and Social Obligation* lays the conceptual foundation by defining social accountability, exploring the profession's evolving role, and stressing the necessity of health sector partnerships. It includes Chap. 1: *Social Accountability in Medical Schools: Concepts, Principles, and Values*, Chap. 2: *The Evolving Role of the Medical Profession and Medical Graduates*, and Chap. 3: *Partnerships to Address Health Needs.*

Part II—*Leadership, Governance, and Institutional Alignment* focuses on leadership as a driver of change. It presents governance structures and faculty empowerment strategies essential for institutional transformation. It includes Chap. 4: *Governance and Leadership for Social Accountability* and Chap. 5: *Empowering Faculty in Socially Accountable Medical Schools.*

Part III—*Community Engagement and the Voice of Society* highlights the role of the community as a partner in co-creating educational relevance and equity. It includes Chap. 6: *The Role of the Community in Medical Education*, Chap. 7: *Engaging with Underserved Communities in the Curriculum*, and Chap. 8: *From Community-Oriented Medical Education to Social Accountability*.

Part IV—*Curriculum Reform for Social Accountability* explores how curriculum design and clinical training can integrate social accountability principles to prepare learners for real-world challenges. It includes Chap. 9: *The Role of Social Accountability in Re-envisioning Medical Education for the 21st Century*, Chap. 10: *Embedding Social Accountability into the Medical Curriculum: Strategies, Insights, and Real-World Applications*, and Chap. 11: *Longitudinal Clerkships to Promote Social Accountability*.

Part V—*Monitoring Outcomes and Measuring Impact* provides tools and approaches for evaluating progress, ensuring accountability, and sustaining long-term change through research and accreditation. It includes Chap. 12: *Socially Accountable Research: An Emerging Framework*, Chap. 13: *Social Accountability in Medical Schools: The Role of Participatory Health Research*, Chap. 14: *Appreciative Inquiry: Catalyzing Progress Towards Social Accountability*, Chap. 15: *Assessing Medical Schools' Compliance with Social Accountability Principles and Values*, and Chap. 16: *Social Accountability and Accreditation of Medical Schools*.

Across these chapters, you will find grounded case examples, reflective insights, and proven models from institutions that are actively reshaping health professions education. This book offers both inspiration and actionable guidance to educators, policymakers, and institutional leaders working to enhance social responsiveness in healthcare systems.

This book is more than a reference. It is a shared commitment and call to action for those determined to align medical education with the health and dignity of all communities.

Limerick, Ireland — Mohamed Elhassan Abdalla
Sharjah, UAE — Mohamed Hassan Taha
SCIEZ, France — Charles Boelen

Contents

About the Editors and Contributors

About the Editors

Mohamed Elhassan Abdalla, MBBS, MSc, PhD, FAcadMEd Dr. Mohamed Elhassan Abdalla is a distinguished leader in Health Professions Education with a career spanning multiple countries and continents. He is Associate Professor of Medical Education at the School of Medicine, University of Limerick, Ireland. A graduate of the Faculty of Medicine at the University of Gezira, Sudan, Dr. Abdalla furthered his education with a master's and PhD in Health Professions Education and is a Fellow of the Academy of Medical Educators (FAcadMEd), UK.

Dr. Abdalla's professional journey reflects a steadfast commitment to aligning medical education with the health needs of communities. He has contributed significantly to the field in Sudan, Saudi Arabia, the UAE, and Ireland, as well as through collaborations in other regions. His leadership in social accountability was recognized with the prestigious Charles Boelen International Award on Social Accountability in 2024.

His affiliations with international organizations, including The Network: Towards Unity for Health (TUFH), the International Reference Group on Social Accountability of Medical Schools, and the Association of Medical Education in the Eastern Mediterranean Region, exemplify his global influence. His research interests span social accountability, teaching and learning, accreditation, and cost and value in Health Professions Education, with numerous impactful publications in these areas.

Mohamed Hassan Taha, MBBS, PhD, FAcadMEd, FAMEE Dr. Mohamed Hassan Taha is an inspirational leader in medical and health professions education. He is known for his transformative vision of linking education to health systems to ensure relevance and improve population health outcomes. With over 15 years of experience, he has consistently driven innovation, collaboration, and social accountability in healthcare education. Dr. Taha is currently the Director of the Medical Education Center and Coordinator of the Master of Leadership in Health Professions

Education at the University of Sharjah, UAE. His leadership extends globally as a Board Director for the EMRO Region at The Network: Towards Unity for Health (TUFH), a member of the ASPIRE Award Panel for Excellence in Health Professions Education in collaboration and partnership, and a member of the AMEE Postgraduate Committee. Throughout his career, Dr. Taha has led curriculum reforms and contributed to developing competency frameworks such as EmiratesMEDs, ensuring healthcare professionals are prepared to meet societal needs. Dr. Taha is a fellow of the Academy of Medical Educators (FAcadMEd) and the International Association for Medical Education (FAMEE). Dr. Taha's work focuses on creating strong linkages between education and health systems. Through research, mentorship, and international collaborations, he empowers future healthcare leaders to drive impactful change and improve healthcare delivery worldwide.

Charles Boelen, MD, DPH, MSC Charles Boelen is a medical doctor (Belgium), specialized in public health (University of Montreal), epidemiology (McGill University), health system management (Harvard and Stanford Universities), and the education of health professionals (University of Paris XIII).

During his thirty years working at the World Health Organization headquarters, regional and country offices, and afterwards as an independent consultant, he developed human resources development strategies with national health and academic authorities in several spots around the world.

His best known works are the creation of the Five-Star-Doctor model, the WHO strategy document Towards Unity for Health, the WHO monograph Defining and Measuring the Social Accountability of Medical Schools, the WHO-UNESCO report "Universities and Health of the Disadvantaged," and the Global Consensus for Social Accountability of Medical Schools.

About the Contributors

Ahmed Maherzi, MD A graduate of the Faculty of Medicine at the University of Tunis El Manar, Dr. Ahmed Maherzi is a pediatrician and was Dean of the Faculty from 2011 to 2017. He is currently a professor in the Faculty of Medicine at the Université de Montréal, where he is Director of the Social Accountability Office. Dr. Maherzi is President of the Strategic Council of the International Conference of Deans and Faculties of Medicine of French-speaking Countries (CIDMEF) and Secretary General of the International Francophone Network for Social Accountability in Health (RIFRESS). He received AFMC-Charles Boelen International Social Accountability Award in 2016 and 2023.

Amy Clithero-Eridon, PhD, MBA Amy Clithero-Eridon is a faculty member in the Department of Family & Community Medicine (FM) at the University of New Mexico School of Medicine. Dr. Clithero-Eridon has a PhD in FM from the University of Kwazulu-Natal in Durban, South Africa; a Master of Business

Administration; and a Master's level certification in Medical Education from the University of New Mexico. In addition to teaching medical students about social determinants of health, health policy, and health services research, Dr. Clithero-Eridon participates in numerous educational research initiatives focusing on educational best practices, health services research, and social accountability within medical education.

Andrew O'Regan, MBBCH, BAO, MICGP, MMedSc, PhD Dr. Andrew O'Regan is a general practitioner and associate professor of general practice. He has played a leading role in the Longitudinal Integrated Clerkship (LIC) at the University of Limerick since 2014. In 2022, he chaired the organization committee for the international consortium of Longitudinal Integrated Clerkships conference in Limerick. The focus of Dr. O'Regan's educational involvement and his research is to ensure delivery of high-quality education whereby students are exposed to all the clinical disciplines in community settings and to foster environments where students can thrive and gain experiences and mentoring relationships that will nurture professional and personal development.

Anne MacFarlane, BA, MA, PhD. Anne is Founder and Co-Director of the Participatory Health Research Unit, School of Medicine, University of Limerick. The Unit is a designated WHO Collaborating Centre for Refugee and Migrant Involvement in Health Research.

Anne is a social scientist with more than 25 years' experience in interdisciplinary, inter-agency primary healthcare research with extensive success in funding competitions and international peer-reviewed publications. Her primary focus is on individual and collective involvement in health decision-making, with specialist expertise in refugee and migrant involvement in decisions about their health.

Anne is an active leader in projects with the WHO, the International Collaboration for Participatory Health Research, and the North American Primary Care Research Group. Her current research interests include the sociological concept of space and how this can enhance understanding of participatory spaces in health.

Anthony Fleg, MD, MPH Anthony Fleg is a family medicine physician at UNM in the Department of Family and Community Medicine and the College of Population Health. Originally from Baltimore, Anthony grounds his healing work in undoing racism, health equity, and with a focus on strengths and holistic health. He also co-founded the Native Health Initiative (NHI), a love grounded partnership, and has dedicated much of his career to improving health in Indigenous communities. Social accountability (of academia, health professions education, conferences, etc.) is a central aspect of his work.

Arindam Sarkar, MD Arindam "Rindy" Sarkar, MD, FAAFP, is a board-certified family physician and an assistant professor at the Baylor College of Medicine. As director of medical student education, Rindy is passionate about delivering high-quality primary care to underserved patients and designing evidenced-based curricula for diverse trainees. His research interests include resistant hypertension and educational innovations to overcome healthcare disparities.

Arthur Kaufman, MD Dr. Kaufman is Distinguished Professor of Family and Community Medicine and Vice President for Community Health. His focus is upon the role of academic health centers in partnering with communities to address adverse social determinants of health including income, education, housing, transportation, food, and safety. The strategy is to create Health Extension Hubs in every county and Tribal community, bringing the resources of the University to the front door of communities. Health Extension agents and Community Health Workers create new community resources. Success is measured by improvement of health in communities, driven by community leadership, priority-setting, and capacity-building.

Bernhard Gaede, MBBCh, MMed(FamMed), PhD Bernhard Gaede is a family physician currently appointed as Associate Professor and Head of Family Medicine at UKZN. Prior to joining the University, he worked in rural hospital settings for well over a decade, the bulk of it in the Bergville area, KwaZulu-Natal. He was deeply involved in the setting up of the anti-retroviral treatment program in the mid-2000s, working with traditional healers, home-based carers, and community structures. He remains engaged in research in healthcare systems, particularly community-level care. In health professional education, he has become increasingly involved in curriculum development, particularly for the medical program, distributed training, and community engagement.

Bridget Kiely, MB BCh BAO, PhD Dr. Bridget Kiely is a GP and Senior Clinical Lecturer in the Department of General Practice in RCSI. She has qualifications in public health, tropical medicine, and clinical leadership. After a brief stint in infectious diseases, she trained as a GP in London. After qualification she worked in Sierra Leone for two years during and after the Ebola epidemic. On return to Ireland, Bridget was the clinical lead in migrant health for a charity providing primary care to marginalized groups and taught on a GP training scheme focused on preparing GPs to work in underserved areas. She completed her PhD on social prescribing in areas of deprivation. Clinically, she works in a GP practice in an underserved diverse urban area.

Cassandra Barber, MA, PhD Dr. Cassandra Barber is a trained demographer and an accomplished researcher, educator, and consultant specializing in health professions education and social accountability. She holds a master's degree in sociology, with a focus on migration and ethnic relations, and earned her PhD from the School of Health Professions Education (SHE) at Maastricht University. Dr. Barber uses a multidisciplinary approach to quantify social problem, with a focus on advancing social accountability in health professions education. Her research explores how large-scale data can reveal connections between educational outcomes and population health, identifying opportunities for systemic improvement.

Charles Boelen, MD, DPH, MSC Charles Boelen is a medical doctor (Belgium), specialized in public health (University of Montreal), epidemiology (McGill University), health system management (Harvard and Stanford Universities), and the education of health professionals (University of Paris XIII).

During his thirty years working at the World Health Organization headquarters, regional and country offices, and afterwards as an independent consultant, he developed human resources development strategies with national health and academic authorities in several spots around the world.

His best known works are the creation of the Five-Star-Doctor model, the WHO strategy document Towards Unity for Health , the WHO monograph Defining and Measuring the Social Accountability of Medical Schools, the WHO-UNESCO report "Universities and Health of the Disadvantaged," and the Global Consensus for Social Accountability of Medical Schools.

Damaris Kiewiets I am the Community Liaison Officer in the Community Engagement Unit_UWC. I am an adult facilitator and learner. I am a passionate health and human rights activist. I was recognized for my work as an activist in 2019. I have held leadership roles in different fields over 3 decades.

David Blane, BSc, MBChB, MPH, PhD David is a GP in Glasgow, Scotland, and Senior Clinical Lecturer at the University of Glasgow. He has been involved in teaching, research, and advocacy related to the social determinants of health since 2010, and is Academic Lead for the "Scottish Deep End Project," a collaboration between academic and frontline practitioners working in the most socioeconomically disadvantaged communities in Scotland. There are now 20 Deep End groups spanning 9 countries and 4 continents. His research explores the role of primary care in mitigating health inequalities. David received the RCGP John Fry Award in 2024.

Debra Klamen, MD, MHPE Debra L. Klamen, MD, MHPE, FAPA, is Professor and Chair of the Department of Medical Education at SIU School of Medicine. She is also the Senior Associate Dean for Education and Curriculum. Dr. Klamen earned her Bachelor's Degree in Genetics at the University of Illinois at Champaign-Urbana, and her medical degree at the University of Chicago–Pritzker School of Medicine. She completed a Psychiatric residency at the University of Illinois at Chicago. She completed a Master's of Health Professional Education at the University of Illinois at Chicago in 1998, and was named a Fellow of the American Psychiatric Association in 1999. Dr. Klamen serves on the Communication Task Force of the National Board of Medical Examiners and has developed and implemented a qualitatively different third year of medical school. Dr. Klamen has written numerous articles on medical school education, particularly in the area of performance evaluation and assessment. She has spoken extensively on the topic of stress management for physicians around the country. She was the author of SIUSOM's successful application for the social accountability ASPIRE award.

Dervla Kelly, PhD Dr. Dervla Kelly is Associate Professor of Medical Education at the University of Limerick and a practicing community pharmacist. She is a leading expert in social pharmacy, with research focused on the societal role of medicines, emerging drug trends, and over-reliance on pharmaceuticals. Since 2018, she has contributed to the University of Limerick's BMBS program, especially in Years 1 and 2. Her responsibilities include problem-based learning (PBL) case development, curriculum review, tutor training, student support, and assessment.

She has a strong background in evidence synthesis, quantitative epidemiological methods, and qualitative research. Her scholarly work in medical education also covers professional identity formation, the assessment of professionalism, and the integration of pharmacy perspectives into medical training. She bridges clinical practice with academic scholarship, contributing to interprofessional education and health systems awareness.

Dina-Ruth Lulua, MBBCh, PG Dr. Dina-Ruth Ayikoru Lulua is an African doctor and medical educationalist who holds an MBBCh and Master's in Health Science Education. She has worked in academic medicine, across institutions, in various roles. Currently, she is the Head of the MBChB program, in the Faculty of Health Sciences, at the University of Cape Town (UCT); in this role she provides strategic leadership for the globally recognized medical curriculum. Dr. Lulua is an emerging researcher, who has presented work locally and internationally, winning awards for her work as well as her leadership. She currently leads multiple research projects and is framing a transdisciplinary PhD.

Erin Cameron, PhD Dr. Cameron is Associate Professor of Medical Education at the Northern Ontario School of Medicine University (NOSMU) in Thunder Bay, Canada, and the inaugural Academic Director of the Dr. Gilles Arcand Centre for Health Equity (formerly the Centre for Social Accountability). As a mid-career educational scientist, Dr. Cameron's research focuses on social justice pedagogies and practices that support the transformation of local education and health systems. In addition to an active research program, Dr. Cameron holds numerous national and international leadership roles with the Association of Faculties of Medicine in Canada (AFMC), the Réseau international francophone pour la responsabilité sociale en santé, and the International Steering Committee of Social Accountability and Accreditation.

Erin Bouquin, MD Dr. Bouquin's work as a physician has centered in communities. She has always held an interest and involvement in global health. She completed her residency at the US-Mexico Border and gained a better understanding of the intersectionality of medicine and healthcare. After her residency she concentrated on direct patient care. She held positions of oversight of other clinicians in direct patient care. Through those positions, she developed skills in teaching clinicians in an interprofessional environment since coming to the University of New Mexico. She is currently the Director of Clinical Preceptorships at the University of

New Mexico School of Medicine. She develops opportunities for clinical immersion and community engagement in rural and underserved communities.

Ghislaine Attema, MA, BEd, PhD(c) Ghislaine Attema is a PhD candidate in the Faculty of Education at Lakehead University, a Researcher at the Arcand Centre at NOSM University, and the Social Accountability Fellowship Coordinator for The Network: Towards Unity for Health (TUFH). Ghislaine's doctoral research focuses on social accountability, teaching, and faculty development and is supported by an SSHRC Banting Doctoral Research Award. Ghislaine is a passionate advocate for teaching, northern and rural communities, and improving access to quality education. She is a mother to three amazing daughters, and calls Thunder Bay, Ontario, Canada, home.

Hannah Herring, BS Hannah Herring is a graduate of the University of New Mexico Biology department and a member of the 2026 MD class. She served as the advocacy chair for the Health Advocacy Initiative of New Mexico, the student conference chair for the National Learning Communities Institute, and was awarded the prestigious Summer Oncology Research Fellowship at the University of Southern California in partnership with the Los Angeles Children's Hospital. She is passionate about creating medical education that leads to quality healthcare for all New Mexicans and the role of physicians in statewide advocacy.

Heidi Honegger Rogers, DNP, FNP-C, APHN-BC Heidi Honegger Rogers is a family nurse practitioner and an advanced practice holistic nurse. She is an associate professor at the University of New Mexico (UNM) College of Nursing. She is a Senior Fellow in Planetary Health with the UNM center for health equity, planetary health, and preparedness and is on the leadership team for UNM's Accelerating Resilience in Drylands institute. She was the Director of Interprofessional Education for the UNM Health Sciences Center 2018–2024 and remains a guide on the IPE team. Her advocacy and scholarship centers in climate change and health, equity and justice, nature connection, well-being, planetary health, and interprofessional education.

Jessica Jurgutis, PhD Jessica is the Manager of the Dr. Gilles Arcand Centre for Health Equity at the Northern Ontario School of Medicine University. Her research and advocacy work are shaped by a commitment to transformative approaches to health equity and health research and by addressing health access and outcome disparities as a feature of settler colonial and carceral violence. Prior to joining the Arcand Centre, Jessica held an academic position at Lakehead University, where she was cross-appointed between the Departments of Gender & Women's Studies, Indigenous Learning, and the Social Justice MA Program. Jessica holds a PhD in Political Science from McMaster University and is a trained Walls-to-Bridges facilitator.

Joseph LeBlanc, PhD Dr. Joseph LeBlanc serves as Associate Dean of Equity and Inclusion and Assistant Professor of Indigenous Health. He is a member of Wiikwemkoong Unceded Territory and a prominent leader in Indigenous health and social accountability in medical education in Canada. He holds a senior advisory role at the Association of Faculties of Medicine of Canada (AFMC), where he oversees the implementation of strategies related to equity, anti-racism, Indigenous health, Francophone inclusion, and planetary health. Dr. LeBlanc has received multiple national awards for his leadership, including the Top 20 under 40 Northwestern Ontario Visionary Award and the Forty under 40 Northern Ontario Business Award. He is widely respected for his community-based approach to health education, with special emphasis on Indigenous food systems, sustainability, and social justice. He brings a strong voice to national conversations on health equity, and his work continues to shape inclusive and community-driven frameworks in Canadian medical schools.

Jyotsna Rimal, MDS, (PhD) Dr. Jyotsna Rimal is an academic with over 20 years' experience in higher education in Nepal. Currently pursuing a PhD in Social Accountability in Medical Education at Griffith University, Australia, she is recognized for her leadership in health professions education and expertise in oral health. As Senior Fellow of the Higher Education Academy (HEA) and FAIMER Fellow, Dr. Rimal has demonstrated commitment to advancing educational standards and promoting social responsibility in medical training. Her career is marked by extensive teaching, curriculum development, and mentorship, making significant contributions to health professions education and shaping future healthcare professionals.

Karen Johnston, PhD, BSc Karen is an early career researcher with a strong interest in advancing health equity through health systems strengthening. Karen is an evidence group member (and formerly research coordinator) for the Training for Health Equity Network (THEnet) which is an international community of practice with a shared mandate for social accountability in health professions education. She currently coordinates the THEnet Graduate Outcomes Study. This is an international longitudinal study being conducted by THEnet partner schools that investigates practice intentions during medical school and outcomes of socially accountable medical education.

Kerri Z. Delaney, PhD Dr. Kerri Delaney is a postdoctoral fellow in knowledge translation at the Dr. Gilles Arcand Centre for Health Equity. Their work is a part of the CREATE Project and focuses on understanding socially accountable research.

Kevin Schroeder, DAT, LAT, ATC, FNAP Kevin M. Schroeder, DAT, LAT, ATC, FNAP, is an experienced athletic trainer, clinical education coordinator, and Director of the University of New Mexico's Interprofessional Education (IPE) Program. With a focus on enhancing collaboration across healthcare disciplines, Kevin integrates principles of social accountability into IPE initiatives to prepare healthcare learners to address community needs effectively. Drawing from his clinical expertise in NCAA sports, military, and Olympic settings, he fosters innovative educational experiences that emphasize teamwork, equity, and community impact. Kevin's leadership ensures that healthcare education aligns with the evolving demands of diverse populations while promoting excellence in interprofessional collaboration.

Kristin Markle, MS, BA Kristin is a fourth-year medical student, with bachelor's degree in biochemistry and a master's degree in bioinformatics. She is the first student with a diagnosed hearing disability to be admitted to the University of New Mexico School of Medicine. She has worked with school leadership, faculty, and staff to change policies related to the basic sciences and clinical curriculum to support students who have disabilities. She has presented her advocacy work at medical educational conferences and in publications.

Lindsey Yelton, B.S., B.A., MD Lindsey is a former Air Force Aerospace/Surgical Technician who received multiple awards; while in active duty, she was nominated for the STFM Conference on Medical Student Education Student Scholarship and was the recipient of the La Tierra Sagrada Scholarship in 2022. She has been on the Dean's Honor List at New Mexico State University numerous times and was a Howard Hughes Medical Research Scholar from 2006 to 2008. She has mentored peers and children in Africa affected by AIDS. She is an avid contributor to the community through various community service projects and has sat on the Albuquerque Early Head Start Policy Council.

Lionel Green-Thompson, MBBCh, PhD C-authored the ASSAf Consensus Report: Reconceptualising health professions education in South Africa. A specialist anesthesiologist who completed a PhD in 2014 on the nature of social accountability in South African medical education and practice. Chairperson of the SA Committee of Medical Deans (SACOMD:2022 -2023). Currently co-chairing a National Steering Committee on development of workplace-based assessments for specialist medical education. Interests include professional identity formation, transformative education, and social accountability.

Board membership: Rural Health Advocacy Project (RHAP) and Towards Unity for Health (TUFH) where he is Vice Secretary General for TUFH in the term 2023–2027. Currently serves on the AMEE Research Committee, chairing the Network for Medical Education in Resource Constrained Environments (MERCS). Co-chairs the International Social Accountability Accreditation Steering Committee (ISAAC).

Marlene P. Ballejos, PhD Dr. Ballejos is a dedicated advocate for integrating social justice and advocacy into medical school admissions. In 2021, she served on the AAMC Group on Student Affairs/Group on Diversity and Inclusion (GSA/GDI) Workgroup on Advocacy and Social Justice in Admissions. Their efforts focused on equipping the admissions community with tools to recognize and value applicants' experiences through an advocacy and social justice lens. Dr. Ballejos led workshops at regional and national meetings and provided guidance on incorporating these principles into interview and secondary application processes, fostering a more equitable admissions landscape that aligns with the values of diversity and inclusion.

Maxwell Kennel, BA, MTS, PhD Dr. Maxwell Kennel is affiliated with the Dr. Gilles Arcand Centre for Health Equity NOSM University, and the Canadian Institute of Far-Right Studies. He is the Director of Pandora Press and editor of its Anabaptist and Mennonite Studies series. His work concerns social bonds of public trust between secularity and religion, and he is the author of *Postsecular History* (Palgrave, 2022) and *Ontologies of Violence* (Brill, 2023) and editor of *Astrid von Schlachta's Anabaptists: From the Reformation to the 21st Century* (Pandora, 2024). His work on Social Accountability is featured in the Fall 2024 issue of the *Social Innovations Journal.*

Melissa Torbey, MHA Melissa Torbey is a medical student at the University of New Mexico, with a Master's in Health Administration (2023) and a Bachelor's in Kinesiology (2021) from the University of Wisconsin-Madison. With a focus on health equity and social accountability, Melissa has conducted research exploring the effects of adverse childhood experiences (ACEs) on children with special healthcare needs and assessing patient-centered care models for post-stroke patients. Her volunteer work with Salud Morena highlights her dedication to creating educational programs and promoting health equity, emphasizing her commitment to improving outcomes for underserved populations.

Mohamed Elhassan Abdalla, MBBS, MSc, PhD, FAcadMEd Recipient of Charles Boelen International Award on Social Accountability 2024. Graduated with an MBBS from the Faculty of Medicine, University of Gezira, Sudan, and then got a master's and PhD degrees in Health Professions Education. He is a fellow of the Academy of Medical Educators, UK.

He has work experience in Medical Education in Sudan, Saudi Arabia, the United Arab Emirates, and Ireland with contributions to Medical Education in other different countries.

Dr. Mohamed Elhassan has memberships and affiliations to regional and international organizations that work in Health Professions Education such as the Network-TUFH, International Reference Group on Social Accountability of Medical Schools, the Association of Medical Education in the Eastern Mediterranean Region, and the Society of Cost and Value in Health Professions Education.

Dr. Mohamed Elhassan's publications and research interests in Medical Education are in the areas of social accountability, teaching and learning, accreditation, and cost and value.

Mohamed Hassan Taha, MBBS, PhD, FAcadMEd, FAMEE Dr. Mohamed Hassan Taha, MBBS, PhD, FAcadMEd, FAMEE, is an expert in Medical and Health Professions Education with over 15 years of experience. He serves as Assistant Professor and Director of the Medical Education Center at the University of Sharjah. Dr. Taha is Fellow of AMEE and the Academy of Medical Educators (UK) and holds leadership roles in curriculum development, faculty training, and social accountability. He collaborates with AMEE and TUFH, contributing to global advancements in Health Professions Education through research, publications, and workshops.

Mohi Eldin Magzoub, MD MSc PhD MFPHM Prof. Magzoub is currently the Chair of the Department of Medical Education, College of Medicine and Health Sciences United Arab Emirates University. Graduated in 1984 from the Faculty of Medicine University of Gezira in the Sudan, he obtained a Master's from London University and PhD in Health Professions Education from Maastricht University in 1994. He published a number of articles in Community-based education which is very relevant to social accountability.

Mona S. Ghaly, MD Mona S. Ghaly is Professor of Rheumatology and Rehabilitation at the Faculty of Medicine, Suez Canal University (FOM/SCU). She previously served as the Vice Dean for Students and Educational Affairs at FOM/SCU from 2018 to 2022. Currently, she holds the position of Vice Dean for Students and Educational Affairs at the Faculty of Medicine, Delta University, a private institution.

Dr. Ghaly is an experienced reviewer for the National Authority for Quality Assurance and Accreditation in Education (NAQAAE) in Egypt and also serves as an external reviewer for the National Center for Academic Accreditation and Assessment (NCAAA) in the Kingdom of Saudi Arabia.

Her areas of interest include quality assurance and accreditation, assessment, and social accountability. She has authored three publications focusing on social accountability.

Natalie Reid, MS4 Natalie is an MS4 at the University of New Mexico School of Medicine and is currently pursuing a career in emergency medicine. She has a specific interest in the intersections between rural, global, and underserved patient populations. She is passionate about creating medical education that uses a social accountability framework to better train physicians to serve these patient populations.

Natasha Dark, BS I am a third-year medical student who co-pioneered a student charter, The Healthcare Advocacy Initiative of New Mexico (HAINM), and created ancillary curriculum opportunities for training in healthcare advocacy and policy-making. I am also a Social Mission Alliance 2024 Health Justice Scholar. I am working on policymaking to protect LGBTQ+ civil rights in New Mexico (NM), as well as advocate for enactment of more comprehensive anti-discriminatory laws in healthcare access in NM. I am also planning the 2025 annual "Med-Law-Psych Day" for case-based interprofessional learning opportunities for medical, law, and psychology students at the UNM Law School.

Nicholas Torres, MEd Nicholas Torres is a seasoned and successful Business, Healthcare and Human Services Executive with over 25 years of experience in C-suite executive leadership, serving in CEO and C-Suite Consulting roles throughout his career in startup, small, and large social sector organizations. Nicholas works at the cross section between the private sector, government, and not-for-profits aligning them toward action on mutually agreed upon strategies and goals. He has designed, founded, and led and managed multiple for-profit, not-for-profit, and cross-organization/system social ventures that are driven by social impact, financial sustainability, and systems change.

Nicholas serves as President of The Network: Towards Unity for Health (TUFH) a non-state actor in official relations with the World Health Organization (WHO); CEO of Social Innovations Partners that publishes the Social Innovations Journal and oversees regional Social Innovations Awards process to drive financial capital to community changemakers; and Faculty at the Fels Institute of Government and Social Policy School at the University of Pennsylvania.

Patrick O'Donnell, MB BCh BAO, MICGP, MSc, PhD Dr. Patrick O'Donnell is General Practitioner who specializes in inclusion health, and he is also Associate Professor of General Practice at the University of Limerick School of Medicine. He has completed his PhD and an associated body of research on social exclusion and health. He is involved in the education and training of undergraduate and postgraduate students in the healthcare professions on topics relating to inclusion health. He has also established and managed primary care services for a range of vulnerable and socially excluded patients across the Mid-West of Ireland.

Pearl Huynh Pearl Huynh is currently a third-year medical student at the University of New Mexico School of Medicine, pursuing her Doctor of Medicine degree. She graduated summa cum laude from the University of New Mexico with a Bachelor of Arts in Health, Medicine, and Human Values, complemented by minors in Chemistry and Psychology. Pearl is deeply committed to mentorship and community engagement, working with underrepresented students and providing healthcare services in underserved communities. Her accolades underscore her dedication to academic excellence and impactful leadership. She is also fluent in Vietnamese, reflecting her commitment to cultural competency in medicine.

Prattama Santoso Utomo, MD, MHPEd Prattama is Assistant Professor in the Department of Medical Education and Bioethics, Faculty of Medicine, Public Health and Nursing, Universitas Gadjah Mada, Indonesia. He is an International FAIMER Institute (IFI) faculty. He was involved in his institution's social accountability task force, and was also part of The Network: TUFH's ISAT team. His research interest is in health professions education and general medicine, particularly social accountability in medical education, teaching-learning in medicine, programmatic assessment, and interprofessional education. He is currently pursuing a PhD in Higher Education with concentration in Health Professions Education, with research focus on social accountability of medical education, at Warner School of Education, University of Rochester, USA.

Robert Woollard, MD, CCFP, FCFP, LM, DHC (Laval) Dr. Woollard is Professor Emeritus of Family Practice at the University of British Columbia, with extensive national and international experience in medical education, social accountability in medical schools, ecosystem health approaches, and sustainable development. He holds leadership positions in several national and international organizations and chairs the IAB of the newly established University of Nepal, a public liberal arts university. His work in East Africa and Asia focuses on social accountability, primary care, rural health, and accreditation systems.

Robyn Preston, BA, PhD Robyn Preston is Senior Lecturer, Public Health at CQUniversity, Queensland, Australia. She is a public health-focused social scientist specializing in qualitative (ethnography, PAR, case study) and mixed-methods research. Dr. Preston's research focuses on access to health and community services for prioritized communities (First Nations; refugees; regional, rural, and remote peoples); Rural Home-based Aged Care; and Socially Accountable Health Professional Institutions. She was an inaugural member of the evaluation and research group of the Training for Health Equity Network (THEnet). Robyn's PhD analyzed how contextual issues influenced social accountability at four medical schools in the Philippines and Australia.

Roger Strasser, MBBS, FRACGP, FACRRM, FCAHS Between 2002 and 2019, Prof. Roger Strasser was NOSM Founding Dean and CEO. He is a leader in the global reform of rural health professional education and research. Recognizing the importance of context and community in medical education and research, Professor Strasser has become one of the world's foremost authorities on rural, socially accountable medical education, and a sought-after speaker and advisor.

Prior to 2002, Roger Strasser was Professor of Rural Health and Head of the Monash University School of Rural Health in Australia and had an international role with the World Organization of Family Doctors (WONCA) as inaugural Chair of the Working Party on Rural Practice from 1992 to 2004.

Rukhsana Zuberi, MHPE, FCPS, MBBS Prof. Rukhsana Zuberi is a senior faculty member at Aga Khan University Medical College in Pakistan with over 35 years of experience in health professions education. She earned her MHPE from the University of Illinois at Chicago and is a Fellow of the College of Physicians and Surgeons Pakistan. She has held multiple leadership roles including Associate Dean for Education, Chair of the Department for Educational Development, and Founding Interim Director of the Center for Innovation in Medical Education (CIME). She currently chairs the university-wide Committee for Strategic Planning for Competency-Based Medical Education (CBME). Her academic contributions include developing and evaluating assessment systems, advancing clinical competence evaluation, and integrating PBL into medical curricula. She is also a longstanding member of the Ethics Review Board and plays a key role in institutional and national policy development related to medical education reform.

Saad Chahine, PhD Saad Chahine, PhD, is Associate Professor and Research Integrity Officer at Queen's University. He is also the founder and director of

Metrein Inc., an assessment, research, and evaluation organization dedicated to using data for meaningful change. Saad has been a teacher, researcher, and evaluator focused on improving policy and practice, with a particular emphasis on health professions education. With over 20 years of experience, he has published more than 50 research papers and consulted across K-12, higher education, regulatory bodies, and NGOs.

Samantha Longley, BSc, BA I grew up in the suburbs of Chicago but have been living in NM for almost a decade. I am from a multiracial family and NM is the first place where I finally felt like we fit in. Diversity is celebrated and something to take pride in. I received my BA and BSc from the University of New Mexico. I'm proud to say that I am attending the University of New Mexico School of Medicine. I look forward to giving back to the state that welcomed me with open arms.

Sarah Larkins, MBBS, BMedSci, MPH&TM, PhD Prof. Sarah Larkins is Dean, College of Medicine and Dentistry at James Cook University, and Founding Member of the Training for Health Equity Network (THEnet). She is a General Practitioner and Health Systems researcher, whose work focuses on making the health system fairer and more accessible for rural, remote, First Nations, and other underserved populations and training a health workforce with skills and attitudes fit for this purpose.

Sarah Nickolich, MD Dr. Sarah Nickolich is Assistant Professor in the Department of Family and Community Medicine at Penn State Health. She received her Doctor of Medicine degree from Case Western Reserve University School of Medicine and then completed residency in Family Medicine followed by a chief residency and a career development fellowship at the University of North Carolina. She is currently the course director for Foundations of Patient-Centered Care at Penn State College of Medicine.

Sarah Strasser, MBBS, FRACGP, FACRRM Emeritus Professor Sarah Strasser graduated from the Royal Free Hospital, University of London, in 1981. She is internationally recognized for developing innovative health professional training programs for undergraduate, postgraduate, and faculty development in medicine and interprofessional health. She has held academic leadership roles in Australia, Canada, Guyana, and New Zealand. Sarah was awarded Member of the Order of Australia in 2019 for her work in medical education and rural practice. She is passionate about general practice/family medicine, health equity, women in medicine, and encouraging youth to consider health as a career.

Shafik Dharamsi, PhD Dr. Shafik Dharamsi is Dean and Professor of the College of Public Health at the University of North Texas Health Science Center. He holds degrees from York University, Medical College of Georgia, and the University of British Columbia. With a distinguished interdisciplinary background and extensive international experience, his teaching and scholarly work spans public health, medical humanities, global health, ethics, and health professions education. A globally recognized scholar, Dr. Dharamsi has published widely in the area of socially accountable approaches to health professions education, and mentored generations of healthcare professionals, fostering compassionate and competent practitioners and scholars.

Siobhán Neville, MB BCh BAO, MSc, MRCPCH, MRCPI Dr. Siobhán Neville is a Consultant Pediatrician at University Hospital Limerick and Associate Professor of Paediatrics at the University of Limerick School of Medicine, Ireland. She has a Master's in Quality and Safety in Healthcare Management from the Royal College of Surgeons Ireland and completed a clinical fellowship in Paediatric Hospital Medicine at the Hospital for Sick Children, Toronto, Canada. Her clinical and research interests are in Inclusion Health and the impact of the social determinants of health on child health and well-being. She is currently leading the implementation of a pilot Inclusion Health service at the University of Limerick Hospitals Group.

Somaya Hosny, PhD Prof. Somaya Hosny is a board member of the National Authority for Quality Assurance and Accreditation in Education, Egypt. She is Professor at the Faculty of Medicine, Suez Canal University, in which she served as the Dean (2010–2014).

She got a master's degree in health Professions Education Leadership from the University of Illinois, Chicago, USA, in 1987. She has publications in leading medical education journals. She is an EMRO/WHO consultant in Medical Education, and Editor in Chief *of the international* journal *HPE*. She is a board member of the International Social Accountability and Accreditation steering committee and coordinator of its standard setting group.

Sookyung Suh, PhD Dr. Sookyung Suh is an educator, coach, and change management expert dedicated to empowering individuals and organizations. At Southern Illinois University School of Medicine, she serves as Assistant Professor of Medical Education, Director of Organizational Change, Equity Transformation Strategist, and Director of the Accelerate Leadership Development Program. With over ten years in management consulting and a background in instructional systems and executive coaching, Dr. Suh brings expertise in guiding strategic change and fostering inclusive growth. She holds a Project Management Professional certification and MS and PhD degrees from Florida State University.

Susan Smith, MD MSc BCh BAO Susan Smith is Professor of General Practice at Trinity College Dublin and works as a General Practitioner at Inchicore Family Doctors in Dublin 8. Her research interests include improving outcomes for patients with multimorbidity and medicines management. She is Associate Director of the HRB Primary Care Clinical Trials Network Ireland and is Clinical Lead for the HRB Evidence Synthesis for Clinical Guidelines program. She also has an interest in health equity and coordinates the Deep End Ireland Group, which advocates for needs-based resource allocation for primary care services for socioeconomically disadvantaged groups.

Tasleem Ras, MBChB, MFamMed, FCFP(SA), PhD I am a clinician with specialist registration in Family Medicine, as well as an educationist, holding a doctorate in Health Sciences Education (HSE). My interests in HSE relate to critical pedagogy, the intersection between clinical and health systems, and socially accountable HSE. My research thus far has focused on health systems in underserved areas, as well as the impact of aspects of HSE on the work experiences of graduates.

Tegan Whitney, BA Tegan is a 4th-year medical student at University of New Mexico, who is planning on going into Family and Community Medicine.

Tom Limanovich, BS I am a second-year medical student at the University of New Mexico School of Medicine interested in pursuing Internal medicine and/or Cardiology.

Tom Markle, PhD Dr. Tom Markle is an educational psychologist who specializes in belief formation and change. He has previously worked as a lead researcher and project director within the defense industry, and now serves as an assistant professor and the director of the Applied Cognition Office at the University of New Mexico's School of Medicine where he focuses on improving student approaches to learning and problem-solving.

Tracey Naledi, MBChB, FCPHM (SA), PhD Tracey Naledi is a collaborative leader focused on health equity and strengthening primary healthcare system. Associate Professor in Public Health Medicine and Deputy Dean Social Accountability and Health Systems at the University of Cape Town, she fosters partnerships between academia, government, and other partners. Her work connects research and policy to improve health outcomes. Naledi has experience in South Africa and Botswana across governmental and non-governmental sectors. She is the founding Chairperson of Tekano: Atlantic Fellows for Health Equity in South Africa. She chairs SHAWCO, the oldest student NGO in Africa, and the Children's Institute. She serves on the boards of the Global Brain Health Institute and the South African Medical Research Council.

Wail Mukhtar, MD Wail Mukhtar, MD, is Associate Professor and Consultant of Otorhinolaryngology Head and Neck Surgery at the Faculty of Medicine, University of Gezira, Sudan. He also serves as a Health Professions Education Specialist and is the current Dean of the Faculty of Medicine at the University of Gezira.

Previously, Dr. Mukhtar was the Director of the Medical Education Development and Research Center at the same institution. He has been a member of several national and regional councils, including the ENT Advisory Council of the Federal Ministry of Health (2021–2023), the ENT Head and Neck Scientific Council of the Sudan Medical Specialization Board (SMSB) since 2012, and the Scientific Committee of the ORL Head and Neck Council under the Arab Board for Health Specializations since 2018. Additionally, he has been a member of the Supreme

Authority of the Sudan Medical Council (SMC) since 2019 and contributed to the National Competency Framework for Medical Graduates in Sudan from 2021 to 2022.

Dr. Mukhtar has published extensively in the fields of otolaryngology and medical education. He has played a pivotal role in advancing social accountability in medical education, including the establishment of a national alliance for social accountability for medical schools in Sudan in 2016. His contributions also include the development of an online course on social accountability, the council of social accountability at FMUG, and Bashir Hamad's Chair for Research in Medical Education and Social Accountability. He led the successful completion of the iSAT self-study, organized and certified by TUFH, and spearheaded numerous university initiatives addressing community needs.

William Ventres, MD, MA Bill Ventres is a family physician with more than 30 years' experience as a community-based family doctor working with underserved and minority populations in safety-net clinics and correctional health settings. His academic interests include the global family medicine, physician–patient communication, and socially accountable medical education. He recently retired as the Ben Saltzman, MD, Distinguished Chair of Rural Family Medicine in the Department of Family and Preventive Medicine at the University of Arkansas for Medical Sciences. He currently resides in San Salvador, El Salvador, where he is a graduate student in Latin American Philosophy at the University of Central America.

Abbreviations

ABRASCO	Associação Brasileira de Saúde Coletiva (Brazilian Association of Collective Health)
ALAMES	Asociación Latinoamericana de Medicina Social (Latin American Social Medicine Association)
AMEE	International Association for Health Professions Education
ASPIRE	A Schools Programme for International Recognition of Excellence in Education
CBE	Community-Based Education
CCC	Comprehensive Community Clerkship
COMET	Community-Oriented Medical Experience Track
COME	Community-Oriented Medical Education
CPU	Conceptualization, Production, Usability
CQI	Continuous Quality Improvement
DCEL	Distributed Community Engaged Learning
ELT	Experiential Learning Theory
EPAs	Entrustable Professional Activities
FAIMER	Foundation for Advancement of International Medical Education and Research
FGDs	Focus Group Discussions
GCSA	Global Consensus for Social Accountability
HLE	Healthy Life Expectancy
ICL	Integrated Clinical Learning
IFMSA	International Federation of Medical Student Associations
IMD	Index of Multiple Deprivation
IPSF	International Pharmaceutical Students' Federation
IADS	International Association of Dental Students
IVSA	International Veterinary Students' Association
JHLES	Johns Hopkins Learning Environment Scale
LASMCH	Latin American Social Medicine and Collective Health
MBChB	Bachelor of Medicine and Bachelor of Surgery
MS-ATU	Medical Student Attitudes Toward the Underserved

MS-IWU	Medical Student Future Intention to Work with the Underserved
NGOs	Non-Governmental Organizations
NO	Northern Ontario
NOSM	Northern Ontario School of Medicine
OSCE	Objective Structured Clinical Examination
PBL	Problem-Based Learning
SA	Social Accountability
SDOH	Social Determinants of Health
SIMD	Scottish Index of Multiple Deprivation
SSCs	Student Selected Components
TUFH	The Network: Towards Unity for Health
UK	United Kingdom
UN	United Nations
USA	United States of America
WHO	World Health Organization
WP	Widening Participation

Part I
Social Accountability: Concepts, Principles, and Social Obligation

Chapter 1
Social Accountability in Medical Schools: Concepts, Principles and Values

Mohamed Elhassan Abdalla

Learning Outcomes

1. Define the concept of social accountability and its relevance across disciplines.
2. Discuss the significance of social accountability in enhancing healthcare delivery through medical schools.
3. Analyze the historical evolution of social accountability in medical education, focusing on its milestones and implications.
4. Examine the core values of social accountability—relevance, equity, quality, and cost-effectiveness.

The Concept of Social Accountability

The Social Accountability (SA) concept was firstly introduced in politics, then moved to economics and business and spread to other disciplines, including medical education. The World Bank, a leading organisation that supports the concept, identify it as part of any organisation's social contract with the societies they serve [1]. The concept starts in politics to describe processes that need government accountability outside the electoral system and also describes the relationships between the government and population relying on civic engagement [2], to improve services for low-income and marginalised people [3].

There are different definitions for the SA concept in the literature; the World Bank has defined SA as the "extent and capability of citizens to hold the state accountable and make it responsive to their needs" [1] this definition stated the main three elements in SA; citizens role, the responsibility of states towards society and

M. E. Abdalla (✉)
School of Medicine, University of Limerick, Limerick, Ireland
e-mail: melhassan.elsayed@ul.ie

M. E. Abdalla et al. (eds.), *Social Accountability of Medical Schools*,
https://doi.org/10.1007/978-3-031-94435-2_1

the accountability to cover society needs. Those elements are the basics of SA when applied to any discipline including medical education. Other literature has emphasised transparency as one of the main elements to enhance citizen participation and hence improve accountability [2].

So in politics -the same can be applied to other disciplines as we are going to discuss below-SA is perceived to encompass strategies, processes or involvements used by citizens to ensure that politicians, policymakers and service providers respond to them and are accountable and responsible for their actions and resolutions [4].

The SA concept is also used in economics and business, but it is called corporate social responsibility (CRS). There is no one agreed on definition for CSR [5, 6], Dahlsrud, 2008 reported an analysis of 37 definitions of CSR in the business world [6]. Some of the definitions reported in that analysis [6] are ' A concept whereby companies integrate social and environmental concerns in their business operations and in their interaction with their stakeholders on a voluntary basis' another definition is 'The commitment of business to contribute to sustainable economic development, working with employees, their families, the local community and society at large to improve their quality of life'. The analysis of the 37 definitions revealed common dimensions in all the definitions which are: stakeholder dimension, social dimension, economic dimension, voluntariness dimension and environmental dimension [6].

In terms of SA application and implementation, the World Bank and other organisations have published different SA models to rely on; the principal-agent model which is seen as a step of the new public management (NPM) theory that supports the idea of client power. The model considers citizens as clients who are served and can be loyal to good service or exit unsatisfactory ones [2]. Loyalty and exit are two of Hirscman's notions that include voice as a third one; the notions were published in 1970 to explain clients' reactions to public service; it is usual to use two of them and rarely can clients use the three [2, 7].

The other model that supports SA is the voice and participation model. This model explains SA as giving an active voice to citizens through different means and encouraging the participation of all citizens in shaping their public world [2]. This model depends heavily on two issues: transparency and availability of information.

Based on the definitions and the discussion above, we can identify the primary goal of social accountability as twofold: first, to enhance organizational actions by fostering greater citizen participation in policy-making and service delivery; and second, to increase the public responsiveness of these organizations [4]. So it is a concept that is tailored towards the political side or the social side of population life. The goal and orientation of the concept is almost the same in all disciplines-Including medical schools- with the changes based on the context of each discipline.

The Landscape of SA of Medical Schools

In the year 1995, the concept of SA has officially entered the world of medical education when the WHO produced the definition of SA of Medical Schools as "the obligation [of medical schools] to direct their education, research and service activities towards addressing the priority health concerns of the community, region, and/or nation they have a mandate to serve. The priority health concerns are to be identified jointly by governments, health care organizations, health professionals and the public" [8]. This definition obligates medical schools to ensure community and other organisations' effective and essential participation in their roles to satisfy the health needs of the community. It encourages partnerships between medical education institutions, health systems, other partners e.g.: NGOs and communities to produce rich and contextualised learning experiences for students [9, 10] besides delivering health services and conducting research that will build on the designed continuous interaction between the education system, partners including communities, and health systems as illustrated by the Fig. 1.1 below. This interaction and collaboration is expected to guide medical schools to form effective partnerships with the communities they serve—and give them a role-to produce the needed doctors who are both person- and community-oriented who work to address health needs [11, 12].

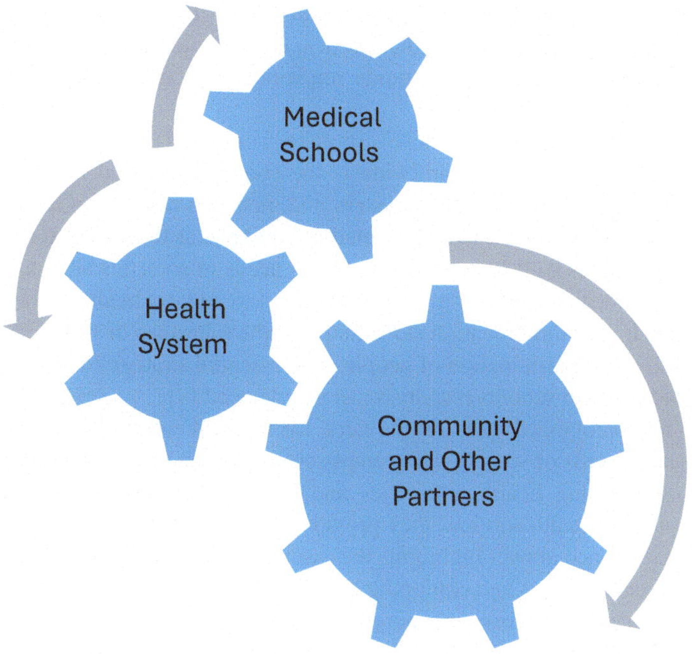

Fig. 1.1 Interaction between the community, medical schools and health system to produce SA

In one of the studies aimed to facilitate understanding of SA in medical schools, community members described SA as a way of their (community) involvement with and empowerment by medical schools; they stated that SA would make medical schools advocators for the community's health and well-being [13]. In another study, stakeholders have identified the functions of a socially accountable medical school under three main headings: developing a health workforce that responds to regional health needs and covers their shortage, providing training for future physicians to deliver quality care for patients and to offer service to the surrounding community [14]. Based on the expectation of communities from those studies, it is anticipated that the ultimate goal SA of medical schools is the training of medical graduates and those already working within the health system to deliver relevant, high-quality, cost-effective and equitable health care within the health and social care systems within the current situation and anticipate future needs [8, 15]. Considering the context in which medical schools are working, one can elicit that the principles of SA of medical schools are the similar to the principles described in politics and business worlds.

Moreover, SA of medical schools is ruled by two principles that need to be considered by all frameworks that explain the SA further or design specific SA-related interventions by medical schools. Those principles are the humanistic principle that relate to the role of society, and the systemic principles that relate to the relation between medical schools and health systems [16] as the presence of external dimensions in SA of medical schools (the need of people and the relation with health system) produce a complexity that necessitate more effort from medical schools such as considering the plans of other parties, etc. in order unify understanding of the concept, its terminologies and guide implementation of any SA activities and frameworks [17].

The complexity mentioned above originate from the fact that the only stable thing within health systems worldwide is the changing societal need for health, which requires a responsive health system and, hence, a responsive health professions education institutions, including medical schools, as the source for the health workforce [18]. It is well-known that changing needs of societies are not related to treatments and health facilities only but expanded to address health workers' competencies such as communication skills and also the relevance of health services. It is believed that the participation of people is an essential strategy for making health systems and medical schools responsive to people need [4].

The WHO recognized early on the need for medical schools to respond to the priority health needs of society. They emphasized that medical schools should contribute to addressing health disparities and inequalities through their curricula, research, and the health services they provide [8]. The definition of SA of medical schools—mentioned above- highlights the essential role of medical schools in tackling workforce shortages and equipping healthcare professionals with the skills and knowledge necessary to drive meaningful changes in health systems to better meet societal health needs [9, 19]. To further explain the roles of medical schools in responding to community health needs, needs of health systems and to build a better understanding of SA, a review of eleven theories, models, and frameworks of SA was conducted by Wood et al., 2022; they reported that most of the current frameworks cited the needs of the underserved communities as the target of social accountability. The study also highlighted that identification of community health needs should consider all the community categories with social justice in mind. If not, SA will be subtracted to serving only one community category [17].

Further elaboration of the roles of medical schools will reveal that proper planning of the education programmes based on health needs will help graduates to function properly towards attaining those needs; some authors claim that linking students to their communities through any of the service learning approaches will provide students with contextual learning that will end in attaining the needed SA impact [9]. Medical schools in some parts of the world develop their educational programmes around health problems in the countries where they exist and train their students in community settings around the medical schools to improve the outcomes of their programmes [20]. For example, clinical placements within underserved communities and the experience of local cultures will make the future health workforce sensitive to the needs of those communities [9, 12].

With ongoing changes in society's health needs and the health system's needs, health professional institutions needs to adapt its programme at all levels undergraduate, postgraduate and continuous professional development (CPD) to fit those expected and anticipated changes. As an example from postgraduate level, the GP training in the UK has set 12 principles for training to accommodate the principles of SA [21]. Further discussion of those principles will be provided in the chapter that discusses SA in the curriculum of medical schools. In CPD, Fleet, et.al 2008, mentioned that in the era of SA, CPD activities must be extended to include personal and social aspects of healthcare and not only aspects of disease management [22].

Furthermore, SA of medical schools must consider society needs, health system needs and challenges and opportunities within health system when planning and providing any health services either though school's health facility or by clinical, academic and other staff; medical schools can be part of the health committees within the health system [23, 24]. On the other hand, In research, medical schools should work with its partners to identify society's current and anticipated health needs and challenges to set research priorities and plans with the aim to improve and have an impact on health system performance and society health status [24].

Historical Evolution of SA in Medical Education

There is an earlier agreement that medical schools are 'moral agents' with a social contract and a responsibility to reduce health disparities in their communities [25]. Based on that agreement, increasing connections between medical schools and the communities they serve is an old concern for medical education and health system personnel. In 1978, the Alma-Ata Declaration made a clear call for medical schools to adopt an education concentrate on common health problems [26]. That declaration led to the development of the Community-Oriented Medical Education (COME) and Community-Based Education (CBE) approaches that were adopted by a group of medical schools around the world who later formed a network to improve implantation of those strategies [26]. This network is currently named the Network-TUFH.

Going in the same direction, in 1988, the Edinburgh Declaration, a final product of the World Federation of Medical Education Conference, called for a reform in medical education to produce doctors who would be promoters of health for all. The declaration also recommended expanding students' training to include community sites and building partnerships with the health system [27]. The movement went on with different recommendations from different medical education and health system assemblies until the Year 1995 which was marked by the WHO publication of the definition of SA of Medical Schools, as the capacity of medical schools to respond to societal needs and health system challenges by asking the medical schools to direct their education, research, and community service activities towards the priority health needs in the communities they are intended to serve [8], from that year the concept of SA increasingly publicized in medical education and transferred to other health professions, as it has been advocated not only the WHO but by other organisations such the THEnet and the Network-TUFH, individual countries and medical schools. Looking at the WHO definition, as explained earlier, readers can realise that it identifies the general outcomes of SA of medical schools as having a positive impact on population health. It has also set the base for outcomes that depend on collaboration with partners, including the community members themselves [28].

With more adoption of SA, a landmark was in 2010 which is the publication of the Global Consensus for SA of Medical Schools (GCSA). The consensus was developed through a rigorous consultation of 131 organisations and leaders in medical education. The GCSA defined a socially accountable medical school as one that "responds to current and future health needs and challenges in society, orientates its education, research and service priorities accordingly, strengthens governance and partnerships with other stakeholders and uses evaluation and accreditation to assess their performance and impact" [29]. Below is an extract of the GCSA introduction.

(The consensus on social accountability embraces a system-wide scope from identification of health needs to verification of the effects of medical schools on those needs. The list of 10 areas reflects this logical sequence, starting with an understanding of the social context, an identification of health challenges and needs and the creation of relationships to act efficiently (Areas 1 and 2). Among the spectrum of required health workforce to address health needs, the anticipated role and competencies of the doctor are described (Area 3) serving as a guide to the education strategy (Area 4), which the medical school, along with consistent research and service strategies, is called to implement (Area 5). Standards are required to steer the institution towards a high level of excellence (Areas 6 and 7), which national authorities need to recognise (Area 8). While social accountability is a universal value (Area 9), local societies will be the ultimate appraisers of achievements (Area 10)).

The 10 strategic directions stated in the GCSA are discussed in depth in different chapters of this book and are presented in Box 1.1 below.

Box 1.1 Strategic Directions of SA of Medical Schools
Area 1: Anticipating Society's Health Needs
Area 2: Partnering with the Health System and other Stakeholders
Area 3: Adapting to the Evolving Roles of Doctors and other Health Professionals
Area 4: Fostering Outcome-Based Education
Area 5: Creating Responsive and Responsible Governance of The Medical School
Area 6: Refining the Scope of Standards for Education, Research and Service Delivery
Area 7: Supporting Continuous Quality Improvement in Education, Research and Service Delivery
Area 8: Establishing Mandated Mechanisms for Accreditation
Area 9: Balancing Global Principles with Context Specificity
Area 10: Defining the Role of Society

Principles of SA of Medical Schools

A common question among medical educators is how a medical school can be socially accountable. Many scholars have worked on this question and provided answers in different directions. Boelen and colleagues attempted to answer this question by describing a distinction between three levels of responding to society's needs in medical education that make a continuum rather than absolute categorisation [24, 30, 31] See Fig. 1.2 below and more elaboration on the scale can be found in chap. 9:

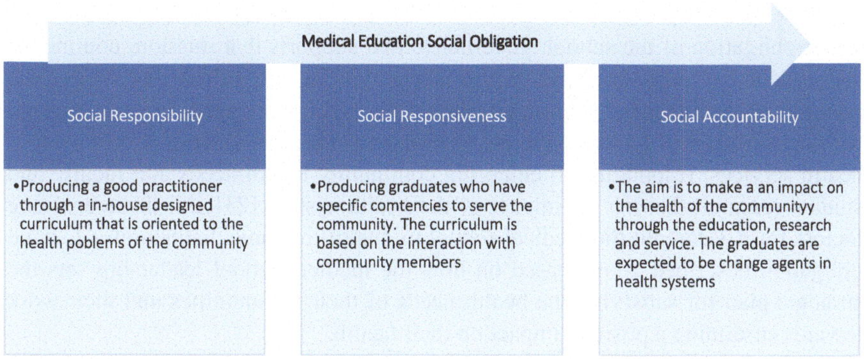

Fig. 1.2 Social Obligation Continuum

- Social Responsibility: Medical schools aim to produce' good practitioners' who work to achieve the expectations of society that the schools identify.
- Social Responsiveness: Medical schools respond by directing their education activities towards explicitly identified societal health priorities. It produces graduates with specific competencies to address peoples' health concerns.
- Social Accountability involves all three functions: education, research, and service activities to achieve the priority health needs of society, as well as partnering with stakeholders to identify those needs. The graduates are expected to be change agents in the health system.

This distinction describes a socially accountable medical school as the one that strives to consider the four values of the health system: relevance, equity, quality, and cost-effectiveness in all three functions: education, research, and service [8]. The relevance value means that the medical school will work towards the jointly identified needs of the community in the curriculum, e.g., the content to address the social determinants of health. In research relevance means conduction and dissemination of research that can be applied to improve the health status of the community and focus of hot issues in the health system while in the service domain, relevance means that the medical school is to provide the needed health service through the schools' staff, students, premises and resources. The equity value is concerned with the involvement and targeting of all community classes in all the work of medical school and to reduce the conscious and unconscious biases towards any individual or a group of individuals that may be deprived from the benefits of any of the functions of medical school e.g.: admission of students from underserved or under privileged areas. Quality is concerned with fitting for purpose; the functions are to be planned and executed to positively impact the health of individuals and the community. Cost-effectiveness alarms the value for money and resources used in medical school functions. It is essential to recognise that the return on investment (ROI) in socially accountable medical education is not only money. The most crucial ROI is the positive impact on the health status of the community the medical school has the mandate to serve.

For the general look of the socially accountable medical school, Abdalla et al., 2022 identified six themes for SA, which are a mission that explicitly defines the social obligation of the school, governance that supports that mission, continuous and productive communication with stakeholders, a curriculum that adopts the community-oriented and community-based as basic approaches in teaching and learning as this will facilitate the move towards social accountability, provision of health services, responding to emerging community health needs and faculty and student research that has an impact of the health system [23]. All those enabling factors for SA can put the medical school in one of the three distinctions of social obligation described above based on how the medical school leadership sets the strategic plan for satisfying the health needs of their communities and their work towards sustaining a positive impact on their health.

On another dimension, Ross and Cameron, 2021 concluded in their narrative review about the SA of Medical schools that the reported outcomes of SA are producing physicians who fit for purpose and reduce inequities in health. They also reported the actions by medical schools to achieve SA, such as adapting the curriculum content to include items such as concentration on primary health care, interprofessional education, and community-based activities. Other actions reported are the change in admission policy to recruit students from underserved areas and the change in the school's governance to make SA explicit in the school governance [28].

Commenting on the education part in medical schools, Khanpoor et al. 2024 have suggested a model for medical education that is responsive to society's health needs by educating graduates capable of taking responsibility for those needs. The model was developed through different steps, including a literature review, expert consultation and confirmatory analysis [18]. The model has four dimensions with different components in each one, as shown below.

- Planning Dimension: alignment of the curriculum with health needs of the community, education for research and education for sustainable development.
- Implementation Dimension: change in attitudes from clinical to community-oriented, skill empowerment with a social perspective on health and modern educational methods.
- Monitoring and Evaluation Dimension: setting community-oriented education indicators will create a move to enhance community-oriented teaching strategies and regulations.
- Intersectoral Collaboration Dimension: cross-organisational project management and university-community interactions

A critical look at the four dimensions above will reveal that they are in alignment with the Extended SA Grid published by the WHO, in which the three functions of medical schools (Education, Research, and Service) are plotted against the four values of SA (Relevance, Equity, Quality, Cost-effectiveness). Each function is viewed in three phases: planning, doing and impacting [8].

The commonality between the descriptions of the dimensions above is that what characterises SA is the role of medical school in responding to health needs and striving to impact this endeavour positively. That matches the discussion of SA based on a common framework suggested by Boelen and Woollard to direct understanding of SA towards having the needed impact on communities; the framework known as the CPU model (Conceptualisation-Usability-Productivity) [16]. The CPU model is used by some medical schools to evaluate their current status and future directions for social accountability [32–34]. As described by the CPU model authors, if we dissect the education function of a medical school concerning social accountability, the framework's three components (Conceptualisation-Usability-Productivity) must be ruled by society's needs. The conceptualisation of the desired professionals (graduate attributes) will depend on the institution's role in fulfilling society's needs. The production of that desired professional will depend on carefully designing what and how to learn with the expectation that the usability of the graduates will be in addressing society's needs [16]. The above dissection can be made to the other two medical education functions; research and health service. To help in using the CPU framework for social accountability, Boelen et al., 2012 have produced a generic list of indicators that can be adopted by medical schools in their movement towards achieving SA [24].

Case Studies

The section below presented two case studies of medical schools conducting different activities to impact their communities' health.

Case Study 1: The University of new Mexico Health Sciences Center's

The University of New Mexico Health Sciences Center's (UNMHSC) development and implementation of Health Extension Rural Offices (HEROs) has developed a plan for community and stakeholder engagement to improve the poor health conditions of the New Mexico population and change the image of the UNMHCO- among the rural community health leaders- the centre is not responding to the community and its needs. As such, the UNMHSC developed a network of HEROs in communities with the mission to work as facilitators of the UNMHSC's works and use its resources to address community health. The HEROs enabled the work to be addressed inside the targeted communities. They identified work areas related to social determinants of health for those communities. Still, the most critical issue is the realisation by the UNMHSC of the mismatch between community priority health needs, which are mainly bio-social issues, and institutional research output, which is mainly biomedical. This work has resulted in a significant change at UNMHSC concerning forming sustainable partnerships with community partners and incorporating social determinants as priority areas in research, education, and clinical service [35].

This case study can be a practical example of the development of partnership to help addressing the society health needs as part of SA in medical education and its conceptualisation as the responsibility mandate of the schools to respond to the priority health needs of the communities they serve and to imply the school resources (human and physical) prove the impact of its plans and activities on the health of those communities [17].

Case Study 2: Faculty of Medicine-University of Gezira (FMUG), Sudan

The Faculty of Medicine-University of Gezira (FMUG), Sudan, which has an early-developed community-based curriculum in the Eastern Meditrenean Region, has a record in addressing its surrounding community health needs through students work in the community. In the period 2000–2014, students covered more than 3750 families in the city where FMUG is located (Wad Medani City), and they conducted more than 50,000 family visits during this period. Students' visits and activities with the families, such as follow-up of children's immunisation and linking pregnant women to antenatal care, have resulted in a positive impact on the health of those families and improved their connection with the health system. During the same period (2000–2014), students covered with their work during the Interdisciplinary field training and rural development programme around 237 villages. Examples of the activities in the villages were health campaigns, planting of trees and establishing Tuberculosis Treatment Units [33].

The case study from the FMUG reflected how the curriculum can be used for service together with equipping learners (future practitioners) with competencies and skills that will help them work properly in health systems to advocate for the health needs of the communities they serve [36].

Take-Home Message

The concept of SA of medical schools emphasize the responsibility to address communities' priority health needs. SA involves active engagement with community members and stakeholders to ensure that education, research, and service activities are aligned with societal needs. The historical evolution of SA has seen significant milestones, such as the Al-Mata declaration, the WHO's 1995 definition and the 2010 Global Consensus. Effective community engagement and collaborative partnerships are crucial, as they enable medical schools to integrate community-oriented and community-based approaches into their curricula, ultimately fostering a health workforce that is both competent and compassionate. By adopting frameworks like the CPU model, medical schools can systematically plan, implement, and evaluate their SA efforts, ensuring a positive impact on community health and reducing disparities. Examples from institutions like the University of New Mexico and the University of Gezira illustrate these principles' practical application and benefits in real-world settings.

References

1. World Bank. Strengthening governance, tackling corruption: the World Bank Group's updated strategy and implementation plan [Internet]. 2012 [cited 2024 Apr 5]. Available from: https://reliefweb.int/report/world/strengthening-governance-tackling-corruption-world-bank-group's-updated-strategy-and
2. Grandvoinnet H, Aslam G, Raha S. Social accountability: a popular yet fuzzy concept. In: Opening the black box: the contextual drivers of social accountability [internet]. The World Bank; 2015. Available from:. https://doi.org/10.1596/978-1-4648-0481-6.
3. Joshi A. Legal empowerment and social accountability: complementary strategies toward rights-based development in health? World Dev [Internet]. 2017;99:160–72. Available from: https://linkinghub.elsevier.com/retrieve/pii/S0305750X17302425
4. Ogbuabor DC, Onwujekwe OE. The community is just a small circle: citizen participation in the free maternal and child healthcare programme of Enugu state, Nigeria. Glob Health Action

[Internet]. 2018;11(1):1421002. Available from: https://www.tandfonline.com/doi/full/10.1080/16549716.2017.1421002
5. Beal BD. What is CSR? In: Beal BD, editor. Corporate social responsibility: definitions, Core issues and recent developments. SAGE Publications Ltd; 2014. p. 1–15.
6. Dahlsrud A. How corporate social responsibility is defined: an analysis of 37 definitions. Corp Soc Responsib Environ Manag [Internet]. 2008;15(1):1–13. Available from: https://onlinelibrary.wiley.com/doi/10.1002/csr.132
7. Fox J. Exit, voice, and Albert O. Hirschman [Internet]. Harv Bus Rev 2012 [cited 2024 Apr 7]. Available from: https://hbr.org/2012/12/exit-voice-and-albert-o-hirsch
8. Boelen C, Heck JE. Defining and measuring the social accountability of medical schools. World Health Organization; 1995.
9. Dubé TV, Cumyn A, Fourati M, Chamberland M, Hatcher S, Landry M. Pathways, journeys and experiences: integrating curricular activities related to social accountability within an undergraduate medical curriculum. Med Educ [Internet]. 2024;58(5):556–65. Available from: https://asmepublications.onlinelibrary.wiley.com/doi/10.1111/medu.15260
10. Wood B, Fitzgerald M, Kendall C, Cameron E. Integrating socially accountable health professional education and learning health systems to transform community health and health systems. Learn Heal Syst [Internet]. 2021;5(3) Available from: https://onlinelibrary.wiley.com/doi/10.1002/lrh2.10277:e10277.
11. Clithero-Eridon A, Ross A, Albright D. Conceptualising social accountability as an attribute of medical education. African J Prim Heal Care Fam Med. 2020;12(1):1–8.
12. Aiyer H, Walling E, Yeo L, Woollard R. Proposing the community triad model to action social accountability in medical schools. Med Teach [Internet]. 2024;13:1–7. Available from: https://www.tandfonline.com/doi/full/10.1080/0142159X.2024.2351585
13. Oriojot L, Rujumba J, Munabi IG, Mubuuke AG, Kiguli S. Implementation of social accountability in undergraduate medical training at a sub-Saharan African medical school. Educ Heal. 2024;37(1):30–8.
14. Reddy AT, Lazreg SA, Phillips RL, Bazemore AW, Lucan SC. Toward defining and measuring social accountability in graduate medical education: a stakeholder study. J Grad Med Educ [Internet]. 2013;5(3):439–45. Available from: https://meridian.allenpress.com/jgme/article/5/3/439/34036/Toward-Defining-and-Measuring-Social
15. A Strategic Framework for Postgraduate Medical Training in Ireland 2021–2030 [Internet]. 2021. Available from: https://www.theforum.ie/wp-content/uploads/2021/11/Strategy-22-10.pdf
16. Boelen C, Woollard B. Social accountability and accreditation: a new frontier for educational institutions. Med Educ. 2009;43(9):887–94.
17. Wood B, Bohonis H, Ross B, Cameron E. Comparing and using prominent social accountability frameworks in medical education: moving from theory to implementation in Northern Ontario, Canada. Can Med Educ J [Internet]. 2022 Jun 7; Available from: https://journalhosting.ucalgary.ca/index.php/cmej/article/view/73051
18. Khanpoor H, Amerzadeh M, Alizadeh A, Khosravizadeh O, Rafiei S. Developing a responsive model to societal needs in medical education. BMC Med Educ [Internet]. 2024;24(1):370. Available from: https://bmcmededuc.biomedcentral.com/articles/10.1186/s12909-024-05355-9
19. Health Canada. Social accountability. A vision for Canadian medical schools [Internet]. 2001. Available from: https://www.afmc.ca/wp-content/uploads/2022/10/sa_vision_canadian_medical_schools_en.pdf
20. Mullan F, Frehywot S, Omaswa F, Buch E, Chen C, Greysen SR, et al. Medical schools in sub-Saharan Africa. Lancet [Internet]. 2011;377(9771):1113–21. Available from: https://linkinghub.elsevier.com/retrieve/pii/S0140673610619617
21. Patterson D, Blane DN. Training for purpose–a blueprint for social accountability and health equity focused GP training. Educ Prim Care [Internet]. 2021;32(6):318–21. Available from: https://www.tandfonline.com/doi/full/10.1080/14739879.2021.1966652

22. Fleet LJ, Kirby F, Cutler S, Dunikowski L, Nasmith L, Shaughnessy R. Continuing professional development and social accountability: a review of the literature. J Interprof Care [Internet]. 2008;22(sup1):15–29. Available from: http://www.tandfonline.com/doi/full/10.1080/13561820802028360
23. Abdalla ME, Taha M, Wadi M, Khalafalla H. What makes a medical school socially accountable? A qualitative thematic review of the evaluation of social accountability of medical schools in the eastern Mediterranean region. East Mediterr Heal J [Internet]. 2022;28(5):381–9. Available from: https://applications.emro.who.int/EMHJ/V28/05/1020-3397-2022-2805-381-389-eng.pdf
24. Boelen C, Dharamsi S, Gibbs T. The social accountability of medical schools and its indicators. Educ Heal [Internet]. 2012;25(3):180. Available from: http://www.educationforhealth.net/text.asp?2012/25/3/180/109785
25. Puschel K, Rojas P, Erazo A, Thompson B, Lopez J, Barros J. Social accountability of medical schools and academic primary care training in Latin America: principles but not practice. Fam Pract. 2014;31(4):399–408.
26. Hamad B. What is community-based education? Evolution, definition and rationale. Handbook of community-based education: theory and practices. Maastricht: Network Publications; 2000.
27. WFME. The Edinburgh declaration. Med Educ [Internet]. 1988;22(5):481. Available from: https://onlinelibrary.wiley.com/doi/10.1111/j.1365-2923.1988.tb00788.x
28. Ross BM, Cameron E. Socially accountable medical education: our story might not be yours. High Educ Stud [Internet]. 2021;11(1):114. Available from: http://www.ccsenet.org/journal/index.php/hes/article/view/0/44539
29. GCSA. Global consensus for social accountability of medical schools [Internet]. Vol. 2011, Global Consensus for Social Accountability of Medical Schools. 2010 [cited 2018 Oct 2]. Available from: http://healthsocialaccountability.sites.olt.ubc.ca/files/2011/06/11-06-07-GCSA-English-pdf-style.pdf
30. Boelen C, Woollard R. Social accountability: the extra leap to excellence for educational institutions. Med Teach. 2011;33(8):614–9.
31. Preston R, Larkins S, Taylor J, Judd J. Building blocks for social accountability: a conceptual framework to guide medical schools. BMC Med Educ [Internet]. 2016;16(1):227. Available from: http://bmcmededuc.biomedcentral.com/articles/10.1186/s12909-016-0741-y
32. Hosny S, Ghaly M, Boelen C. Is our medical school socially accountable? The case of Faculty of Medicine, Suez Canal University. Med Teach. 2015;37(S1):S47–55.
33. Elsanousi S, Elsanousi M, Khalafallah O, Habour A. Assessment of the social accountability of the faculty of medicine at University of Gezira, Sudan. East Mediterr Heal J. 2016;22(4):258–66.
34. Alrebish SA, Taha MH, Ahmed MH, Abdalla ME. Commitment towards a better future for medical education in Saudi Arabia: the efforts of the college of medicine at Qassim university to become socially accountable. Med Educ Online [Internet]. 2020;25(1):1710328. Available from: https://www.tandfonline.com/doi/full/10.1080/10872981.2019.1710328
35. Fitzgerald M, Shoemaker E, Ponka D, Walker M, Kendall C. Global health and social accountability: An essential synergy for the 21 st century medical school. J Glob Health [Internet]. 2021;11:03045. Available from: http://jogh.org/documents/2021/jogh-11-03045.pdf
36. Abdalla ME, Taha MH, Mukhtar WN, Elsanousi M. Impact of community-based medical education on graduate performance: a qualitative study using a critical incident technique. Heal Prof Educ [Internet]. 2022;8(1):38–44. Available from: https://hpe.researchcommons.org/journal/vol8/iss1/6

Chapter 2
The Evolving Role of the Medical Profession and Medical Graduates

Mohamed Hassan Taha, Wail Nuri Osman Mukhtar, and Robyn Preston

Learning Outcomes

1. Identify the expanding roles and responsibilities of medical professionals in addressing societal and systemic healthcare challenges.
2. Discuss the essential competencies required for socially accountable physicians to fulfill their evolving roles.
3. Analyze the significance of interdisciplinary collaboration and patient advocacy in reducing health disparities.
4. Evaluate the ethical considerations and challenges surrounding technological advancements in healthcare.
5. Understand the role of Health System Science education in preparing future physicians for their diverse responsibilities.

Introduction

The Changing Landscape of Medical Practice

In recent years, the landscape of medical practice has expanded significantly due to rapid technological advancements, substantial policy reforms, and increasing public

M. H. Taha (✉)
College of Medicine and Medical Education Center, University of Sharjah, Sharjah, UAE
e-mail: mtaha@sharjah.ac.ae

W. N. O. Mukhtar
Faculty of Medicine, University of Gezira, Wad Madani, Sudan

R. Preston
School of Health, Medical and Applied Sciences, CQUniversity,
Norman Gardens, QLD, Australia

M. E. Abdalla et al. (eds.), *Social Accountability of Medical Schools*,
https://doi.org/10.1007/978-3-031-94435-2_2

expectations. Where physicians were once primarily focused on direct patient care, their roles now encompass broader responsibilities, including engagement with social determinants of health, systemic healthcare reform, and the promotion of health equity [1]. Social accountability (SA) has emerged as a guiding principle in modern medicine, urging future and current physicians to address the complex needs of contemporary healthcare systems while considering the broader community [2, 3].

Frenk et al. (2010) emphasize the importance of adaptability, suggesting that future physicians must be prepared to navigate dynamic healthcare environments that reflect contemporary societal values and priorities [4]. Physicians are now encouraged to extend their influence beyond clinical encounters, adopting roles that contribute to community well-being and systemic reform [5]. This chapter explores the evolving roles of medical professional and medical graduates and how social accountability reframes the physician's role, preparing practitioners not only to meet individual patient needs but also to contribute to community health and advocate for systemic equity.

Defining Social Accountability at Different Levels of Medical Practice

Social accountability in the medical schools represents a commitment to aligning healthcare services, research, and education with the primary health needs of the communities served [2]. Social accountability in medical practice is an approach where physicians and healthcare institutions prioritize the well-being of underserved populations, integrating community engagement, health equity, and policy advocacy into their roles [6].

While socially accountable physicians acknowledge that health outcomes are influenced by a range of factors outside traditional clinical boundaries, such as socioeconomic status, education, and environmental conditions [1, 7]. They actively engage with these determinants through advocacy, collaboration across sectors, and policy reforms that promote health equity. Medical schools play a crucial role in instilling these values, fostering a commitment to social responsibility and equitable care in their graduates [8]. By embedding SA principles into medical curricula, educational institutions help shape physicians who are prepared to address real-world health challenges facing diverse populations.

The Evolving Roles of Medical Professionals

Physicians are now tasked with bridging clinical practice with broader societal, technological, and systemic responsibilities, ultimately contributing to improved healthcare outcomes on multiple levels. This evolving role encompasses patient advocacy, system integration, technological innovation, and collaboration—requiring physicians to adapt continually to meet the needs of individual patients, communities, and the healthcare system at large.

Patient Advocacy and Health Equity

One of the most significant expansions in the physician's role is patient advocacy, particularly in promoting health equity. Physicians are increasingly recognized not only as healers but as advocates for justice within healthcare. The socially accountable physician is one who sees beyond the exam room, actively addressing barriers to care that many patients face, particularly marginalized groups. These barriers often stem from social determinants of health, including socioeconomic status, education, and environmental factors. Through advocacy, physicians work to dismantle these obstacles, ensuring that all patients, regardless of their background, have fair access to quality healthcare [9].

Physicians committed to health equity go beyond treating individual cases; they engage in public health initiatives, support healthcare reforms, and collaborate with community organizations to improve health outcomes for vulnerable populations. This requires a deep sense of empathy, cultural competence, and a dedication to justice. Socially accountable physicians prioritize the well-being of their patients while acknowledging and working to rectify the broader inequalities that impact health on a community level.

System Integration and Collaborative Care

The complexity of modern healthcare requires physicians to be adept system integrators. Physicians today are increasingly expected to collaborate with interdisciplinary teams, navigating complex healthcare systems to provide comprehensive care that addresses both clinical and psychosocial aspects of health [10, 11]. This role necessitates a broader understanding of healthcare systems and an ability to coordinate across various levels of care, from primary to specialized services.

As system integrators, physicians work alongside a wide array of healthcare professionals—nurses, social workers, mental health specialists, and community health workers—to create holistic care plans tailored to the unique needs of each patient. This collaborative approach is essential for ensuring that patient care is cohesive, efficient, and attuned to a patient's broader context, thereby promoting better health outcomes and more effective resource utilization. System integration demands not only clinical acumen but also skills in teamwork, communication, and systems navigation, positioning physicians as facilitators of a seamless, patient-centered healthcare experience.

Technological Innovation and Ethical Integration

The rapid advancements in healthcare technology, such as telemedicine, artificial intelligence, and data analytics, are reshaping the physician's role in unprecedented ways. The socially accountable physician must now be able to incorporate these technologies into their practice while maintaining a strong ethical foundation [12]. Technologies like AI-driven diagnostics and remote monitoring devices have the potential to improve access to care, especially for underserved populations, but they also present ethical challenges related to privacy, equity, and the potential for bias in machine-learning algorithms.

Socially accountable physicians are tasked with ensuring that technological innovations are utilized in ways that enhance patient care without compromising ethical standards. This includes advocating for policies that promote equitable access to healthcare technology and addressing biases inherent in AI-driven tools. Physicians must balance the efficiency of technology with a commitment to ethical integrity, ensuring that these innovations serve all patients fairly. This expanded role requires a nuanced understanding of both technological possibilities and their limitations, coupled with a commitment to patient privacy, informed consent, and transparency.

Health System Science Education: A Foundation for the Evolving Roles of Medical Graduates

Health System Science (HSS) education has become a crucial element in medical education, preparing Health System Science (HSS) has become a crucial element in medical education, preparing future physicians to meet the demands of an evolving healthcare landscape. HSS encompasses key areas such as healthcare policy, quality improvement, and social determinants of health, equipping graduates with the competencies needed to navigate complex healthcare systems and address structural health disparities [13].

Integrating HSS into medical curricula ensures that graduates are not only clinically proficient but also skilled in understanding and engaging with the broader systems that impact health outcomes [14]. This systems-based approach reflects the need for physicians who can lead systemic improvements, advocate for population health, and work toward equitable healthcare. Graduates trained in HSS are thus well-prepared to address the interconnected challenges of modern healthcare, making them valuable contributors in both clinical practice and public health initiatives.

Models of Accountability in Healthcare

Emanuel and Emanuel (1996) introduce a comprehensive framework for accountability in healthcare that highlights the evolving roles and responsibilities of healthcare professionals, including new graduates [15]. This structured approach includes three main components: *loci of accountability* (who is responsible), *domains of accountability* (areas of responsibility), and *procedures of accountability* (mechanisms to enforce accountability). Together, these elements work to enhance transparency, ethical conduct, and quality of care, aligning both individual and institutional actions with the larger goals of healthcare and societal well-being.

The framework also distinguishes three accountability models: Professional Accountability, Economic Accountability, and Political Accountability, which guide how healthcare professionals fulfill their responsibilities. Together, these models highlight the expanding roles of medical graduates, who must now consider ethical decision-making, cost-effective practices, and community health advocacy as integral to their practice.

Professional Accountability

Professional accountability lies at the heart of SA in healthcare. It requires physicians to uphold high standards of clinical and ethical conduct, recognizing that their responsibilities extend beyond patient care to include public welfare and community health. Socially accountable physicians demonstrate patient-centered care, cultural competence, and a commitment to equity in healthcare delivery, regardless of socioeconomic status or background [6].

Economic Accountability

Economic accountability underscores the importance of resource stewardship in healthcare, ensuring that care remains accessible and affordable. Physicians committed to SA advocate for fair healthcare policies, practice cost-effective care, and consider the economic impact of their decisions on patients and communities [16]. This approach demands an understanding of healthcare economics and sustainable funding, aligning financial practices with the best interests of society.

Political Accountability

Political accountability positions physicians as catalysts for social change, advocating for policies that promote public health and equity. Physicians in this role actively participate in health policy development, public health initiatives, and community health campaigns [15]. By leveraging their expertise, socially accountable physicians work to influence policy, support inclusive healthcare delivery, and remove systemic barriers to care.

The Multi-Dimensional Accountability of the Socially Accountable Physician

Today's healthcare landscape requires a multi-dimensional accountability framework for physicians, encompassing a broad range of stakeholders and demands. Physicians are accountable to patients, government bodies, legal and professional associations, private payers, and the larger community. This accountability is structured across multiple domains Fig. 2.1:

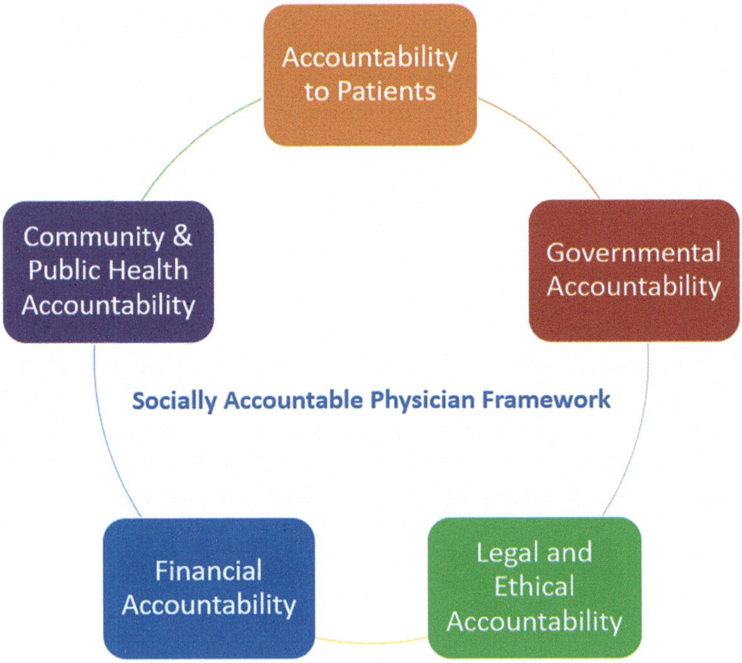

Fig. 2.1 Socially accountable physician framework

1. **Accountability to Patients**: Physicians are primarily responsible for delivering high-quality, patient-centered care. Socially accountable physicians engage with patients as advocates, ensuring care accessibility and affordability, and adapting practices to meet the diverse needs of patient populations [17].
2. **Governmental Accountability**: Physicians must comply with healthcare standards, legal mandates, and public health goals established by government bodies. Socially accountable physicians align their practices with national health priorities, promoting equity and justice in healthcare [18].
3. **Legal and Ethical Accountability**: Physicians answer to legal and professional entities that monitor ethical standards and clinical quality. Socially accountable physicians uphold transparency, ethical integrity, and adherence to established codes of conduct, maintaining the profession's highest standards [1].
4. **Financial Accountability**: Physicians are accountable to private payers and employers, advocating for cost-effective, high-quality care while using healthcare resources responsibly [19]. Socially accountable physicians practice economic efficiency, balancing patient welfare with fiscal responsibility.
5. **Community and Public Health Accountability**: Physicians have a societal responsibility to engage in public health efforts, preventive care, and address social determinants of health [20]. Through partnerships with public health agencies, community organizations, and government bodies, socially accountable physicians work to improve population health and advance health equity, especially for underserved communities.

This comprehensive approach to accountability establishes the core principles of socially accountable medical schools. Graduates from such programs are equipped not only with clinical expertise but also with a strong foundation in ethical practice, resource stewardship, and community advocacy. This preparation empowers them to manage the complexities of modern healthcare, drive systemic improvements, and champion equitable healthcare that benefits all stakeholders (Boelen et al., 2012). This framework enables medical graduates to navigate the healthcare landscape adeptly, advocate for vulnerable populations, and advance an inclusive, fair healthcare system.

Community Expectations from Doctors: Competencies for Socially Accountable Physicians

The "Five-Star Doctor" model proposed by the World Health Organization provides a foundational framework for the socially accountable physician, outlining key roles such as caregiver, decision-maker, communicator, community leader, and manager [21]. This model highlights the diverse responsibilities that physicians now fulfill, emphasizing not only patient-centered care but also the need to address social determinants of health, advocate for public health initiatives, and work collaboratively within multidisciplinary teams. International competency frameworks build upon this foundation, preparing physicians to respond effectively to evolving community needs and complex healthcare challenges.

As societal expectations of physicians expand, communities increasingly view doctors as advocates, educators, and leaders whose influence reaches beyond individual patient care to impact broader public health. The public now anticipates that physicians will engage in policy advocacy, consider the social factors affecting health, and support public health initiatives. This evolving perspective aligns closely with the role of the socially accountable physician—one who is proactive in addressing community health needs, committed to health equity, and dedicated to the overall well-being of society.

Competencies Required for Medical Graduates for their Evolving Roles

The competencies needed for evolving roles expand upon traditional clinical skills to encompass advocacy, policy engagement, and community health. This approach aligns with global frameworks that outline the skills physicians require to meet the changing expectations of the communities they serve.

1. **Clinical Expertise and Patient-Centered Care** At the core of clinical competence. Physicians are expected to provide safe, high-quality, evidence-based care, focusing on individual patient needs and delivering patient-centered services. This means understanding patients' backgrounds, preferences, and cultural contexts, ensuring that care is both respectful and responsive to the unique needs of each individual [22].
2. **Advocacy and Health Equity** Communities look to physicians as advocates for health equity and social justice. Medical graduates should actively engage with vulnerable populations and work to address social determinants of health, such as income, education, and access to healthcare [20]. By championing these issues within healthcare systems and at policy levels, physicians play a crucial role in reducing health disparities and ensuring equitable care for all community members.
3. **Community Engagement and Leadership** medical graduates need to be trained to be leaders in their communities, working collaboratively with local organizations, public health agencies, and government bodies. Community engagement involves listening to and understanding community needs, building partnerships, and working toward shared health goals [23]. Through this role, physicians become trusted figures who drive health promotion, engage in preventive care, and contribute to building healthier communities. Physicians must also recognize when to step back and allow the community or other health professionals to take on these leadership roles.
4. **Ethics and Professionalism** Ethical practice and professionalism are fundamental to medical practice. Physicians are expected to uphold the highest ethical

standards, demonstrating integrity, respect, and empathy. Professionalism also involves being accountable to diverse stakeholders, including patients, healthcare institutions, and society at large [24]. By adhering to ethical principles, socially accountable physicians build trust with their communities, maintaining the credibility and integrity of the medical profession.

5. **System-Based Practice and Interprofessional Collaboration** Modern healthcare systems are complex, requiring physicians to work within multidisciplinary teams. Learning about System-based practice enables medical graduates to navigate these systems effectively, ensuring continuity of care and resource efficiency [25]. By collaborating with other healthcare professionals, physicians can offer comprehensive care that addresses the full spectrum of a patient's needs, from clinical treatment to social and psychological support.
6. **Policy Engagement and Public Health Promotion** Medical graduates need to understand the importance of healthcare policies and participate in policy reform to promote health equity. This includes contributing to policy discussions, advocating for fair healthcare practices, and supporting public health initiatives. Physicians who engage in policy work help shape healthcare systems that better serve all community members, particularly those from marginalized backgrounds.

Examples from International Competency Frameworks and Evolving Roles of Medical Graduates

Global competency frameworks increasingly focus on developing socially accountable physicians who can respond to evolving community expectations. These frameworks expand traditional clinical skills to include competencies in advocacy, policy engagement, and community health, reflecting the growing role of medical graduates in addressing social determinants of health and supporting population well-being. Notable frameworks include:

- **CanMEDS Framework**: Developed by the Royal College of Physicians and Surgeons of Canada, CanMEDS outlines seven essential roles: medical expert, communicator, collaborator, leader, health advocate, scholar, and professional. The "health advocate" role is particularly relevant, encouraging physicians to take on a proactive role in addressing social determinants of health and advocating for patients within healthcare systems and society, meeting community expectations for socially responsible healthcare [26].
- **ACGME (Accreditation Council for Graduate Medical Education)**: In the United States, the ACGME framework defines six core competencies: patient care, medical knowledge, professionalism, communication, practice-based learning, and systems-based practice [27]. This framework is essential in training physicians to be patient-centered, ethical, and aware of social and systemic factors impacting healthcare, aligning with the growing community expectation for physicians to act as advocates and ethical leaders.

- **Tomorrow's Doctors**: Developed by the General Medical Council in the UK, the "Tomorrow's Doctors" framework emphasizes competencies in teamwork, communication, and understanding the social context of health [28]. This framework prepares graduates to navigate ethical complexities and actively engage with social determinants of health, promoting equity and meeting the public's expectation for compassionate, socially aware healthcare professionals.
- **International Medical University (IMU) Competency Framework**: The IMU framework in Malaysia emphasizes producing culturally aware and socially accountable physicians. By focusing on communication, ethical practice, and community service, the IMU framework equips graduates to address health disparities in Southeast Asia through advocacy and interprofessional collaboration, responding to the community's call for greater engagement in public health and social equity.
- **SaudiMEDs**: Saudi Arabia's competency framework, SaudiMEDs, highlights the roles of "collaborator" and "community advocate," encouraging physicians to engage in preventive care, health promotion, and public health [29]. With an emphasis on cultural competence, SaudiMEDs prepares graduates to address the nation's healthcare needs and evolving expectations, particularly in preventive and public health.
- **EmiratesMEDs**: In the UAE, the Emirates Medical Education Competencies framework aligns with national health priorities, emphasizing leadership, patient-centered care, and public health. This framework highlights the importance of cultural sensitivity and adaptability, preparing physicians to meet the expectations of a diverse and multicultural society while upholding high standards of social responsibility and healthcare quality [30].

Collectively, these frameworks underscore the global commitment to evolving medical education that meets shifting community expectations. They prepare physicians to be not only clinicians but also advocates, collaborators, and leaders who contribute to public health, social equity, and responsive, patient-centered healthcare.

Conclusion

The evolving role of the physician is both a response to and a driver of the changes taking place in healthcare today. Socially accountable physicians are no longer limited to traditional clinical roles; they are advocates, leaders, and collaborators committed to addressing health disparities and promoting public health. By integrating social accountability into medical education, the healthcare system can prepare a new generation of physicians equipped to meet these diverse challenges, ensuring that future physicians are not only clinically proficient but also socially conscious and community-focused.

The competencies outlined in this chapter—spanning patient advocacy, system integration, technological ethics, and community engagement—highlight the multifaceted nature of the modern physician's role. SA redefines this role, challenging physicians to extend their impact beyond clinical care and engage in initiatives that advance public health and healthcare equity. In this expanded role, the socially accountable physician becomes a catalyst for positive change, fulfilling the healthcare needs of individuals and communities alike while advancing the principles of equity, compassion, and social justice.

Take-Home Message

The evolving role of the medical profession calls for physicians who are more than just clinical experts; they are advocates, leaders, and active contributors to public health and social justice. This chapter underscores the importance of socially accountable medical practice, where physicians address social determinants of health, engage in ethical use of technology, and collaborate across disciplines to improve healthcare equity. By developing these competencies, future physicians can impact individual patient outcomes and advance the health of communities at large. As socially accountable professionals, physicians are empowered to promote a healthcare model that prioritizes empathy, inclusivity, and systemic progress for all.

References

1. Clithero-Eridon A, Albright D, Ross A. Conceptualising social accountability as an attribute of medical education. African J Prim Heal Care Fam Med. 2020;12(1):1–8.
2. Boelen C, Heck J. Defining and measuring social accountability of medical schools. Vol. WHO/HRH/95. 1995.
3. Markham R, Graham S, Hunt M, Betkus G, Woollard B, Snadden D, et al. Social accountability in practice: breathing and weaving together to build relationships and transform rural health services. Soc Innov J. 2022:14.
4. Frenk J, Chen L, Bhutta ZA, Cohen J, Crisp N, Evans T, et al. Health professionals for a new century: transforming education to strengthen health systems in an interdependent world. Lancet. 2010;376(9756):1923–58.
5. Abdalla ME, Taha MH, Onchonga D, Magzoub ME, Au H, O'Donnell P, et al. Integrating the social determinants of health into curriculum: AMEE Guide No. 162. Med Teach. 2023;1–13.
6. Green-Thompson LP, McInerney P, Woollard B. The social accountability of doctors: a relationship based framework for understanding emergent community concepts of caring. BMC Health Serv Res. 2017;17:1–7.
7. Buchman S, Woollard R, Meili R, Goel R. Practising social accountability: from theory to action. Can Fam Physician. 2016;62(1):15–8.
8. Abdalla ME, Taha MH, Onchonga D, Preston R, Barber C, Green-Thompson L, et al. Instilling social accountability into the health professions education curriculum with international case studies: AMEE Guide No. 175. Med Teach. 2024;1–14.

9. Abdalla M, Taha M, Mukhtar WNO, Elsanousi M. Impact of community-based medical education on graduate performance: a qualitative study using a critical incident technique, vol. 8; 2022. p. 38–44.
10. Grady CM. Can complexity science inform physician leadership development? Leadersh Health Serv. 2016;29(3):251–63.
11. Al-Fraihat D, Joy M, Masa'deh R, Sinclair J. Evaluating E-learning systems success: An empirical study. Comput Human Behav. 2020;
12. Murphy K, Di Ruggiero E, Upshur R, Willison DJ, Malhotra N, Cai JC, et al. Artificial intelligence for good health: a scoping review of the ethics literature. BMC Med Ethics. 2021;22:1–17.
13. Gonzalo JD, Chang A, Dekhtyar M, Starr SR, Holmboe E, Wolpaw DR. Health systems science in medical education: unifying the components to catalyze transformation. Acad Med. 2020;95(9):1362–72.
14. Singh MK, Gullett HL, Thomas PA. Using Kern's 6-step approach to integrate health systems science curricula into medical education. Acad Med. 2021;96(9):1282–90.
15. Emanuel EJ, Emanuel LL. What is accountability in health care? Ann Intern Med. 1996;124(2):229–39.
16. Guerzovich F, Poli M. How social accountability strengthens cross-sector initiatives to deliver quality health services? Glob Partnersh Soc Account Note. 2020;17
17. Chen J, Mullins CD, Novak P, Thomas SB. Personalized strategies to activate and empower patients in health care and reduce health disparities. Heal Educ Behav. 2016;43(1):25–34.
18. Dharamsi S, Ho A, Spadafora SM, Woollard R. The physician as health advocate: translating the quest for social responsibility into medical education and practice. Acad Med. 2011;86(9):1108–13.
19. Brett AS. Physicians have a responsibility to meet the health care needs of society. J Law Med Ethics. 2012;40(3):526–31.
20. National Academies of Sciences and Medicine E. A framework for educating health professionals to address the social determinants of health. 2016;
21. Boelen C. Frontline doctors of tomorrow. Indian J Pediatr. 1995;62(5):592.
22. Sopoaga F, Zaharic T, Kokaua J, Covello S. Training a medical workforce to meet the needs of diverse minority communities. BMC Med Educ. 2017;17(1):19.
23. Thach S, Hodge B, Cox M, Parlier-Ahmad A, Galvin S. Cultivating country doctors: preparing learners for rural life and community leadership. Fam Med. 2018;50(9):685–90.
24. Harden RM. Trends and the future of postgraduate medical education. Emerg Med J. 2006;23(10):798–802.
25. Gonzalo JD, Dekhtyar M, Starr SR, Borkan J, Brunett P, Fancher T, et al. Health systems science curricula in undergraduate medical education: identifying and defining a potential curricular framework. Acad Med. 2017;92(1):123–31.
26. Frank JR, Danoff D. The CanMEDS initiative: implementing an outcomes-based framework of physician competencies. Med Teach. 2007;29(7):642–7.
27. Day SH, Nasca TJ. ACGME international: the first 10 years. J Grad Med Educ. 2019;11(4s):5–9.
28. Rubin P, Franchi-Christopher D. New edition of tomorrow's doctors. Med Teach. 2002;24(4):368–9.
29. Zaini R, Al-Rumayyan A, Abdulghani H, AlQumaizi K, Al-Kadi A, Al-Hayani A, et al. Saudi medical education directives (MEDs) framework Saudi MEDs framework. Heal Prof Educ. 2023;9(4):7.
30. 3 Emirates MEDs Scientific Committee 202. UNITED ARAB EMIRATES Competency Framework For Medical Education [Internet]. Available from: https://www.caa.ae/PORTALGUIDELINES/2023-04-27 UAE Competency Framework For Medical Education, EmiratesMeds.pdf.

Further Reading

Benner P, Sutphen M, Leonard V, Day L. Educating nurses: a call for radical transformation, vol. 15. John Wiley & Sons; 2009.

Bleakley A, Bligh J, Browne J. Medical education for the future: identity, power and location, vol. 1. Springer Science & Business Media; 2011.

Rupert D. The evolving role of the physician: leading in care, leading in health care system change. 2018.

Chapter 3
Partnerships to Address Health Needs

Roger Strasser and Shafik Dharamsi

Learning Outcomes

1. Define partnership models that enhance social accountability in health professions education and public health.
2. Analyze the features of effective partnerships using case studies from Northern Ontario and North Texas.
3. Discuss strategies to leverage partnerships for achieving social accountability in diverse settings.

Partnerships in Healthcare, Public Health, and Health Professions Education

In this section, we highlight partnerships that have shaped health professions education, the delivery of health services, and the establishment of public health to meet population health needs.

Historical Context Historically, physicians have been solo practitioners who provide care for individual patients, although group medical practices began to emerge in the late nineteenth century. By the early twenty-first century, studies showed that group practices have many benefits for patients, physicians, and health systems [1].

R. Strasser (✉)
Northern Ontario School of Medicine (NOSM) University, Sudbury, ON, Canada

University of Waikato, Hamilton, New Zealand
e-mail: roger.strasser@nosm.ca

S. Dharamsi
University of North Texas Health Science Center School of Public Health, Fort Worth, TX, USA

M. E. Abdalla et al. (eds.), *Social Accountability of Medical Schools*,
https://doi.org/10.1007/978-3-031-94435-2_3

For institutional care, there historically has been a symbiotic relationship between physicians and hospitals based on an implicit agreement to work together to provide quality patient care [2].

Expansion of Medical Specialties and Public Health Programs Through the twentieth century, there was rapid expansion in medical specialties, public health programs, and health professional disciplines, as well as growing complexity in HSD systems [3]. These trends contributed to calls for and the development of partnership models to enhance the quality and effectiveness of health care while managing rising costs. Examples include intensive care units in hospitals [4] and community health centres [5], all of which feature interprofessional collaboration involving various health professionals and health administrators.

For HPE, partnerships between universities and hospitals were a key recommendation in the 1910 Flexner Report [6]. Flexner recommended that medical schools should be university based with the first half of undergraduate medical education programs focussed on the basic sciences and the second half involving students learning clinical medicine in teaching hospitals. Teaching hospitals or Academic Health Centres (AHC) are founded on partnerships between the universities/medical schools and the hospitals/health services. By the end of the twentieth century, AHCs were the predominant site of clinical education for most health professions [3].

Similarly, in 1915, Milton Rosenau's article in the Journal of the American Medical Association (JAMA) [7] and the subsequent Welch-Rose Report [8] were instrumental in shaping the landscape of public health education and the establishment of the first school of public health at Johns Hopkins University.

Rosenau advocated for a specialized approach to public health education and practice as distinct from medical education:

> The medical curriculum, already overcrowded, has little time for sanitation and hygiene, much less for epidemiology, public health administration, quarantine, management of epidemics, food adulteration, sewage disposal, water purification, housing, social service work, infant mortality, public health laboratory methods….

He called for specialized training in public health, including epidemiology, biostatistics, sanitation, and health policy. This article, along with other voices advocating for improved public health infrastructure and education, contributed to a growing awareness of the importance of public health as a distinct field of study and practice.

Shift Towards Social Determinants of Health In the 19th and early 20th centuries, schools of public health primarily focused on training in epidemiology, biostatistics, and environmental health to tackle issues like sanitation, hygiene, and infectious diseases. However, with the onset of the twenty-first century, there was a noticeable shift towards recognizing the impact of social and structural determinants of health and the importance of partnering across multiple sectors to advance health and health equity [9, 10]. This shift also highlighted a problem with the historical separation between the public health and healthcare sectors, leading to a disconnect between individual patient care and the broader well-being of communities and populations, and often neglecting crucial social determinants of health. The need for multisectoral partnerships involving health services organizations, public health entities, civil society, business and industry, and governmental organizations became evident to improve health outcomes on a larger scale.

Intersecting Medicine and Public Health In response to these challenges, the American Medical Association and the American Public Health Association collaborated to establish the Medicine/Public Health Initiative [11, 12]. This initiative examined why public health and medicine functioned as "separate and virtually independent components of the American health system" and explored opportunities for closer collaboration between them. The resulting report recommended strategies for reuniting public health and primary care medicine, emphasizing enhanced collaboration, closer working relationships, and a holistic approach to address both individual patient care and community health needs. Recognizing the critical role of connecting primary care with public health was seen as key to establishing more effective and equitable healthcare delivery systems.

In 2003, the Institute of Medicine (IOM) issued a critical analysis of the public health sector through its report, "Who Will Keep the Public Healthy?" [13] The report highlighted the growing disconnect between academic public health, the persistent inequities in health outcomes and addressing community-identified needs. Academic public health is now being called upon to help lead the transformation from siloed, disease-centric models focused on individuals to a collaborative, community-centered, population health model. This will necessitate robust partnerships across sectors between academia, civil society, government, and non-governmental agencies to effectively tackle emerging health challenges.

In 2010, 100 years post-Flexner, several published reports advocated for a new paradigm for HPE that focused on the priority health concerns of the community, region and/or nation they have the mandate to serve [14–18]. The most comprehensive and influential report was published by the Lancet Global Independent Commission entitled *Health Professionals for a New Century: Transforming Education to Strengthen Health Systems in an Interdependent World* [19]. It recommended a series of instructional and institutional reforms and enabling actions to address "fragmented, outdated, and static curricula that produce ill-equipped graduates; the mismatch of competencies to patient and population needs; poor teamwork; persistent gender stratification of professional status; narrow technical focus without broader contextual understanding; episodic encounters rather than continuous care; predominant hospital orientation at the expense of primary care; quantitative and qualitative imbalances in the professional labour market; and weak leadership to improve health-system performance." [19] Partnerships and Social Accountability were highlighted as pivotal principles for addressing these challenges and advancing health equity.

The Global Consensus for Social Accountability (GCSA) of medical schools was another landmark document published in 2010 documenting results from a

Delphi process involving 130 organizations including international health organizations, medical schools, professional associations, regulatory bodies, and government agencies, representing a broad spectrum of stakeholders in health education and policy-making.

The GCSA calls attention to quality, equity, relevance, and cost-effectiveness to guide the evolution of health professions education for the twenty-first century, with particular emphasis on partnerships with local communities and the health sector to identify and address local health needs and prioritize research and service activities accordingly [20]. For more details on the GCSA, see chaps. 1 and 9.

Beyond Voluntary Association to Binding Agreement

In general, the initial impetus for partnerships may be: locally driven or bottom-up; policy driven or top-down; or incentive driven in which there is money available for certain types of activities [21]. Partnerships within Health Professions Education and Health Services Delivery can emerge from tightly integrated alliances to more loosely connected associations [22]. Successful partnerships require agreement amongst all partners to include: a shared purpose and benefits; a clear sense of responsibilities and obligations; and agreement on the source and distribution of funding, expertise, and personnel. In HPE and HSD, the form of these partnerships varies considerably including public-private partnerships, inter-institutional collaborations in and between HSD and HPE institutions, partnerships to integrate individual and population health care, and government and non-government organization participation [23]. These health partnerships occur at the local, regional, national, and international levels shaped by identified needs, health system parameters, government policies, and funding sources [24].

At the global level, there has been a particular focus on partnerships that aim to address the global commitments to Universal Health Coverage (UHC) [25] and the Sustainable Development Goals (SDGs) [26]. Public-private partnerships have emerged as a key form through which healthcare and education are defined, delivered, and developed in low- and middle-income countries. These partnerships connote three fundamental themes: relative equality between partners; a mutual commitment to agreed objectives; and a mutual benefit for the participants involved [23]. There are many challenges associated with these partnerships including a tendency to focus on specific diseases which can distort planned health system development due to piecemeal interventions [24, 27].

For-profit business partnerships, including amongst health professionals, place legal obligations on partners that may not occur amongst and between HSD and HPE institutions. Collaborative initiatives between these institutions may be established with a shared vision, principles, and consensus decision-making; however, consensus decision-making may not deliver desired outcomes when participating organizations have overlapping mandates and hierarchical structures [28]. Successful partnerships require formal collaboration agreements that specify common purpose, partner contributions, and agreed goals and activities for mutual benefit.

Another recent HSD trend is person-centered care promoted globally in the WHO Framework on integrated people-centered health services (IPCHS) [29]. The IPCHS Framework calls for a fundamental shift in the way health services are funded, managed, and delivered [30]. Person-centered care is reflected in efforts to ensure patient participation in the design and implementation of healthcare towards the co-production of HSD [31]. Similarly, a people-centered approach to public health is intended to advance primary care, address the social determinants of health, and integrate the Sustainable Development Goals into essential public health functions and services through meaningful engagement and co-creation with communities [32]. There are calls also for co-production in HPE recognising the interconnections between HSD and HPE [33]. Co-production may be defined as "making better use of each other's assets, resources, and contributions to achieve better outcomes or improve efficiency". Social accountability provides a way for HPE to contribute to effective, equitable, and sustainable HSD improvements focussed on people's health needs [34].

Partnerships for Social Accountability

The 2000 WHO Working Paper *Towards Unity for Health: Challenges and Opportunities for Partnership in Health Development* [35] set out the principles and practicalities of implementing integration of individual and population health care, both in HSD and in HPE, towards achieving social accountability. This working paper introduced the Social Accountability Partnership Pentagram (SAPP) that specifies five key partners in determining and addressing people's health needs: policy makers; health managers; health professionals; academic institutions; and communities (see Fig. 3.1). Consistent with person-centredness and people-centered public health, the working paper highlights the importance of community participation acknowledging that the community partner perspective is often missing in developing HSD systems and public health programs. In this context, Community Engagement in the form of active community participation that values people's local knowledge and expertise is a key strategy for achieving social accountability and transformative change.

The SAPP provides a practical framework for collaborations focussed on HSD and HPE to address people's needs at the local, regional, provincial/state, and national levels. In British Columbia, Canada, the Rural Coordination Centre (RCC) adapted the SAPP to include a sixth partner, "linked sectors" (commercial and not-for-profit organizations) to the Partnership Pentagram Plus (PPP). Working with remote, rural, and Indigenous communities, the RCC convened PPP groups at local, regional, and provincial levels in Appreciative Inquiry to bring about practical and positive change to health services in these communities [36] (Fig. 3.2).

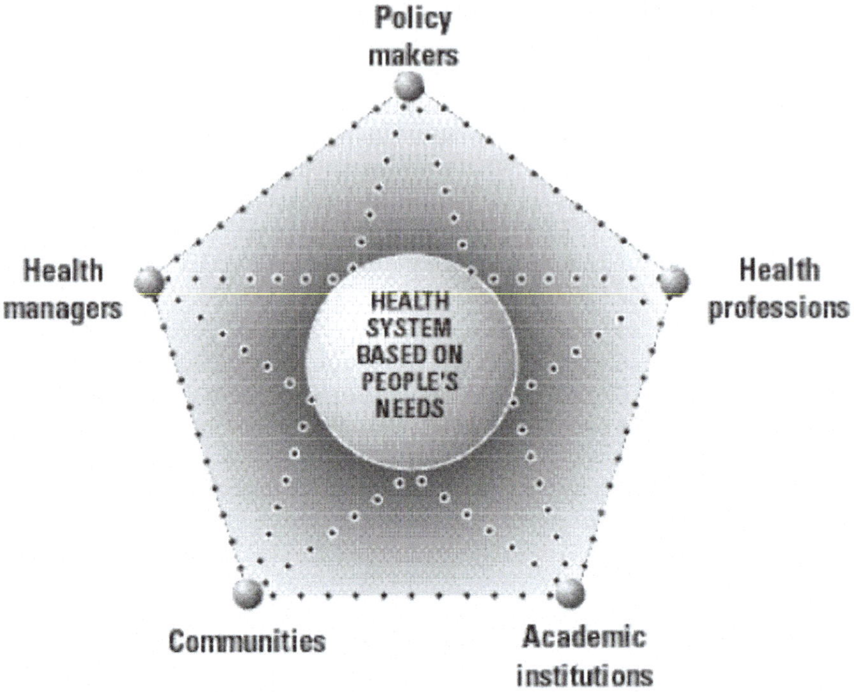

Fig. 3.1 Social accountability partnership pentagram (SAPP) (Partnership pentagram for a people-centered health system)

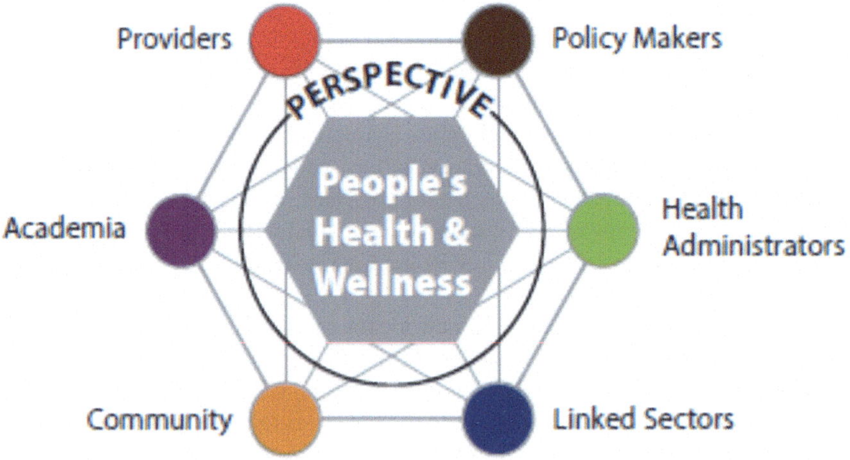

Fig. 3.2 Social accountability partnership pentagram plus (SAPPP) (Expanded partnership framework for people's health and wellness)

Case Studies

– Northern Ontario School of Medicine (NOSM) University

Northern Ontario, Canada is geographically vast (>800,000 km2) with a volatile resource-based economy and 40% of the population living in rural and remote areas including diverse communities and cultural groups, most notably Indigenous and Francophone peoples. The health status of people in the region is much worse than the province as a whole, and there is a chronic shortage of physicians and other health professionals. In this context, a widespread community movement advocated for the Ontario government to create a standalone Northern Ontario School of Medicine (NOSM). NOSM (now NOSM University) was established in 2002 with an explicit social accountability mandate focussed on improving the health of the people and communities in Northern Ontario [37].

Curriculum Model Consistent with its social accountability mandate, NOSM developed Distributed Community Engaged Learning (DCEL) as its distinctive model of medical education and health research [38]. Distributed learning occurs in over 90 sites and relies heavily on information and communications technology to connect the sites in real-time or asynchronously. The NOSM Health Sciences Library provides an extensive digital library service which, via the Internet, provides access to educational resources and information similar to that in urban teaching hospitals [39].

DCEL involves Immersive community-engaged education (ICEE) [40] whereby students are living and learning in a range of community and clinical settings during their 4 years of undergraduate medical education, most notably during the third year Comprehensive Community Clerkship (CCC). During this year, students live in one community away from the University centers and are based in family practice where they learn their core clinical medicine from the community, family practice perspective. The CCC is an example of a Longitudinal Integrated Clerkship (LIC—see Chap. 14) and it is the intense interaction with patients that motivate students to study hard and do the best they can for "their patients". Within 2 months, students have joined the health team and speak about going to work, rather than going to study. They have the social accountability orientation (focus on the health needs of the people they are serving) and a service mindset. In addition, their principal clinical teachers and role models are rural generalist physicians and other members of the health team [41].

Another feature of DCEL is Integrated Clinical Learning (ICL) which involves a team of clinical teachers from a range of health professions teaching a team of students learning together in common community and clinical settings. It is a balanced integration of educational strategies to develop healthcare providers and team-based competencies focused on improving the quality of care. Learning outcomes are developed with and in consideration of the goals of patients or the community through relational learning that mirrors person-centred care. Integrated Clinical Learning, team teaching and team learning, is Interprofessional Education in practice and has many advantages and substantial benefits for all involved, the patients and wider community, the clinicians and the learners [42].

Community Partnerships Community Engagement, the central feature of DCEL and ICEE, occurs through inter-dependent partnerships between the School and the communities for mutual benefit [43]. This form of community engagement is based on recognition that community members are experts on themselves and their community context, so that the partnership involves sharing expertise. Community Engagement in HPE involves active community participation in curriculum development and delivery, as well as hosting learners and helping them to appreciate the social determinants of health at the local level.

NOSM engaged Northern Ontario communities in the development of its academic programs from the outset, starting with a three-day *Getting Started in the North* workshop in January 2003 in preparation for the development of the NOSM curriculum, attended by over 300 participants drawn from communities across the region. Community engagement has continued through regular gatherings involving a wide range of community partners, including members of the local Indigenous and Francophone communities. NOSM community engagement aims to achieve co-creation, co-development co-delivery, and co-evaluation of NOSM's programs and activities [39].

Community engagement contributes throughout the career pathway stages of preadmission, admission, undergraduate medical education, postgraduate education, and beyond. Examples include high school students from Northern Ontario communities participating in NOSM's week-long Health Sciences Summer Camps; community volunteers participating in the MD admissions process, including as raters of written submissions and as interviewers; community members as standardized patients participating in clinical skills teaching; community members in over 90 communities, including Indigenous communities, hosting medical and other HPE students; and advocating for provincial government resources to enhance NOSM's programs and effectiveness [39].

Practicalities of Community Engagement In reality, implementing community engagement for mutual benefit is quite challenging. Communities often view academic institutions as distant "ivory towers" that only approach communities when they are looking to benefit the institution. This preconception has been the case, particularly for Indigenous communities. Consequently, engaging communities as genuine contributors and as shared decision-makers requires considerable effort. Effective strategies that promote mutually beneficial partnerships involve frequent discussions and regular face-to-face contact between NOSM personnel and community members in the communities. Relationships are formalized in written collaboration agreements and also by organizational structures such as the Local NOSM Groups (LNG) that function as steering committees in communities and are a mechanism by which NOSM is a part of the communities and the communities are a part of the School, particularly in the communities that host third-year medical students for the CCC.

Membership of LNGs is decided locally but usually includes local clinical faculty members, hospital/health service leaders, local government nominees, members of the physician recruitment committee, and representatives of local secondary and post-secondary institutions in these communities. NOSM funds a local Site Administrative Coordinator (SAC) in each CCC community with responsibility for the organization of all local NOSM-related activities, including student scheduling, and connecting students with local community activities and with NOSM support services [39].

In addition, there are two Reference Groups that are advisory committees on the health needs of Indigenous and Francophone populations in Northern Ontario, and staff in the communities are hired to work for the School (such as Regional Indigenous Coordinators for the Indigenous community experience and SACs in the CCC communities). It is an ongoing challenge to facilitate meaningful, reciprocal collaboration and ensure that suggested improvements are made while meeting accreditation criteria and other external constraints.

NOSM has hundreds of collaboration agreements with hospitals and health services, with community groups and organizations, and with other agencies across Northern Ontario. Each Collaboration Agreement begins by outlining NOSM's objectives and those of the partner organization, and is followed by an outline of the basis for collaboration, then the list of the responsibilities and expectations of both partners, and mechanisms whereby the partners will work together to achieve common goals facilitated by regular meetings. There are also a series of clauses that provide legal protection to both partners.

In addition to undergraduate medical education, NOSM offers postgraduate medical education (residency training) in family medicine and eight other major general specialties, as well as clinical education for future dietitians, physician assistants, physiotherapists, occupational therapists, speech-language pathologists, audiologists, and pharmacists. Like the MD program, these programs provide DCEL in a range of community and clinical settings in the region. NOSM's residency training is targeted on practising in Northern Ontario or similar rural/remote areas. Once in practice, NOSM provides continuing education/professional development to support and maintain Northern Ontario physicians and other health professionals. In addition, graduate studies programs encourage these health professionals to pursue academic careers with NOSM.

NOSM Outcomes It is 20 years since NOSM accepted its first students and there have been many positive outcomes for Northern Ontario and beyond.

Consistent with its Social Accountability mandate, NOSM aims to reflect the population distribution of Northern Ontario in each MD program class. A 10-year review of NOSM admissions showed that each year there were over 2000 applicants for 64 places with 20% of applicants called to interview and 15% of interviewees enrolled in the MD program. Overall, 92% of NOSM medical students have grown up in Northern Ontario with 40% from remote or rural backgrounds and 22% Francophone backgrounds, both of which are consistent with Northern Ontario demographics [38]. On the other hand, an average of 7% of each class were

Indigenous which is below the 12% target [44]. Subsequent changes to the NOSM admissions processes have raised the proportion of Indigenous students to around 12%. It is worth noting that the average Grade Point Average (GPA) of NOSM students on enrolment was 3.7 (out of 4) which is comparable to the academic scores of students admitted to other Canadian medical schools.

From the first graduation, NOSM MD students compared favourably with conventional medical schools in their Medical Council of Canada (MCC) qualifying examination results, including outperforming students from other schools in clinical decision-making. In most years, all NOSM MD students have been matched to residency in the first round of the national residency match known as Canadian Resident Matching Service (CaRMS). By contrast, there has been concern in recent years about Canadian students remaining unmatched to any residency program at the end of the CaRMS process.

Ten years after the first NOSM MD graduation, 77% of the graduates were in family practice and 14% were practising in other general specialties including general internal medicine, general surgery and paediatrics. 92% of the family practitioners who completed NOSM undergraduate and postgraduate training were practising in Northern Ontario [45].

Students, clinical teachers and communities report that their NOSM ICEE experiences are generally positive. Comments about the students' experiences include: "you won't be it, if you don't see it"; "the students learn from the patients"; "I like how much variety that can be in the doctor's role" and "you don't know it until you live it". A study of NOSM students' and graduates' experience of generalism in rural practice concluded that rural generalist medicine is not an alternative to urban specialist care, but an explicit provision of quality health care within geographic, demographic and cultural context, and human and material resource constraints of rural communities. Also, NOSM students and graduates reported that their NOSM experience shaped their career choices including specialty, scope of practice and location of practice [46].

Clinical teachers speak about the LIC experience as professionally rewarding and personally energising, with some physicians indicating that they delayed retirement or departure because of their renewed enthusiasm. They enjoy the relationships with students and other learners recognising the parallel between the patient-doctor and learner-teacher processes. Also, clinical teachers comment on the rewards of ICL collegiality and of patient involvement. Feedback from patients is summed up in the phrase "you're a better doctor when you have a student" because of the additional discussion and explanation involving the patient and the student [47].

Active community participation with NOSM fosters greater social connectedness and a collective community pride in educating future physicians. Research into the CCC identified the community contribution to the student's professional identity formation summed up by the phrase "it takes a community to train a future physician" [41]. In addition, studies of the impact of NOSM on Northern Ontario have shown benefits in terms of recruiting physicians and other health professionals, particularly to rural communities, as well as community capacity and capability building in terms of economic and social benefits including in the small communities [48]. The studies of NOSM's economic impact have shown a multiplier effect such that for every dollar of government funding spent, there are more than two dollars of new economic activity that would not be there without NOSM in the community [49]. The social impact reflects a sense of collective community empowerment summed up by the phrase "If we can do a successful medical school, we can do anything".

Facilitated Generalist Pathways From the beginning, NOSM focused on the life cycle of a physician in Northern Ontario based on evidence that students who have grown up in remote or rural communities followed by rural-based undergraduate and postgraduate education are much more likely to choose a career in rural practice. Subsequently, the life-cycle approach has been redeveloped as the Facilitated Generalist Pathway (FGP). This is a "cradle-to-grave" approach that begins with encouraging young people in Northern Ontario communities, including Indigenous communities, to see a career in health including studying medicine in their future. NOSM holds health sciences summer camps every year that bring high school students to the University sites for a week of activities that make the connection between their school studies and health careers [38]. More generally, the FGP involves visible and supported pathways into and through undergraduate and postgraduate medical education featuring ICEE, followed by support during the transition into unsupervised clinical practice. Once in practice, the FGP continues with continuing professional development, and opportunities for enhanced skills and other training including academic training while staying in their community. The NOSM Rural Generalist Pathway [50] is now established and similar pathways have developed for Indigenous and Francophone generalist careers as well.

Beyond Northern Ontario, other medical schools in Canada and elsewhere have drawn on the NOSM experience to introduce NOSM education innovations, including distributed medical education and rural family practice-based LICs.

In April 2022, NOSM transitioned to full university status as Canada's only medical university. This development has opened opportunities for NOSM to offer a wider range of HPE, and graduate studies and to be more involved in research focused on improving the health of the people of Northern Ontario.

- **University of North Texas Health Science Center School of Public Health (UNTHSC SPH)**

The School of Public Health (SPH) at the University of North Texas Health Science Center (HSC) was established in 1999 to address the region's health challenges, including high rates of chronic diseases and growing disparities in health outcomes. The new SPH was expected to focus on advancing health equity by protecting and promoting community well-being and improving population health outcomes in North Texas.

Although the United States spends over $4 trillion on health annually, more than other high-income countries, life expectancy is lower and health outcomes have deteriorated further since the start of the COVID-19 pandemic. Persistent underfunding has also led to a public health system that struggles to meet the country's population health needs and address growing disparities in health outcomes within and between communities. Texas, in particular, lags in avoidable deaths, maternal care, and healthcare accessibility according to the Commonwealth Fund's State Health System Performance Scorecard. These challenges have contributed to a growing mistrust in public health institutions (governmental, non-governmental, and community organizations) and public health systems (infrastructures, policies, and resources that support public health efforts). A joint report by the Robert Wood Johnson Foundation (RWJF) and Harvard TH Chan School of Public Health, released during the pandemic, highlighted this 'crisis of trust' in public health institutions. The report indicated lower trust levels among the public for key governmental institutions such as CDC (52%), state/local health departments (41%), NIH (37%), FDA (37%), and DHHS (33%) regarding recommendations made to improve health [51].

SPH Strategic Plan Despite its critical role in fostering trust and addressing health inequities and the social determinants of health, social accountability remains underemphasized in academic health science centers, including schools of public health. At the core of a socially accountable public health system lies the imperative to foster trust by prioritizing authentic, transparent, and meaningful community-centered engagement. This priority provided the foundation for a more compelling strategic plan for the SPH in the twenty-first century: *IMPACT 2030—Commitment to Community* [52], with a mission to advance health equity by collaboratively creating solutions for healthier communities and equitable health systems through socially accountable, community-centered and globally relevant education, research and service. To realize this mission, the SPH created a unique model—the *SPH Community Corps* [53]—to position community and health sector partners as an integral part of the shared governance process and the continuous refinement of curricula and research priorities for identifying and addressing the root causes of health inequities in the region.

Community Partnerships Developed by a task force comprised of community members, alumni, faculty, and students, the *Community Corps* aims to ensure that all partners have a meaningful and enduring voice in informing and transforming teaching, research, and service activities in ways that will prepare a community-responsive workforce, undertake scholarly activities that help to close the know-do gap, and collaboratively co-create solutions for healthier communities. The *SPH Community Corps* ensures that SPH's academic efforts are impactful and transformative toward improving the quality and conditions of life in the communities the SPH has a mandate to serve. Students are exposed to extended practical, real-world learning experiences and are actively involved in community-driven projects that have a meaningful impact. This approach prepares them for the challenges of public health practice and also nurtures a sense of social accountability and health advocacy [54].

Community Collaborative Research Regarding research, the SPH recognizes that historically, research within schools and programs of public health often overlooked non-academic partners as collaborators, limiting their involvement to supporting predefined research agendas. There is a growing recognition of the benefits of community-centered engagement in research, both in identifying key research questions and equitably engaging with community partners [55]. Fostering better health outcomes in our communities requires us to bridge the gap between scientific discovery and its effective translation and implementation into practice and policy [56]. This requires partnerships with community members, community-based organizations, and public health agencies throughout the research process, from conceptualization to dissemination to application. Community-Based Participatory Research (CBPR) and the Consolidated Framework for Implementation Research have served as fruitful models for bridging public health research and practice [57–59]. The SPH brings experience in supporting community-driven research and is institutionalizing this approach through the *Community Corps* model through collective capacity-building sessions with researchers, students, and community organizations.

Key to the SPH's continued success is recognizing and engaging the expertise and lived experience of local communities to help improve health outcomes, emphasizing trust, respect, shared decision-making, and acknowledging the strengths each partner brings [60]. This approach ensures relevance and fosters trust and sustainability in collaborative initiatives [61]. Members of the *Community Corps* serve in a variety of roles within the SPH. They serve as co-educators to help advance high-impact educational practices, partner in participatory research, contribute to strategic direction, facilitate special projects, and collaborate in workforce development. These roles integrate community perspectives, expertise, knowledge, and resources into SPH activities.

The establishment of the *Community Corps,* as a participatory framework within the academic shared governance model, is a key driver of change toward social accountability in public health education and research that fosters health equity.

SPH Priorities: As a result, transforming the SPH into a socially accountable and community-centered institution also required revising the academic promotion and tenure criteria. Extensive input from faculty led to the inclusion of assessment criteria based on engagement activities, seeking external reviews from community partners, and recognizing faculty leading community-partnered efforts. The following guidelines inform the SPH's approach to socially accountable partnerships:

- *Establish a Clear Mission*: Define a mission that explicitly addresses local health challenges and emphasizes community well-being and health equity.
- *Recognize Regional Health Needs*: Identify and prioritize specific health issues within the region, including inequities in health outcomes, and tailor joint efforts to create collaborative solutions.
- *Address Underfunding Challenges*: Acknowledge the impact of underfunding on public health systems and leverage collective resources to meet population health needs effectively.

- *Operationalize Social Accountability through Shared Governance*: Facilitate active participation of community and health sector partners in shared governance activities and setting research agendas, developing curricula, and informing resource allocation decisions, with a focus on collective capacity building and sustainable impact.
- *Prioritize Transformative Learning*: Design educational programs that offer transformative learning experiences, combining theoretical knowledge with practical, real-world projects to prepare students for public health practice and instil a sense of social responsibility.
- *Leverage Community Expertise*: Recognize and utilize the expertise within local communities by collaborating closely with community members and health sector partners to inform research, curriculum development, and strategic initiatives for co-creating and implementing solutions that are relevant, sustainable, and impactful.

– **Partnerships for Social Accountability around the World**

Although the two in-depth case studies are in North America, there are many examples of successful community partnerships to achieve HPE social accountability in other parts of the world, including low- and middle-income countries, particularly focused on rural health workforce [62]. Larkins et al [63] reviewed evidence from 14 THEnet schools with social accountability missions around the world to identify key factors that contribute to producing a fit-for-purpose rural health workforce, including community partnerships. The systematic literature review by Reeve et al [64] focused on the impact of socially accountable HPE highlighted community partnerships, equitable selection criteria, and community engaged placements in underserviced areas positively impact the learning and attitudes of students. In sub-Saharan Africa, Danhoundo et al. found that effective social accountability interventions involve leveraging partnerships and building coalitions, along with: being context appropriate; integrated data and information collection and analysis; clearly defined roles standards and responsibilities of leaders and meaningful citizen engagement [65].

The Patan Academy of Health Sciences (PAHS) in Nepal stands out as a successful model of HPE founded on partnerships including community participation in curriculum design, student selection, rural education teaching-learning processes and student assessment [66].

Similarly, Public Health and Health Policy social accountability initiatives have been implemented around the world. These initiatives have been tailored to address specific local needs and contexts, demonstrating the versatility and adaptability of social accountability principles. Examples include: in South Africa, the District Health System (DHS) has implemented a social accountability framework to improve healthcare delivery and outcomes [67]; in India, the National Rural Health Mission (NRHM) has incorporated social accountability principles to improve healthcare services in rural areas, including community-based monitoring, village health committees, and citizen-led planning and budgeting [68]; in Croatia, Serbia and Ghana, the Kybele partnership model built on strong champions, stakeholder engagement, and partners co-creating solutions has brought improvements in maternal and neonatal health [69]; in Nigeria, community health committees have been established to pursue health improvements through social accountability with particular emphasis on community engagement [70]; and, in Malawi, the CARE Community Score Card has been used to facilitate improvements in reproductive health-related social accountability outcomes [71]. These examples demonstrate the potential of social accountability initiatives to improve healthcare services and health outcomes in diverse contexts. By engaging communities, promoting participatory planning, and fostering collaborative monitoring and evaluation, social accountability initiatives can help achieve health equity and social justice [72, 73].

Conclusion

This chapter has highlighted the importance of partnerships to achieve social accountability and health equity. The Socially Accountability Partnership Pentagram (SAPP) adapted to the Partnership Pentagram Plus (PPP) provides a framework to ensure active community participation (Community Engagement). The Global Consensus for Social Accountability (GCSA) highlights quality, equity, relevance, and cost-effectiveness as key criteria for measuring social accountability. There are two in-depth case studies and many other examples of partnerships for social accountability in health professions education and on public health around the world.

Take Home Messages

- Partnerships are integral to the achievement of social accountability and health equity.
- Successful long-term partnerships require formal collaboration agreements that specify a common purpose, partner contributions, and agreed goals and activities for mutual benefit.
- Authentic community engagement is founded on interdependent partnerships between communities and academic institutions, clinical and public health professionals, healthcare institutions, and government and non-government organizations.

Acknowledgments The authors express sincere gratitude to Dr. Emily Spence and Dr. Misty Smethers for providing an insightful review and constructive feedback on the University of North Texas Health Science Center School of Public Health case study. Their contribution has greatly enriched the content and quality of this work.

The Community Corps model was developed by a task force of community partners, faculty, and staff under the leadership of Dr. Spence to consider how the UNTHSC School of Public Health can build an infrastructure that would center community partners in everything we do—It honors their expertise, their lived experiences, and their vital role in driving solutions for a healthier community. The task force sought to move from having a collection of projects and activities that depend on individual relationships, to an architecture that centers community partnerships as the default way of doing business.

References

1. Zwiep T, Ahn S(H), Brehaut J, et al. Group practice impacts on patients, physicians, and healthcare systems: a scoping review. BMJ Open. 2021;11:e041579. https://doi.org/10.1136/bmjopen-2020-041579.
2. Hariri H, Prestipino AL, Rubash HE. The hospital-physician relationship: past, present, and future. Clin Orthop Relat Res. 2007;457:78–86. https://doi.org/10.1097/BLO.0b013e31803372a7.
3. Green LA, Fryer GE Jr, Yawn BP, Lanier D, Dovey SM. The ecology of medical care revisited. N Engl J Med. 2001;344:2021–5. https://doi.org/10.1056/NEJM200106283442611.
4. Kelly FE, Fong K, Hirsch N, Nolan JP. Intensive care medicine is 60 years old: the history and future of the intensive care unit. Clin Med. 2014;14(4):376–9.
5. Community Health Centers: Chronicling Their History and Broader Meaning. Chcchronicles. https://www.chcchronicles.org/stories/community-health-centers-chronicling-their-history-and-broader-meaning
6. Flexner A. Medical education in the United States and Canada: a report to the Carnegie Foundation for the Advancement of Teaching. In: Bulletin number four. New York, NY: Carnegie Foundation for the Advancement of Teaching; 1910.
7. Rosenau MJ. Courses and degrees in public health work. JAMA. 2015 Mar 17;313(11):1172. https://doi.org/10.1001/jama.2015.1736.
8. Thomas KK. Cultivating hygiene as a science: the Welch-rose report's influence at Johns Hopkins and beyond. Am J Epidemiol. 2016 Feb 17;183(5):345–54. https://doi.org/10.1093/aje/kwv331.
9. DeSalvo KB, Wang YC, Harris A, Auerbach J, Koo D, O'Carroll P. Public health 3.0: a call to action for public health to meet the challenges of the 21st century. Prev Chronic Dis [Internet]. 2017 Sep 7;14(E78) Available from: cdc.gov/pcd/issues/2017/17_0017.htm
10. Walker B. The future of public health: the Institute of Medicine's 1988 report. J Public Health Policy [Internet]. 1989;10(1):19–31. Available from: pubmed.ncbi.nlm.nih.gov/2715336/
11. Lasker RD, Committee on Medicine and Public Health NYA of M, Abramson D. Medicine & Public health: the power of collaboration [internet]. NYU scholars. New York, NY: Center for the advancement of collaborative strategies in health, the New York Academy of Medicine; 1997. [cited 2024 Apr 15]. Available from: nyuscholars.nyu.edu/en/publications/medicine-amp-public-health-the-power-of-collaboration
12. Lasker RD. Broadening participation in community problem solving: a multidisciplinary model to support collaborative practice and research. J Urban Health: Bull NY Acad Med. 2003 Mar 1;80(1):14–60. https://doi.org/10.1093/jurban/jtg014.
13. Institute of Medicine (US) Committee on Educating Public Health Professionals for the 21st Century. Who Will Keep the Public Healthy?: Educating Public Health Professionals for the 21st Century [Internet]. nap.nationalacademies.org. 2002. Available from: nap.nationalacademies.org/catalog/10542/who-will-keep-the-public-healthy-educating-public-health-professionals
14. Ludmerer KM. Understanding the Flexner report. Acad Med. 2010;85:193–6. https://doi.org/10.1097/ACM.0b013e3181c8f1e7.
15. Boelen C. A new paradigm for medical schools a century after Flexner's report. Bull World Health Organ. 2002;80:592–3.

16. Cooke M, Irby DM, O'Brien BC. Educating physicians: a call for reform of medical school and residency. Stanford, Calif: Jossey-Bass; 2010.
17. Association of Faculties of Medicine of Canada. The future of medical education in Canada: a collective vision of MD education. Ottawa, Ontario, Canada: Association of Faculties of Medicine of Canada; 2010.
18. Prislin MD, Saultz JW, Geyman JP. The generalist disciplines in American medicine one hundred years following the Flexner report: a case study of unintended consequences and some proposals for post-Flexnerian reform. Acad Med. 2010;85(2):228–35. https://doi.org/10.1097/ACM.0b013e3181c877bf.
19. Frenk J, Chen L, Bhutta ZA, et al. Health professionals for a new century: transforming education to strengthen health systems in an interdependent world. Lancet. 2010;376:1923–58. https://doi.org/10.1016/S0140-6736(10)61854-5.
20. GCSA (Global Consensus for Social Accountability of Medical Schools). 2010. Available at: https://healthsocialaccountability.sites.olt.ubc.ca/files/2011/06/11-06-07-GCSA-English-pdf-style.pdf
21. Brandstetter R, de Bruijn H, Byrne M, et al. Successful partnerships: a guide. OECD LEED. 2006; https://www.oecd.org/cfe/leed/36279186.pdf
22. Allen PM, Finnerty MJ, Gish RS, et al. Guide to Health care partnerships for population health management and value-based care. 2016. Chicago, IL: Health Research & Educational Trust and Kaufman, Hall & Associates, LLC. Accessed at www.hpoe.org
23. Gideon J, Unterhalter E. Exploring public private partnerships in health and education: a critique. Journal of International and Comparative Social Policy. 2017;33(2):136–41. https://doi.org/10.1080/21699763.2017.1330699.
24. Abeykoon P. Partnerships in health development. J Health Manag. 2021;23(1):143–54. https://doi.org/10.1177/0972063421995007.
25. WHO. The world health report: health systems financing: the path to universal coverage. World Health Organization. 2010. Geneva, Switzerland. https://www.who.int/publications/i/item/9789241564021
26. United Nations. Sustainable development goals. 2015. https://sdgs.un.org/goals
27. Strasser R, Kam SM, Regalado SM. Rural health care access and policy in developing countries. Annu Rev Public Health. 2016;37:395–412. https://doi.org/10.1146/annurev-publhealth-032315-021507.
28. Herbert CP, Busing N, Nasmith L. Collaborative governance of postgraduate medical education: can it be achieved? Med Teach. 2021;43(12):1413–8. https://doi.org/10.1080/0142159X.2021.1951691.
29. WHO Framework on integrated people-centred health services (IPCHS) https://www.who.int/health-topics/integrated-people-centered-care#tab=tab_1
30. Elan A, McCormack B, Dewing J, et al. Review of developments in person-centred healthcare. International Practice Development Journal. 2020;10(Suppl):1–29. https://doi.org/10.19043/ipdj.10Suppl2.003.
31. Batalden M, Batalden P, Margolis P, et al. Coproduction of healthcare service. BMJ Qual Saf. 2016;25:509–17. https://doi.org/10.1136/bmjqs-2015-004315.
32. Canchihuaman FA, Leyns CC, Mezzich JE. People-centered public health. In: Mezzich JE, Appleyard WJ, Glare P, Snaedal J, Wilson CR, editors. Person centered medicine. Cham: Springer; 2023. https://doi.org/10.1007/978-3-031-17650-0_38.
33. Englander R, Holmboe E, Batalden P, et al. Coproducing health professions education: a prerequisite to coproducing health care services? Acad Med. 2020;95(7):1006–13.
34. Boelen C. Coordinating medical education and health care systems: the power of the social accountability approach. Med Educ. 2018;52:96–102. https://doi.org/10.1111/medu.13394.
35. Boelen C. Towards Unity for health: challenge and opportunities for partnership in health development. Geneva, Switzerland: World Health Organization; 2000.
36. Markham R, Hunt M, Woollard R, et al. Addressing rural and indigenous health inequities in Canada through socially accountable health partnerships. BMJ Open. 2021;11:e 048053. https://doi.org/10.1136/bmjopen-2020-048053.

37. Tesson G, Hudson G, Strasser R, Hunt D. The making of the northern Ontario School of Medicine: a case study in medical education. Montreal: McGill Queens University Press; 2009.
38. Strasser R, Lanphear J, McCready W, et al. Canada's new medical school: the northern Ontario School of Medicine–social accountability through distributed community engaged learning. Acad Med. 2009;84:1459–64.
39. Strasser R, Hogenbirk J, Jacklin K, et al. Community engagement: a central feature of NOSM'S socially accountable distributed medical education. Can Med Educ J. 2018;9(1):e33–43. https://doi.org/10.36834/cmej.42151.
40. Strasser R. Immersive community engaged education: More CEL than WIL. Chapter 12 in Pretti J, Stirling A (ed). WIL in Canada. eBook: World association for co-op and work-integrated education (WACE) and Co-operative education and work-integrated learning (CEWIL) Canada, 2021.
41. Dube TV, Schinke RJ, Strasser R. It takes a community to train a future physician: social support experienced by medical students during a community-engaged longitudinal integrated clerkship Canadian medical. Educ J. 2019;10(3):e55–60. Available at http://www.cmej.ca
42. Strasser R, Berry S. Integrated clinical learning: team teaching and team learning in primary care. Educ Prim Care. 2021;32(3):130–4. https://doi.org/10.1080/14739879.2021.1882886.
43. Strasser R, Worley P, Cristobal F, Marsh DC, Berry S, Strasser S, Ellaway R. Putting communities in the driver's seat: the realities of community engaged medical education. Acad Med. 2015;90:1466–70.
44. Mian O, Hogenbirk J, Marsh DC. Tracking indigenous applicants through the admissions process of a socially accountable medical school. Acad Med. 2019;94:1211–9. https://doi.org/10.1097/ACM.0000000000002636.
45. Hogenbirk JC, Strasser RP, French MG, Ten years of graduates: a cross-sectional study of the practice location of doctors trained at a socially accountable medical school. PLoS ONE. 2022;17(9):e0274499. 1–15
46. Strasser R, Cheu H. The needs of the many: NOSM students' experience of Generalism and rural practice. Can Fam Physician. 2018;64:449–55.
47. Strasser RP, Herbert CP, Ventres WB. *Learning in Urban and Rural Communities*. In: Dent J, Harden R, Hunt D, editors. A practical guide for medical teachers. 6th ed. Elsevier; 2021.
48. Mian O, Warry W, Strasser R. How underserviced rural communities approach physician recruitment: changes following the opening of a socially accountable medical school in northern Ontario. Can J Rural Med. 2017;22(4):139–47.
49. Hogenbirk HC, Robinson DR, Strasser RP. Distributed education enables distributed economic impact: the economic contribution of the northern Ontario School of Medicine to communities in Canada. Heal Econ Rev. 2021;11(20):1–10. https://doi.org/10.1186/s13561-021-00317-z.
50. NOSM Rural generalist pathw ay. https://www.nosm.ca/our-community/nosm-physician-workforce-strategy/rural-generalist-pathway/
51. Harvard University, Robert Wood Johnson Foundation. The public's perspective on the United States public health system. May 2021. Accessed April 5th 2024. cdn1.sph.harvard.edu/wp-content/uploads/sites/94/2021/05/RWJF-Harvard-Report_FINAL-051321.pdf.
52. UNT HSC School of Public Health Strategic Plan. https://www.unthsc.edu/school-of-public-health/impact-2030-commitment-to-community/
53. Spence E. Twenty-five years of community engagement and the development of the Community Corps. American Association of Schools & Programs of Public Health (ASPPH). ASPPH Presents Webinar: Advancing Public Health Practice: Strategic Partnerships for a Healthier Tomorrow [Webinar]. 2024. Retrieved from https://aspph.org/event/aspph-presents-webinar-advancing-public-health-practice-strategic-partnerships-for-a-healthier-tomorrow/
54. Dharamsi S, Ho A, Spadafora S, Woollard R. The physician as health advocate: translating the quest for social responsibility into medical education and practice. Acad Med. 2011;86(9):1108–13. https://doi.org/10.1097/ACM.0b013e318226b43b.
55. Schiavo R. What is true community engagement and why it matters (now more than ever)? J Commun Healthc. 2021;14(2):91–2. https://doi.org/10.1080/17538068.2021.1935569.

56. Odeny B. Closing the health equity gap: a role for implementation science? PLoS Med. 2021;18(9):e1003762. https://doi.org/10.1371/journal.pmed.1003762.
57. Damschroder LJ, Aron DC, Keith RE, Kirsh SR, Alexander JA, Lowery JC. Fostering implementation of health services research findings into practice: a consolidated framework for advancing implementation science. Implement Sci. 2009;4:50. https://doi.org/10.1186/1748-5908-4-50.
58. Israel BA, Coombe CM, Cheezum RR, Schulz AJ, McGranaghan RJ, Lichtenstein R, et al. Community-based participatory research: a capacity-building approach for policy advocacy aimed at eliminating health disparities. Am J Public Health. 2010 Nov;100(11):2094–102. https://doi.org/10.2105/AJPH.2009.170506.
59. Jull J, Giles A, Graham ID. Community-based participatory research and integrated knowledge translation: advancing the co-creation of knowledge. Implementation Sci. 2017;12:150. https://doi.org/10.1186/s13012-017-0696-3.
60. Tsai E, Allen P, Saliba LF, et al. The power of partnerships: state public health department multisector collaborations in major chronic disease programme areas in the United States. Health Res Policy Sys. 2022;20(1):80. https://doi.org/10.1186/s12961-021-00765-3.
61. Di Ruggiero E, Papadopoulos A, Steinberg M, et al. Strengthening collaborations at the public health system-academic interface: a call to action. Can J Public Health. 2020; 111(6):921–5. https://doi.org/10.17269/s41997-020-00436-w.
62. Johnston K, Guingona M, Elsanousi S, et al. Training a fit-for-purpose rural health workforce for low- and middle-income countries (LMICs): How do drivers and enablers of rural practice intention differ between learners from LMICs and high income countries? Front Public Health. 2020;8:582464. https://doi.org/10.3389/fpubh.2020.582464.
63. Larkins SL, Cristobal F, Hogenbirk, et al. Mission and role modelling in producing a fit-for-purpose rural health workforce: perspectives from an international community of practice. Med J Aust. 2023;219(3 Suppl):s20–6.
64. Reeve C, Woolley T, Ross SJ, et al. The impact of socially-accountable health professional education: a systematic review of the literature. Med Teach. 2017;39(1):67–73.
65. Danhoundo G, Nasiri K, Wiktorowicz ME. Improving social accountability processes in the health sector in sub-Saharan Africa: a systematic review. BMC Public Health. 2018;18(417):1–8.
66. Baral K, Allison J, Upadhyay, et al. Rural community as context and teacher for health professions education. Cureus. 2016;8(11):e866. https://doi.org/10.7759/cureus.866.
67. Tshabalala K, Rispel LC. Piercing the veil on the functioning and effectiveness of district health system governance structures: perspectives from a south African province. BMC Health Research Policy and Systems. 2023;21(89):1–23.
68. Vellakkal S, Gupta A, Khan Z, et al. Has India's national rural health mission reduced inequities in maternal health services? A pre-post repeated cross-sectional study. Health Policy Plan. 2017;32(1):79–90.
69. Ramaswamy R, Kallam B, Kopic D, et al. Global health partnerships: building multinational collaborations to achieve lasting improvements in maternal and neonatal health. BMC Globalization and Health. 2016;12(22):1–8.
70. Abimbola S, Drabarek D, Molemodile SK. Self-reliance or social accountability? The raison d'être of community health committees in Nigeria. Int J Health Plann Mgmt. 2022;37:1722–35.
71. Gullo S, Galavotti C, Sebert Kuhlmann A, et al. Effects of a social accountability approach, CARE's community score card, on reproductive health-related outcomes in Malawi: a cluster-randomized controlled evaluation. PLoS One. 2017;12(2):e0171316.
72. Guerzovich F, Poli M. How social accountability strengthens cross-sector initiatives to deliver quality health services? Global Partnership for Social Accountability Note 17. Washington DC: World Bank Group; 2020.
73. Hilber AM, Doherty P, Nove A, et al. The development of a new accountability measurement framework and tool for global health initiatives. Health Policy Plan. 2020;35:765–74.

Further Reading

ASPPH. Framing the Future 2030s: Fostering Community Partnerships for a Healthier World [Internet]. Available from: https://aspph.org/framing-the-future-2030s-fostering-community-partnerships-for-a-healthier-world-report/

Dharamsi S, Ho A, Spadafora SM, Woollard R. The physician as health advocate: translating the quest for social responsibility into medical education and practice. Acad Med. 2011;86(9):1108–13. https://doi.org/10.1097/ACM.0b013e318226b43b.

Frenk J, Chen L, Bhutta ZA, et al. Health professionals for a new century: transforming education to strengthen health systems in an interdependent world. Lancet. 2010;376:1923–58. https://doi.org/10.1016/S0140-6736(10)61854-5.

Forum on Public-Private Partnerships for Global Health and Safety. Board on Global Health; Institute of Medicine; National Academies of Sciences, Engineering, and Medicine. The role of public-private partnerships in health systems strengthening: workshop summary. Washington (DC): National Academies Press (US); 2016 Jun 1.

National Academies of Sciences, Engineering, and Medicine; Health and Medicine Division; Board on Population Health and Public Health Practice; Committee on community-based solutions to promote health equity in the United States. Editors: Alina Baciu, Yamrot Negussie, Amy Geller, and James N. Weinstein. Washington (DC): National Academies Press (US); 2017 Jan 11.

Strasser R, Strasser S. Reimagining primary health care workforce in rural and underserved settings (English). Health, nutrition, and population (HNP) Discussion Paper. Washington, DC: World Bank Group; 2020. http://documents.worldbank.org/curated/en/304851606975759118/Reimaging-Primary-Health-Care-Workforce-in-Rural-and-Underserved-Settings

Part II
Leadership, Governance, and Institutional Alignment

Chapter 4
Governance and Leadership for Socially Accountability

Ahmed Maherzi and Mohamed Hassan Taha

Learning Outcomes

1. Describe leadership models that facilitate the promotion of social accountability in medical schools.
2. Develop strategies to apply leadership principles in guiding medical faculties toward social accountability in diverse contexts.
3. Understand the key characteristics of governance structures that support socially accountable medical education.
4. Draw lessons from case studies on how leaders have successfully promoted social accountability within medical schools.

Background

Social accountability has evolved from a conceptual aspiration into a core operational standard in health professions education. Introduced by the World Health Organization in the 1990s, it has become a defining benchmark for how medical schools contribute to public good. Today, social accountability is not optional—it is essential for institutions seeking to remain relevant, credible, and impactful. This shift reflects growing societal expectations that health professions education

A. Maherzi
Faculté de médecine de l'Université de Montréal (Canada), Conférence Internationale des Doyens et des Facultés de Médecine d'Expression Française (CIDMEF) and Réseau International Francophone pour la Responsabilité Sociale en Santé (RIFRESS), Québec City, Canada

M. H. Taha (✉)
College of Medicine and Medical Education Center, University of Sharjah, Sharjah, UAE
e-mail: mtaha@sharjah.ac.ae

M. E. Abdalla et al. (eds.), *Social Accountability of Medical Schools*,
https://doi.org/10.1007/978-3-031-94435-2_4

responds directly to local, national, and global health needs. Within this evolving context, leadership has emerged as a central lever for translating institutional mission into measurable social impact. Leadership shapes strategic direction, institutional culture, curriculum reform, stakeholder relationships, and research priorities. It is the mechanism by which social accountability moves from rhetoric to reality. Yet, despite its importance, leadership development remains inconsistently addressed. Many institutions lack structured strategies to develop the leadership required for socially accountable education. Where leadership programs do exist, they often emphasize administrative functions or personal traits over systems-level change and social. This chapter explores the critical role of governance and leadership in embedding Social Accountability (SA) within medical education institutions.

Importance of Leadership for Social Accountability of Medical Schools

In an era where healthcare systems worldwide face significant challenges in ensuring universal health, addressing social inequalities, and tackling environmental issues, the role of academic leaders in advancing Social Accountability (SA) in healthcare is paramount [1]. These leaders are crucial in establishing goals, fostering a culture of SA, and serving as role models, thereby influencing the entire medical school's dedication to this cause [2]. Social Accountability must transcend mere rhetoric; it should be integral to the identity of the school. Here, the leadership of senior management, notably the Dean, is pivotal in championing SA. The Dean sets the tone by defining the school's vision [3].

Committed and visionary leadership is essential for the Dean to lead their faculty towards achieving recognition for excellence in SA. By actively promoting SA, the Dean will establish clear sustainability goals, align them with the school's mission, and effectively communicate these objectives to the entire institution. Additionally, the Dean must inspire and persuade various stakeholders—senior faculty leaders, department heads, teachers, students, and community members. Their ability to rally diverse groups around a shared vision is crucial for implementing meaningful change towards SA. This endeavor demands boldness, courage, humility, and a receptive attitude, all of which are pivotal in advancing SA initiatives. The collective commitment to SA will enhance the institution's visibility, credibility, and impact, gradually ingraining SA into the school's DNA.

Dimensions of Leadership in Advancing Social Accountability

Vision and Cultural Leadership Leaders define the organization's vision and values, fostering a culture that prioritizes SA in healthcare. They inspire and motivate staff to integrate SA into their daily practices. For example, a dean may develop a strategic plan that includes specific SA objectives, such as integrating community health projects into the curriculum or emphasizing service-learning opportunities.

Policy and Strategy Development Leaders spearhead the development of policies and strategies that support SA in health. This encompasses initiatives to reduce health disparities, enhance healthcare accessibility, and promote sustainability in medical practices. An example of this in practice would be establishing policies that require all medical students to complete rotations in underserved communities, ensuring they gain first-hand experience with health disparities.

Stakeholder Engagement Leaders mobilize diverse stakeholders—healthcare professionals, patients, policymakers, and community groups—to collaborate on advancing SA in health. They facilitate cooperation to maximize collective impact on public health. Practically, this might involve forming partnerships with local health organizations to co-create community health interventions, ensuring that the medical school's activities are aligned with the needs of the community.

Resource Management Leaders allocate resources strategically to bolster initiatives promoting SA. This involves funding for prevention programs, community health services, and research on social determinants of health. For instance, a dean could secure funding to support student-led community clinics that provide free or low-cost care to underserved populations, thus addressing immediate health needs and offering practical learning experiences.

Accountability Leaders ensure accountability by overseeing the organization's societal impact and health outcomes. They establish mechanisms to evaluate performance and drive continual improvement in SA practices. This might include implementing a framework for regular assessment of SA initiatives, using metrics such as community health outcomes, student engagement in SA activities, and feedback from community partners.

In summary, effective leadership is essential for promoting Social Accountability of medical schools through vision setting, policy development, stakeholder engagement, resource allocation, and accountability. Leaders' decisions and actions significantly influence population health and societal well-being. Their commitment to these principles ensures that Social Accountability becomes an enduring and intrinsic part of the medical faculty's identity and operations. By linking theoretical models of leadership to practical applications, leaders can create a culture of Social Accountability that not only improves health outcomes but also fosters a more equitable and just healthcare system.

Leadership Models that Promote Social Accountability of Medical Schools

Leadership models that emphasize Social Accountability (SA) in healthcare and health professions education prioritize collaboration, values-driven approaches, and stakeholder engagement. These models are instrumental in fostering environments where ethical principles and community needs drive decision-making and action

[4]. This section explores key features of these models, drawing from literature in medical education and providing practical examples.

Transformative Leadership

Transformative leadership aims to inspire and motivate team members towards shared goals, fostering creativity, innovation, and commitment to Social Accountability (SA). Transformative leaders position themselves as agents of positive change, driving significant and enduring improvements within the healthcare sector by prioritizing ethical values, equity, and community commitment [5]. Givens, R. J. (2008) describe transformational leaders as those who inspire followers by creating a vision and encouraging innovation [6]. Transformational leadership is characterized by four components: idealized influence, inspirational motivation, intellectual stimulation, and individualized consideration [7]. Transformative leaders serve as exemplars, guided by principles such as health equity, social justice, and respect for human rights [8]. In medical schools, transformative leaders inspire their teams by clearly articulating a vision for SA and encouraging faculty and students to engage in innovative community health projects [9, 10]. For example, a dean who leads the development of a community health initiative that integrates service learning into the curriculum demonstrates transformational leadership. This approach addresses community needs while fostering a commitment to SA among students and faculty.

By integrating these characteristics, transformative leadership in SA serves as a catalyst for reshaping medical practices and health policies, ultimately advancing the health and well-being of vulnerable populations. This holistic approach ensures that future healthcare professionals are well-equipped to serve diverse populations and address complex social determinants of health.

Box 4.1 Example of Transformative Leadership and Social Accountability

A Dean at a medical school recognizes significant health disparities in the local community, particularly among low-income and minority populations. To address this, the Dean articulates a vision for the school to become a leader in community health and Social Accountability (SA). By inspiring faculty, students, and community members through town hall meetings and social media, the Dean fosters a collective commitment to this vision. They develop new curriculum components that integrate service learning and community-based research, and form partnerships with local health organizations to create joint initiatives such as free health clinics and health education programs. By providing resources and empowering students and faculty to pursue innovative projects, and establishing a committee to track outcomes and refine strategies based on evidence, the Dean ensures that the medical school's efforts are effective and sustainable, ultimately transforming both the institution and the community it serves.

Participative Leadership

Participative leaders actively engage their team members in decision-making processes [11]. By creating an environment where everyone's voice is heard and valued, these leaders stimulate creative and innovative solutions that address community healthcare needs. Participative leadership, rooted in democratic leadership theories, emphasizes collaboration and inclusivity [12]. Yukl (2019) notes that participative leaders enhance decision quality and subordinate commitment by involving team members in decision-making processes [13]. In practice, participative leadership in medical education involves the creation of advisory boards that include faculty, students, and community representatives [14]. These boards can provide input on curriculum design, ensuring it addresses local health issues. An example is a medical school that involves local community members in developing health promotion programs, ensuring the initiatives are culturally relevant and effectively address community needs.

Box 4.2 Example of Participative Leadership and Social Accountability
A medical school might establish a community advisory board composed of local residents, healthcare providers, and public health officials. This board could meet regularly to provide feedback on the medical curriculum and suggest improvements based on the community's health needs. This inclusive approach ensures that the education provided is relevant and beneficial to the community, thereby promoting SA. By integrating these characteristics, participative leadership in SA ensures that medical education is aligned with the needs of the community and that all stakeholders are actively engaged in the process. This collaborative approach enhances the effectiveness and sustainability of SA initiatives, ultimately leading to better health outcomes and more equitable healthcare delivery.

Ethical Leadership

Ethical leaders base their actions and decisions on sound moral principles. By prioritizing respect, reciprocity, and justice, healthcare leaders ensure that their practices and policies promote SA and enhance the well-being of individuals and communities [15]. Lawton, A., & Páez, I. (2015) define ethical leadership as the demonstration of normatively appropriate conduct through personal actions and interpersonal relationships [16]. Ethical leaders promote fairness, honesty, and integrity. Ethical leadership in medical education involves establishing admissions policies that promote diversity and inclusion, ensuring equal opportunities for all applicants. For instance, a Dean who implements a holistic admissions process that considers socioeconomic background and life experiences exemplifies ethical leadership, as this approach promotes equity and diversity within the student body.

Box 4.3 Example of Ethical Leadership and Social Accountability
A Dean who revises the admissions criteria to include assessments of candidates' commitment to serving underserved communities, life experiences, and socio-economic backgrounds demonstrates ethical leadership. By doing so, they ensure that the medical school attracts a diverse cohort of students who are not only academically qualified but also possess the empathy and commitment necessary to address health disparities. By integrating these characteristics, ethical leadership in SA ensures that medical education is aligned with moral principles that promote justice, equity, and respect for all individuals. This leadership model creates a foundation for trust and integrity, essential for fostering a socially accountable healthcare system.

Collaborative Leadership

Collaborative leaders work closely with other organizations, agencies, and stakeholders to achieve common health objectives [17]. By fostering partnerships and coordination among different parties, these leaders enhance the effectiveness of SA initiatives. Collaborative leadership is based on principles of shared power and collective decision-making [18]. It emphasizes the importance of partnerships and teamwork in achieving organizational goals. Collaborative leadership can be seen in medical schools that form partnerships with local public health departments and non-profit organizations to conduct joint health assessments and interventions [19]. An example is a medical school that collaborates with a local health department to provide free health screenings and education programs, demonstrating a commitment to addressing community health needs through teamwork and partnership.

Box 4.4 Example of Collaborative Leadership and social accountability
A medical school collaborates with the local health department and several non-profit organizations to address high rates of diabetes in the community. The Dean, exemplifying collaborative leadership, brings together a team of public health experts, medical students, and community health workers to design and implement a comprehensive diabetes prevention and management program. This program includes free health screenings, educational workshops, and support groups for patients and their families. By leveraging the strengths and resources of each partner, the initiative not only provides immediate health benefits but also builds a sustainable framework for ongoing community health improvement. This collaborative approach ensures that the program is well-rounded, culturally sensitive, and capable of addressing the complex factors contributing to diabetes in the community.

In addition to transformative, participative, ethical, and collaborative leadership, other effective models that promote Social Accountability (SA) include charismatic leadership, pedagogical leadership, and inspirational mentorship. These models each bring unique strengths that can significantly enhance SA initiatives in medical education.

Charismatic Leadership

Charismatic leaders use their personal charm and persuasive communication to inspire and motivate others [20]. According to Tucker, R. C. (2017), charismatic leadership is characterized by the ability to articulate a compelling vision and evoke strong emotional responses from followers [21]. Charismatic leadership involves a high level of emotional engagement and the ability to influence others through personal appeal. Conger, etal (2000) emphasize that charismatic leaders are often seen as extraordinary individuals who can create a strong sense of commitment and enthusiasm [22]. In the context of medical education, a charismatic leader might rally the school around a new SA initiative by effectively communicating its importance and potential impact. For example, a Dean who passionately advocates for integrating SA principles into the curriculum can inspire faculty and students to embrace these values. Their ability to connect emotionally with their audience can lead to a heightened collective commitment to SA. A Dean who leads a campaign to promote community engagement in medical education by sharing personal stories of impact and success can inspire faculty and students to participate actively in these initiatives. By using their charisma to highlight the tangible benefits of SA, they can foster a culture of enthusiasm and dedication.

Pedagogical Leadership

Pedagogical leadership focuses on teaching and development. Leaders in this model prioritize the educational growth of their faculty and students, ensuring that teaching practices align with the principles of SA [23]. Male, T., & Palaiologou, I. (2015) describe pedagogical leadership as an approach that emphasizes the development of teaching and learning processes [24]. It involves mentoring, coaching, and providing professional development opportunities to enhance educational practices. A Dean who mentors faculty in developing community-based curricula embodies pedagogical leadership. This approach ensures that the curriculum is not only academically rigorous but also socially relevant, preparing students to address real-world health disparities. A Dean might organize workshops and training sessions for faculty on how to integrate social determinants of health into their teaching. By providing resources and support, they help faculty develop new courses and modules that focus on SA, thereby enriching the educational experience for students.

Inspirational Leadership

Inspirational leaders guide their fellow by sharing their experiences and values. This form of leadership is particularly effective in fostering a deep commitment to SA among future leaders in medical education [25]. Inspirational leadership is part of mentorship, Clutterbuck, D. (2005). defines mentorship as a developmental relationship where a more experienced individual provides guidance and support to a less experienced person [26]. Inspirational mentorship involves not only skill development but also the transfer of values and ethical principles. In the context of SA, a senior faculty member who mentors junior faculty and students in conducting community-based research projects demonstrates inspirational mentorship. This mentorship helps build a new generation of educators and healthcare professionals who are committed to addressing social inequities.

By adopting these leadership models and integrating SA principles into their practice, leaders in medical education can significantly enhance the health and well-being of individuals and communities. Effective leadership in SA involves not only addressing immediate health needs but also building a sustainable culture of equity, justice, and community engagement in healthcare education and practice. This holistic approach ensures that future healthcare professionals are well-equipped to serve diverse populations and address the complex social determinants of health [27].

How Can Leaders' Characters and Models Affect Medical Schools to Become Socially Accountable?

The character and role modeling of leaders within medical schools are crucial in promoting Social Accountability (SA). Leaders achieve this by exemplifying exemplary behaviors, effectively communicating values, creating supportive environments, investing in training and professional development, and cultivating meaningful community partnerships.

1. **Exemplary Leadership**: Leaders must embody the values of SA, such as health equity, social justice, human rights, ethics, empathy, and integrity. By consistently demonstrating these values in their actions, leaders inspire faculty members to adopt similar behaviors, thereby reinforcing a culture of SA within the institution.
2. **Effective Communication**: Clear and regular communication about the importance of SA in medical practice enables leaders to raise awareness and mobilize their teams. Leaders set expectations for ethical behavior and SA, providing guidance that supports a shared understanding across the faculty.
3. **Creating Supportive Environments**: Structuring the faculty environment to support SA initiatives is essential. This may involve implementing institutional policies that encourage participation in community service, research on health disparities, and integrating ethics and social justice education into the medical curriculum.

4. **Training and Professional Development**: Investing in training and ongoing professional development enhances faculty members' understanding, ownership, and commitment to SA. Programs focusing on medical ethics, social determinants of health, health promotion, and community service internships highlight the societal challenges patients face and empower faculty to address them effectively.
5. **Community Partnerships**: Collaborating with community organizations is a strategic approach to addressing local health needs and improving population health. Leaders engage faculty in co-constructive partnerships based on trust, dialogue, and collaboration, centered on community needs and expectations. These partnerships provide concrete opportunities for medical students and faculty to engage in social service and demonstrate the institution's commitment to community involvement.

Ultimately, leaders serve as catalysts in transforming medical schools into socially accountable institutions by fostering cultures of ethics, community engagement, inclusiveness, and SA. Their actions and leadership set the tone for the entire institution, influencing faculty, students, and staff to uphold these values in their professional endeavors. By modeling these behaviors and creating supportive structures, leaders ensure that SA becomes an integral part of the medical school's identity and mission.

Governance of Socially Accountable Medical School

To effectively embody Social Accountability (SA), a medical school must establish robust governance structures, systems, and processes that are closely aligned with SA principles and objectives [28]. By implementing the governance structures, systems, and processes, a medical school can effectively realize its SA principles and demonstrate a genuine commitment to societal health and well-being. Continuous assessment and evaluation ensure that these principles are not merely aspirational but translate into concrete, measurable actions [29, 30]. Incorporating SA into accreditation standards for medical faculties has been crucial in advancing these goals, highlighting the role of medical schools in promoting broader societal health [31, 32].

These elements ensure that the institution's commitment to SA is integrated into every aspect of its operations. The key components of governance for a socially accountable medical school include:

1. **Vision and Values**: A clear vision and set of values that emphasize community service, health equity, accessibility of care, diversity, and inclusion are essential. Faculty leaders, including the dean and council members, must embody this vision and demonstrate a steadfast commitment to ethical principles that support the school's social mission. This vision should be explicitly stated in the Faculty of Medicine's mission, aligning with strategic plans such as those outlined by The Association of Faculties of Medicine of Canada (AFMC) [33]. For instance,

the University of Gezira Faculty of Medicine (FMUG) in Sudan articulates a vision that prioritizes community-based education and health equity, evident in their mission statement emphasizing serving underserved populations and integrating social determinants of health into their curriculum.

2. **Dedicated SA Governance Structure**: Establishing a dedicated governance structure specifically for SA is crucial. This could involve creating a vice deanship or a directorate that includes representatives from faculty, staff, students, and community members. This group is responsible for developing, implementing, monitoring, and evaluating socially accountable initiatives. Effective leadership within this structure should come from SA champions—individuals who exemplify principles of health equity and social justice and have led early efforts in medical education. For instance, at the Northern Ontario School of Medicine (NOSM) in Canada, a dedicated vice dean oversees social accountability initiatives, ensuring that community engagement and health equity are integral parts of the school's operations.
3. **Objectives of SA Governance**: The SA governance structure should aim to:

   - **Develop Institutional Policies**: Create policies that reflect the Faculty's commitment to SA, including diversity, research ethics, community engagement, and environmental sustainability. The University of New Mexico School of Medicine has policies that promote the recruitment of diverse student populations and emphasize community-based research to address local health disparities.
   - **Foster Interdisciplinary Collaboration**: Promote collaboration across health sciences, public health, social sciences, and related fields to support holistic health approaches. The University of Dundee's Medical Education Centre fosters interdisciplinary projects involving public health, social sciences, and medical students to create comprehensive health interventions.
   - **Integrate SA into the Curriculum**: Ensure that SA principles are embedded in the medical curriculum, focusing on health equity, community medicine, cultural diversity, and the social determinants of health. Hull York Medical School (HYMS) in the UK integrates SA into its curriculum by incorporating modules on health inequalities and community-based placements that provide students with real-world experience in diverse settings.
   - **Provide Training and Support**: Offer training and professional development for faculty and staff on SA issues such as diversity awareness, cultural competence, ethics, and community involvement. The Ateneo de Zamboanga University School of Medicine (ADZU-SOM) in the Philippines provides ongoing training for faculty on cultural competence and community engagement, ensuring they are well-equipped to teach and model these principles.
   - **Cultivate Community Partnerships**: Develop strong partnerships with community organizations, local health facilities, government agencies, and other stakeholders for collaborative public health initiatives and community service programs. NOSM and Université de Montréal's Faculty of Medicine (FMUM) collaborates with First Nations communities to develop health programs that address specific health challenges faced by these populations, ensuring that initiatives are culturally appropriate and effective.

- **Engage Students in SA**: Encourage student participation in SA through volunteer programs, community research projects, and awareness campaigns. The University of Gezira requires medical students to participate in community service projects, which are integral to their education and promote a deep understanding of local health needs.
- **Establish Evaluation Mechanisms**: Implement mechanisms to monitor and evaluate progress toward SA goals, including metrics on student diversity, community partnerships, outreach initiatives, and contributions to public health solutions. Regular reporting on SA performance is essential to ensure transparency and accountability. The University of New Mexico School of Medicine uses comprehensive evaluation tools to assess the impact of their community engagement programs, with regular reports to stakeholders on outcomes and areas for improvement.

Case Studies

These case studies illustrate the critical role of leadership and governance in driving social accountability in medical education. By adopting various leadership models and change management approaches, these institutions have successfully integrated social accountability principles into their curricula, community services, and research initiatives, creating impactful educational models that address community health needs and foster a commitment to public service among future healthcare professionals.

Case Study 1 A Leader's Role in Driving Social Accountability in a Medical School and example of transformative leadership

The first author reflects on his pivotal role in advancing social accountability (SA) at medical schools in both Tunis and Montreal. Central to his life's journey is a steadfast commitment to community engagement, which he seeks to impart to future doctors and healthcare professionals, particularly within the French-speaking world [34]. His dedication to SA in healthcare has evolved over a lifetime, shaped by personal and professional experiences that continually challenge his perspectives for progress. His involvement in diverse activities, such as being a national-level volleyball player and vice-president of the municipal council in La Marsa, has deeply sensitized him to social disparities and the critical role of community and civil society in addressing these challenges.

A turning point in his dedication to healthcare SA occurred in October 2011, when he encountered Dr. Charles Boelen at a CIDMEF gathering. Inspired by the "Global Consensus for Social Accountability of Medical Schools," he pledged his faculty's commitment to this vision. He persuaded the faculty council in Tunis to realign priorities towards SA, thereby launching his journey in SA on national and international stages.

During his tenure as dean, his primary focus was to position the Faculty of Medicine of Tunis (FMT) as a linchpin in Tunisia's healthcare strategy [35]. He emphasized the pivotal role universities and medical faculties play in mitigating social inequalities and fostering equitable healthcare access. This commitment led him to coordinate an international research-action project under CIDMEF'S auspices, engaging 56 medical faculties across 18 French-speaking countries in initiatives spanning training adaptation, faculty-territory contracts, primary healthcare, and interdisciplinary collaboration [36]. In Tunisia, the four faculties of medicine collaborated with government authorities, each responsible for developing training and healthcare services in specific territories [10]. His efforts were recognized in 2016 with the AFMC Charles Boelen international award for SA.

Three key events solidified SA as a strategic approach to healthcare in Tunisia and globally:

- The 50th anniversary of the FMT in 2015, themed "A socially accountable faculty of medicine," which galvanized the nation's healthcare stakeholders.
- The World Summit on Social Accountability in April 2017 in Hammamet, Tunisia, which advanced global consensus on SA through accreditation, partnerships, leadership, and defining competencies for health professional graduates, resulting in the Tunis Declaration.
- The establishment of the Réseau international francophone pour la Responsabilité Sociale en santé (RIFRESS) in 2018, co-founded to mobilize diverse stakeholders in achieving universal health and Well-being goals beyond medical schools [37].

In September 2017, he assumed leadership of the Office of Social Accountability at the Université de Montréal's Faculty of Medicine (FMUM), a pivotal role in institutionalizing SA principles locally and globally. He prioritized initiatives addressing the needs of marginalized populations and established a dedicated SA committee. Together, they initiated transformative changes, including enhanced training access for underrepresented groups and community engagement through action research and interdisciplinary initiatives. This collaborative approach significantly contributed to the Faculty's strategic plan for 2021–2026 [38].

Under his stewardship, FMUM structured SA activities, tailored programs, revised admission criteria, and supported marginalized student communities, fostering a new generation of healthcare professionals capable of addressing diverse community needs. The combined efforts of the Office of Social Accountability team enabled FMUM to achieve ASPIRE international recognition in social accountability in 2019.

His international engagements with CIDMEF and RIFRESS aimed to share expertise and reinforce FMUM'S leadership in global networks promoting SA in health across the French-speaking world [39, 40]. His career exemplifies a committed, visionary leader catalyzing institutional and societal transformation through education, research, advocacy, and support amid formidable societal challenges. His recognition includes the AFMC-Charles Boelen international recognition in 2023, underscoring FMUM'S impact in advancing SA across Quebec, Canada, Tunisia, and worldwide.

Case Study 2 Northern Ontario School of Medicine (NOSM), Canada
Pioneering Social Accountability through Leadership and Governance
The Northern Ontario School of Medicine (NOSM) in Canada exemplifies how strategic leadership and governance can promote social accountability [41]. The NOSM developed an innovative curriculum focused on Distributed Community Engaged Learning (DCEL), integrating classroom and clinical learning across over 70 communities. This approach ensured that students understood local health challenges while engaging directly with communities. NOSM's governance structure supported extensive community service initiatives, such as collaborations with First Nations communities on Manitoulin Island to develop health research programs tailored to local needs. Additionally, NOSM's research efforts, including the Northern Health Research Conference and various health research partnerships, have significantly contributed to improving healthcare outcomes in Northern Ontario [42].

NOSM has embedded social accountability into its core mission and operational framework, ensuring that leadership and governance play a pivotal role in promoting this mandate. The leadership at NOSM has aligned the school's vision and mission with its social accountability goals, demonstrating a commitment to improving the health of Northern Ontario communities by recruiting students from the region and training them to serve rural and remote areas. The governance structures at NOSM, including the Academic Council and various committees, are designed to support the school's social accountability objectives. These structures ensure that decision-making processes are guided by the principles of community engagement, cultural competency, and addressing the health priorities of Northern Ontario [43].

Community engagement is a key aspect of NOSM'S leadership approach. The school actively engages with northern Ontario communities to understand their health needs and incorporate these insights into the curriculum. This engagement occurs at both policy and operational levels, involving community members in various aspects of the educational process. The curriculum at NOSM is developed with a focus on the health context of northern Ontario. The leadership ensures that the curriculum is responsive to the region's health priorities, including aboriginal and francophone health issues, and that it prepares students to practice in rural and remote settings.

NOSM promotes interprofessional education to enhance collaborative practice and improve health outcomes. The leadership's commitment to this approach reflects a broader understanding of healthcare that emphasizes teamwork and integrating various health professions. To evaluate the school's progress in fulfilling its social accountability mandate, NOSM'S leadership has implemented mechanisms to track graduates' career paths, assess the socioeconomic impact of the school, and participate in the training for health equity network (THEnet), which provides a framework for evaluating socially accountable health professional education.

Partnerships and collaborations are vital for NOSM'S success. The school's leadership fosters partnerships with local communities, health services, and other educational institutions to strengthen its ability to meet social accountability goals. These partnerships are essential for the success of distributed community-engaged learning and for enhancing the school's educational resources.

In summary, leadership and governance at NOSM are instrumental in promoting social accountability by ensuring that the school's policies, curriculum, and operations align with the health needs of northern Ontario. Through community engagement, interprofessional education, and a commitment to evaluating and improving its impact, NOSM'S leadership demonstrates a proactive approach to fulfilling its social accountability mandate.

Case Study 3 Ateneo de Zamboanga University School of Medicine (ADZU-SOM), Philippines

Transformative Leadership in Community-Engaged Medical Education

The Ateneo de Zamboanga university School of Medicine (ADZU-SOM) is a socially accountable medical school located in Zamboanga City, Philippines. It has been at the forefront of addressing the health workforce needs of the Zamboanga peninsula by focusing on social accountability and community engagement. This case study examines how leadership and governance at ADZU-SOM have enhanced social accountability, contributing to the improvement of health services and health equity in the region [44].

ADZU-SOM'S leadership and governance are guided by a strategic policy framework that emphasizes collaboration with local leaders and stakeholders. The school's faculty and administration are committed to realizing the vision of addressing the health workforce needs of the Zamboanga peninsula. This commitment is reflected in the school's core values, which include equity, quality, relevance, justice, community engagement, and cost-effectiveness.

The school's governance structure integrates these values, ensuring that the management and decision-making processes are aligned with the mission of serving the community. Faculty members are not only educators but also role models for students, demonstrating a strong inclination to serve society. This commitment to service is evident in the early years of the school, where faculty members taught pro bono to support the school's vision.

The leadership and governance at ADZU-SOM have had a significant impact on enhancing social accountability. The school has led the way in social accountability even before the term became widely known, making medical education more accessible and addressing the shortage of physicians in the region. ADZU-SOM'S focus on training doctors in the region to retain them and decrease the region's high infant mortality rate are key priorities that align with socially accountable principles.

The school's leadership has facilitated partnerships with various stakeholders, including the Department of Health, local government, and community stakeholders. These partnerships have resulted in the implementation of projects that support local community policies, reinforce existing laws, and ensure the sustainability of health programs.

Moreover, ADZU-SOM'S leadership has ensured that the curriculum is responsive to the needs of communities and sensitive to the social and cultural realities of the Zamboanga peninsula. The school's "sandwich" model for clinical rotations and the combined MD-MPH program are examples of how the curriculum integrates community-based learning and public health education.

The case of ADZU-SOM demonstrates that strong leadership and effective governance are essential for enhancing social accountability in health professional education. By fostering a culture of service and integrating community engagement into the curriculum, ADZU-SOM has successfully trained a medical workforce that is committed to addressing the health needs of the underserved populations in the Zamboanga peninsula. The school's approach to leadership and governance has not only improved health service delivery but also contributed to the development of health infrastructure and the promotion of health equity in the region.

Case Study 4 Nelson R. Mandela School of Medicine (NRMSM), South Africa

Cultivating Social Responsibility through Ethical Leadership

The Nelson R. Mandela School of Medicine (NRMSM) in South Africa highlights the role of ethical leadership and robust governance in nurturing socially accountable medical professionals. Leadership at NRMSM integrated social determinants of health into the curriculum, particularly through the Department of Public Health Medicine and Family Medicine [45]. The "Making a Difference" module engages students in community service and primary care clinics, fostering practical experience in addressing community health issues. NRMSM's governance supports these initiatives by partnering with NGOs and local health facilities, enhancing both educational outcomes and community health. The inclusion of the Making a Difference (MaD) community service activity in the first-year curriculum indicates that the college's leadership recognizes the importance of early exposure to community-based learning. This decision reflects a commitment to the principles of social accountability, which align with the college's mission to increase social accountability among students [46].

The governance of the college likely supports the MaD activity by providing policies and resources that facilitate its implementation. For example, allocating curriculum time for students to complete the activity and providing faculty members to facilitate the process demonstrate a governance structure that prioritizes experiential learning and community engagement.

Case study 5 The University of Gezira Faculty of Medicine (FMUG) Holistic Healthcare Education: The Transformative Leadership of Professor Bashir Hamad

The University of Gezira Faculty of medicine (FMUG) in Sudan is a testament to the profound impact of transformative leadership, driven by the vision of its founder, professor Bashir Hamad. His leadership emphasized the integration of social and biomedical sciences into a comprehensive curriculum, with a strong focus on community-based education [47]. Under his guidance, FMUG implemented community-based education (CBE) activities across all courses, providing students with practical experiences directly linked to community needs [12]. This approach ensured that students received an education that was not only theoretical but also practical and socially relevant [48].

The leadership and governance at the University of Gezira's Faculty of Medicine are instrumental in driving its social accountability. The faculty's approach is underpinned by strong political commitment, exemplified by the state coordination council led by the governor, which enhances collaboration between academic and health sectors. Partnerships with local health providers and community sectors are forged to effectively address health priorities.

The curriculum integrates social and biomedical sciences, emphasizing a holistic view of health that considers socioeconomic factors. The faculty actively engages in health system development and regularly evaluates the impact of its educational programs on community health. Research is guided by joint criteria from the faculty and health ministries to ensure relevance and influence on healthcare decision-making. The usability of graduates is ensured through their placement in rural health settings, where they are most needed [49, 50].

Additionally, the faculty's strong leadership history provides a cohesive institutional memory, which is vital for maintaining a culture of social accountability. These elements collectively ensure that the faculty's activities are responsive to community health needs and contribute to health system development.

Take Home Messages

- Committed and visionary leadership is essential for embedding a culture of social accountability within a medical school.
- Various leadership models can significantly impact a medical school's progress toward social accountability and should be tailored to fit the local context.
- Robust social accountability governance, backed by inspirational leaders and champions, is crucial for transforming the vision of social accountability into tangible outcomes within medical education.

References

1. Boelen C, Sibilia J, Maherzi A, De Munck P. Le recours à la stratégie de responsabilité sociale pour refonder le système de santé. Rev du Prat [Internet]. 2024;74(2):129–32. Available from: https://www.larevuedupraticien.fr/article/recours-la-strategie-de-responsabilite-sociale-pour-refonder-le-systeme-de-santé
2. Walling E, Lachance E, Yeo L, Koepke K, Wasik A, Woollard R. Key drivers of social accountability in nine Canadian medical schools. Med Teach. 2020:1–7.
3. Koepke K, Walling E, Yeo L, Lachance E, Woollard R. Exploring social accountability in Canadian medical schools: broader perspectives. MedEdPublish. 2020:9.
4. Sciences U of SA for health. 12 Leadership Models That Can Define Your Style. [Internet]. 2022. Available from: https://www.usa.edu/blog/leadership-models/%0D%0A
5. Chai DS, Hwang SJ, Joo B. Transformational leadership and organizational commitment in teams: the mediating roles of shared vision and team-goal commitment. Perform Improv Q. 2017;30(2)
6. Givens RJ. Transformational leadership: the impact on organizational and personal outcomes. Emerg Leadersh Journeys. 2008;1(1):4–24.
7. Montuori A, Donnelly G. Transformative leadership. Handb Pers Organ Transform. 2017:1–33.
8. Shields CM. Leadership for social justice education: a critical transformative approach. In: International handbook of educational leadership and social (in) justice. Springer; 2013. p. 323–39.
9. Anderson JA, Crutcher RA. Driving change through diversity and globalization: transformative leadership in the academy. Routledge; 2008.
10. Boelen C, Pearson D, Kaufman A, Rourke J, Woollard R, Marsh DC, et al. Producing a socially accountable medical school: AMEE Guide No. 109. Med Teach. 2016;38(11):1078–91.
11. Bouwmans M, Runhaar P, Wesselink R, Mulder M. Fostering teachers' team learning: an interplay between transformational leadership and participative decision-making? Teach Teach Educ. 2017;65:71–80.
12. Pless N, Maak T. Building an inclusive diversity culture: principles, processes and practice. J Bus ethics. 2004;54:129–47.
13. Yukl G, Mahsud R, Prussia G, Hassan S. Effectiveness of broad and specific leadership behaviors. Pers Rev. 2019;48(3):774–83.
14. Committee F of FMPL. The future of family medicine: a collaborative project of the family medicine community. Ann Fam Med. 2004;2(suppl 1):S3–32.
15. Knights J. Ethical leadership: how to develop ethical leaders. In: Transpersonal leadership in action. Routledge; 2022. p. 35–46.
16. Lawton A, Páez I. Developing a framework for ethical leadership. J Bus Ethics. 2015;130:639–49.

17. Markle-Reid M, Dykeman C, Ploeg J, Kelly Stradiotto C, Andrews A, Bonomo S, et al. Collaborative leadership and the implementation of community-based fall prevention initiatives: a multiple case study of public health practice within community groups. BMC Health Serv Res. 2017;17:1–12.
18. Orchard C, Rykhoff M. Collaborative leadership within interprofessional practice. In: Leadership and collaboration: further developments for interprofessional education. Springer; 2015. p. 71–94.
19. Garrettson M, Walline V, Heisler J, Townsend J. New medical school engages rural communities to conduct regional health assessment. Fam Med. 2010;42(10):693.
20. House RJ, Howell JM. Personality and charismatic leadership. Leadersh Q. 1992;3(2):81–108.
21. Tucker RC. The theory of charismatic leadership. In: Leadership perspectives. Routledge; 2017. p. 499–524.
22. Conger JA, Kanungo RN, Menon ST. Charismatic leadership and follower effects. J Organ Behav Int J Ind Occup Organ Psychol Behav. 2000;21(7):747–67.
23. Contreras TS. Pedagogical leadership, teaching leadership and their role in school improvement: a theoretical approach. Propósitos y Represent. 2016;4(2):6.
24. Male T, Palaiologou I. Pedagogical leadership in the 21st century: evidence from the field. Educ Manag Adm Leadersh. 2015;43(2):214–31.
25. Mistry J, Hule MA. Inspirational leadership. Prin LN Welingkar Inst Manag Dev Res. 2015;8
26. Clutterbuck D. Establishing and maintaining mentoring relationships: an overview of mentor and mentee competencies. SA J Hum Resour Manag. 2005;3(3):2–9.
27. Abdalla ME, Taha MH, Onchonga D, Magzoub ME, Au H, O'Donnell P, et al. Integrating the social determinants of health into curriculum: AMEE Guide No. 162. Med Teach. 2024;46(3):304–16.
28. Woollard RF. Caring for a common future: medical schools' social accountability. Med Educ. 2006;40(4):301–13.
29. Abdalla S, Elamin E, Ahmed A, Ahmed H, Mohammed H, Sovla MK, et al. Community-based medical education from Gezira medical students' perspective. J Med Educ. 2019;17(4):215–21.
30. Matte MC. Social accountability of medical schools: examining the perceptions of a medical schools' stakeholders on the achievement of the school's specific social accountability mandate. Capella University; 2009.
31. Boelen C, Woollard B. Social accountability and accreditation: a new frontier for educational institutions. Med Educ. 2009;43(9):887–94.
32. Boelen C, Blouin D, Gibbs T, Woollard R. Accrediting excellence for a medical school's impact on population health. Educ Heal. 2019;32(1):41–8.
33. The Association of Faculties of Medicine of Canada (AFMC). 2021–2023 strategic plan. 2021; Available from: https://www.afmc.ca/about/
34. Abdulrahman KA Bin, Mennin S, Harden R, Kennedy C. Routledge international handbook of medical education. Routledge; 2016.
35. Maherzi A. The new mission of the Faculty of Medicine of Tunis (FMT) based on principles of social accountability. Routledge Int Handb Med Educ Ed Bin Abdulrahman K A, Mennin S, Harden R, Kennedy C. 2016; 4-5
36. Ladner J, Maherzi A, Poitevien G, Pestiaux D, Grand'Maison P, Gomès J, Nawar T, Neusy AJ, Roland M, Boelen C. Responsabilité sociale des facultés de médecine francophones : organisation, résultats et leçons apprises du projet de recherche-action international des facultés de médecine francophones. Pédagogie Médicale [Internet]. 2015;16(3):189–200. Available from:. https://doi.org/10.1051/pmed/2016004.
37. RIFRESS (Réseau international francophone pour la responsabilité sociale en santé). Available from: https://rifress.org/
38. Faculte de médecine de l'Université de Montréal. Responsabilité sociale: notre engagement envers la population [Internet]. 2023. Available from: https://medecine.umontreal.ca/faculte/departements-ecoles-unites/responsabilite-sociale/

39. Maherzi A, Ladner J, De Rouffignac S, Boelen C, Cheickna S, Gresenguet G, Dumas JL. Pandémie COVID-19: le défi de la responsabilité sociale des facultés de médecine. Pédagogie Médicale [Internet]. 2020;21(4):195–8. Available from:. https://doi.org/10.1051/pmed/2020054.
40. Maherzi A, Andraos J. Addressing the challenge of medical deserts. Soc Innov J [Internet]. 2023:23. Available from: https://socialinnovationsjournal.com/index.php/sij/article/view/6786
41. Strasser R, Peltier I. From the community to the classroom: the Aboriginal health curriculum at the Northern Ontario School of Medicine. Can J Rural Med. 2014;19(4):143.
42. Strasser R, Hogenbirk JC, Minore B, Marsh DC, Berry S, Mccready WG, et al. Transforming health professional education through social accountability: Canada's Northern Ontario School of Medicine. Med Teach. 2013;35(6):490–6.
43. Rourke J. Social accountability: a framework for medical schools to improve the health of the populations they serve. Acad Med. 2018;93(8):1120–4.
44. Guignona M, Halili S, Cristobal F, Woolley T, Reeve C, Ross SJ, et al. A curriculum for achieving Universal Health Care: a case study of Ateneo de Zamboanga University School of Medicine. Front Public Heal. 2021;9:612035.
45. Clithero-Eridon A, Albright D, Ross A, Crandall C. Contribution of the Nelson R. Mandela School of Medicine to a socially accountable health workforce. African J Prim Heal Care Fam Med. 2019;11(1):1–7.
46. Van Wyk JM, Naidoo SS, Esterhuizen TM. Will graduating medical students prefer to practise in rural communities? South African Fam Pract. 2010;52(2):149–53.
47. Hamad B. Problem-based education in Gezira. Sudan. Med Educ. 1985 Sep;19(5):357–63.
48. Choulagai BP. Community-based education in the institute of medicine, tribhuvan university, nepal: a qualitative assessment. Adv Med Educ Pract. 2019;10:469–78.
49. Osman WN, Diaa-eldin EA, Elsanousi M. The impact of the faculty of medicine, University of Gezira, innovative programme on its. Gezira J Heal Sci. Graduates. 2013;9(2)
50. Abdalla M, Taha M, Mukhtar WNO, Elsanousi M. Impact of community-based medical education on graduate performance: a qualitative study using a critical incident technique. Health Professions Education. 2022;8:38–44.

Chapter 5
Empowering Faculty in Socially Accountable Medical Schools

Maxwell Kennel, Ghislaine Attema, Jyotsna Rimal, Prattama Santoso Utomo, and Nicholas Torres

Learning Outcomes

1. Understand the principles and importance of faculty empowerment within the context of socially accountable medical schools.
2. Identify and implement strategies for faculty empowerment using frameworks like the Primary Healthcare Approach and the ISAT.
3. Recognize the role of cultural shifts in institutions to support faculty development in socially accountable practices.
4. Learn from case studies about how empowered faculty can transform medical education and community health outcomes.

M. Kennel
Dr. Gilles Arcand Centre for Health Equity, Northern Ontario School of Medicine University, Thunder Bay, ON, Canada

G. Attema
PhD Candidate Lakehead University Faculty of Education, Research Assistant, Dr. Gilles Arcand Centre for Health Equity, NOSM University, Thunder Bay, ON, Canada

J. Rimal
B.P. Koirala Institute of Health Sciences, Dharan, Nepal

School of Medicine and Dentistry, Griffith University, Gold Coast, Australia

P. S. Utomo
Faculty of Medicine, Public Health and Nursing, Universitas Gadjah Mada, Yogyakarta, Indonesia

Warner School of Education, University of Rochester, Rochester, NY, USA

N. Torres (✉)
The Network: Towards Unity for Health, Philadelphia, PA, USA

University of Pennsylvania, Fels Institute of Government and School of Social Policy, Philadelphia, PA, USA
e-mail: nicktorres@thenetworktufh.org

M. E. Abdalla et al. (eds.), *Social Accountability of Medical Schools*,
https://doi.org/10.1007/978-3-031-94435-2_5

Introduction

At its core, Social Accountability (SA) is a social movement centered on helping both individual professionals and entire institutions to address the priority health needs of the communities they are tasked to serve. The oft-cited definition of SA from the WHO remains essential, even as it has been revised and extended. SA in medical schools, when it is done well, ought to mirror SA done in the health sector as illustrated through our inclusion of the Primary Healthcare Approach (PHC) in this chapter.

The Social Accountability of medical schools is a concept that underscores the responsibility and responsiveness of medical schools and their faculty to address the health needs of society. For these goals to be met, we assert that faculty must be empowered. What empowerment looks like will vary by institution and geography, yet the core principles of this empowerment hold constant. In this section, we outline a series of nine core concepts that contribute to faculty empowerment.

Important Considerations for Faculty Development and Faculty Empowerment

Faculty are often regarded as the universities' most valuable asset, and faculty development in educational institutions is an important part of continued training in the context of healthcare education. However, faculty development and faculty empowerment are not the same thing. For faculty to be empowered, there must first be an intentional investment in their development. Faculty development programs are necessary, and they offer considerable value in empowering faculty, but faculty empowerment requires more than just faculty development programs—it requires larger cultural shifts in the institution. Empowering faculty involves preparing them to adapt to changing educational landscapes, to embrace interdisciplinary approaches, and to prioritize responsiveness to social and environmental determinants of health. Empowered faculty are better equipped to drive innovation, inspire students, and engage with communities.

The goal of faculty empowerment in the context of SA is to produce compassionate and competent health care professionals who are committed to serving the needs of their communities. Medical schools can fulfill their mission of producing graduates who are equipped to address the evolving healthcare challenges of the future by investing in faculty empowerment and a culture of SA.

The needs of faculty empowerment can be broadly discussed under following headings (Fig. 5.1):

Understanding Organizational Culture Understanding organizational culture is a crucial driver for faculty empowerment [1]. A culture that values both the personal and professional development of faculty members will promote empowerment

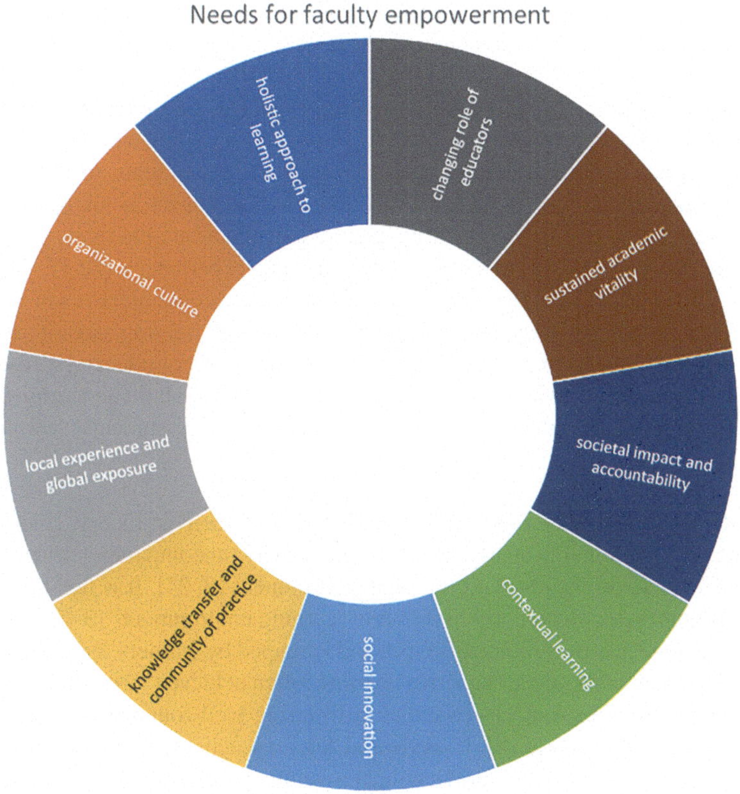

Needs for faculty empowerment
holistic approach to learning
changing role of educators
sustained academic vitality
societal impact and accountability
contextual learning
social innovation
knowledge transfer and community of practice
local experience and global exposure
organizational culture

Fig. 5.1 Emerging needs for faculty empowerment

activities [2–8] from leadership to teaching. Organizational culture impacts institutional commitments and resource allocations, which are key drivers in faculty empowerment [3, 5, 9]. A supportive organizational culture with a commitment to equally valuing teaching, research, and clinical service, is instrumental in advancing the SA of medical schools [2, 5, 10–13].

Following the Changing Role of Educators As the practice of medicine is transforming from the information age to the age of artificial intelligence, medical educators have to keep pace with these changes in critical ways [14, 15]. Faculty development in medical education offers a venue for hospital-based educators to become societal change agents, influencing health care while demonstrating the values of SA [5, 16, 17]. The typical culture in medical education focuses on performance and may encourage a fixed mindset in a way that is at odds with newer educational models such as competency-based education, which centre on continued development and the mastery of skills throughout one's career [6, 7, 18]. Faculty need to be prepared for teaching and role-modelling social and environmental accountability in educational practice and within health care systems [5, 7, 14, 16,

19, 20] fostering a supportive learning environment conducive to the personal and professional growth of both student and teacher [2, 7, 8, 14, 18, 21].

Fostering a Holistic Approach to Learning Students, like patients, often have similar fears, anxieties, and feelings of uncertainty. By adopting a holistic approach to teaching, educators can emulate the principles of holistic care in their role as medical educators [2, 5, 8, 9, 21–23]. Effective medical educators are described as embodying a balance between nurturing mentorship and academic rigor, fostering a culture of inquiry, and promoting holistic learning experiences [2, 17, 23, 24]. Faculty empowerment plays a vital role in advancing the core objectives of medical education, enhancing patient and community care through training and education of skilled medical professionals. This hinges on nurturing adept educators, researchers, and administrators who dedicate themselves to fostering holistic learning environments to develop healthcare professionals and enhancing students' learning [5, 20, 23].

Promoting Contextual Learning According to constructivist theory, context is a dynamic and relational property arising from activity, encompassing what people do, their roles, relationships, and physical environment [8, 24]. It is flexible, emergent, and interpreted differently in different learning environments [3–5, 7, 14, 18, 21, 23]. In active learning, context shapes and is shaped by learners' engagement [5, 6, 23, 25]. In medical education, active learning, often achieved through the integration of experiential learning, is essential in fostering well-rounded and competent healthcare professionals [5, 8]. Experiential learning actively engages students in real-world clinical scenarios, allowing them to apply theoretical knowledge in practical settings [3, 12, 15, 24]. Through hands-on experiences, students develop critical thinking skills, clinical reasoning abilities, and interpersonal competencies crucial for effective patient care [4, 5, 20, 23, 26]. Experiential learning also encourages reflection on practice, promoting self-awareness and continuous improvement [5, 8, 18, 27, 28]. Faculty empowerment can focus on contextualizing teaching skills, staying updated with pedagogical advancements, and aligning with institutional mission and standards [5, 9, 12, 21]. Integrating both professional and personal development into these empowerment activities is crucial for nurturing well rounded educators [5, 11, 12, 14, 19, 26, 29]. Personal development aims at fostering individual growth, wellbeing, and resilience, which are equally important for effective teaching roles and overall workplace wellbeing [5, 22, 29]. All the above concept are essential when implementing of social accountability principles and values in medical schools.

Sustaining Academic Vitality Stress and burnout are prevalent among medical educators [5, 18]. The rise in student enrolment, evolving healthcare management, administrative duties, and research obligations contribute to the shifting roles and responsibilities within academic medicine [5, 8–10, 14, 22–24, 26]. One crucial factor influencing individuals' ability to navigate the demands of academia is their ability to adaptively respond to educational challenges [1, 8, 25, 29, 30]. Academic vitality manifests as spontaneous actions, devoid of frustration and fatigue, accompanied by a sustained sense of vigour and increased energy [1, 29, 30]. Vitality is expressed through its capacity to influence the outside world and advocate change among various other health stakeholders. Furthermore, it correlates with heightened feelings of self-efficacy and empowerment when confronting challenges, reduced levels of anxiety and depression, a heightened sense of responsibility in managing academic tasks, and ultimately, improved academic success [8, 11, 29]. Academic vitality is a key component in facilitating adaptation to the diverse circumstances encountered throughout their academic pursuits [5, 29]. In fostering academic vitality, implementing faculty empowerment activities tied to rewards and incentives, can aid in retaining educators, clinicians, researchers, and administrators [5, 8, 9, 11]. These activities serve as visible demonstrations of institutional confidence in their workforce [5, 29].

Cultivating Local Experience and Transnational Education Medical educators play a vital role in promoting social accountability by ensuring that medical education aligns with the needs of society [3, 11, 15, 17, 22, 26]. This involves fostering a shared commitment to address health disparities, community needs and ethical responsibilities [9, 16, 26, 28, 31]. Medical educators must navigate global perspectives and challenges to advance social accountability at international levels [2, 12, 20, 22, 24]. This includes promoting culturally sensitive healthcare practices, advocating for health equity and collaborating across borders to tackle global health issues [5, 21, 31]. Local contexts are unique to particular geographic locations, regions, nations, continents depending on the cultural norms [3, 10]. Passionate and dedicated medical educators acquire the innovation and creativity to enhance the quality of learning, both locally and globally [3, 9, 10, 14, 15, 28]. They actively engage with the community to address pertinent challenges, advocate for progress, and drive advancement through various initiatives [10, 11, 15, 21]. Faculty empowerment requires a tailored approach to accommodate the unique requirements of institutions, disciplines and individual educators including scholars and leaders [5, 10, 15]. As medical education expands globally, these needs may become increasingly specialized, such as a demand for international assessors or accreditors [2, 5, 9, 13, 24, 32]. Empowering faculty members involves considering their diverse perspectives and providing them with necessary support and resources to thrive in their roles, ultimately contributing to the enhancement of accountability of medical education on a broader scale [5, 13]. International experiences are indispensable for faculty in medical schools, enabling them to comprehend the diverse needs of the global community and foster equitable opportunities [5, 12, 13]. Moreover, international experiences facilitate cross-cultural collaboration and networking, promoting the exchange of knowledge and best practices [2, 4, 10, 15, 20]. By embracing internationalization, medical schools can cultivate a more inclusive and globally competent faculty who are better equipped to address the complex healthcare landscape [2, 5, 8, 14, 15].

Engaging in Social Innovation Empowered faculty members are catalysts for driving innovation, inspiring students, and engaging communities, all of which are fundamental aspects of SA of medical schools [10, 14, 15]. By empowering educators with autonomy, resources, and support, institutions can foster an environment conducive to creativity and innovation in teaching and research [5, 18]. Empowered faculty can serve as role models who ignite passion and curiosity in their students, motivating them to actively contribute to addressing societal health needs [5, 8, 14, 16, 20]. Through community engagement initiatives, empowered faculty bridge the gap between academia and the public, promoting collaboration to address health disparities and improve access to healthcare services [10–12, 15, 19, 28].

Considering Societal Impact and Individual Accountability As medical schools' curricula have been evolving to encompass topics like social accountability and community engagement, it is imperative that faculty empowerment activities incorporate considerations for social responsibility and accountability [3–6, 19, 22]. In situations where there is a lack of institutional support, empowered faculty can advocate for resources, policies, and initiatives that prioritize professional growth [5, 6, 21, 29]. By empowering teachers, institutions can also challenge misconceptions and attitudes that hinder development, fostering a culture of continuous improvement and openness to change [2, 7, 9, 10, 19]. Empowered faculty are more likely to engage in and contribute to research on effective teaching practices, bridging the gap in knowledge and promoting evidence-based approaches to teaching enhancement [5, 10, 15]. Faculty empowerment efforts should also focus on preparing faculty to become societal change agents, influencing healthcare delivery and promoting social accountability in medical practice [5, 16, 17]. This aligns with the broader goal of medical education to improve patient care and community health [4–6, 20, 23, 26], providing avenues for hospital-based faculty to participate and observe social accountability in practice [5, 8, 14, 16, 23, 24].

Forming Knowledge Networks and Communities of Practice Building capacity is not just found in a single intervention, but it is as a process that starts with an intervention, and then continues with evaluation and dialogue over time [2, 5, 6, 8, 9, 12, 15, 17, 18, 24, 29]. Medical educators' curiosity, commitment to excellence and willingness to explore innovative pedagogies are essential for advancing and ensuring the future healthcare professionals are prepared to meet the needs of diverse communities [2, 21]. This involves the exchange and dissemination of knowledge, skills, and best practices among stakeholders, including students, faculty, researchers, healthcare professionals, and community members [2, 4, 10, 15, 20]. Building capacity and community for social accountability is not a one-time intervention but a continuous process. It involves ongoing evaluation, reflection, and dialogue among stakeholders to identify areas for improvement and innovation [2, 5, 12, 15, 28]. Medical schools strengthen their commitment to social accountability to ensure that their educational programs remain responsive to evolving societal needs [5, 8, 10, 19, 20, 22, 24, 27]. Academic partnerships and collaborations with other institutions, organizations, and communities help medical schools leverage their collective expertise and resources to address and knowledge-sharing initiatives [2, 3, 5, 7, 8, 10, 12, 13, 19, 20, 28, 31]. This way medical schools can contribute to the development of innovative solutions and approaches that promote social accountability and improve population health outcomes [2, 3, 9, 10, 12, 15, 17, 20, 26]. By nurturing a culture of inquiry, collaboration and lifelong learning, medical educators can inspire others to embrace the principles of social accountability and make meaningful contributions to health and wellbeing of society [2, 5, 10, 21].

Guided Strategies for Empowering Faculty: Using the Primary Healthcare Approach and the ISAT Tool

Social Accountability of Medical Schools is both a goal and a process. Its successful trajectory requires efforts across and within systems and institutions, with all involved working towards a common mission. While there are many enablers and enactors involved, faculty have a crucial role, as they work within and across these systems and institutions. Empowered faculty are agents of change, and while there is agreement that faculty should be empowered in socially accountable medical education, not all institutions have knowledge of or access to the tools that can help them on their journey. In response to this need, below we focus on two useful tools: the Primary Healthcare Approach Primer (PHC) from the World Health Organization, and the Indicators for Social Accountability Tool (ISAT) from The Network Towards Unity for Health. The next part of the chapter begins with a brief overview of each, and then points to specific areas in each where they can aid in empowering faculty.

The Primary Healthcare Approach

As part of their global health strategies, the World Health Organization (WHO), has supported efforts to achieve quality health care for everyone. The "right to health" is the foundational goal of these efforts, with the mechanism for achieving this goal through a **Primary Healthcare Approach** (https://www.who.int/publications/i/item/9789240090583)—An evidence based tool and reflecting lessons from 50 countries and all WHO Regions (Primer page 4). This approach is grounded in six core principles; Universal access; Solidarity and equity; Holistic approach; Multisectoral policy and action; Community engagement to co-create health; and Care which is of good quality and affordable (Primer, page 5). The following passage provides a useful overview of this approach:

> The **Primary Healthcare Approach** (PHC) is the cornerstone of strong and resilient health systems. It shapes them so that they respond to people; offer quality, affordable care close

to communities; and engage people in their own health and well-being. The key messages include:

- PHC is fundamentally about delivering holistic, integrated health services.
- Person-centred primary care services and the population focus of public health are linked by PHC, which makes PHC a tool for stronger UHC, health security, health, and well-being.
- PHC acts as a bridge between health care and community engagement and so supports access, participation and quality.
- Different sectors are brought together by PHC on policy and for action, fostering whole-system, whole society thinking.(Primer)

The Primary Healthcare Approach is a broader concept than 'primary care' because it recognizes that health is more than just the treatment of diseases. The PHA encompasses an holistic, community-centred care model, rooted in equity, human rights and justice (Primer, page ix), and the components of this model are visualized through a triangle pyramid (See Fig. 5.1). It is through this approach where we find useful implementation strategies and approaches for empowering faculty. The rest of this chapter section concentrates on section two of the Primary Healthcare Approach Primer, which focuses on implementation, highlighting relevant sections pertaining to faculty empowerment (Fig. 5.2).

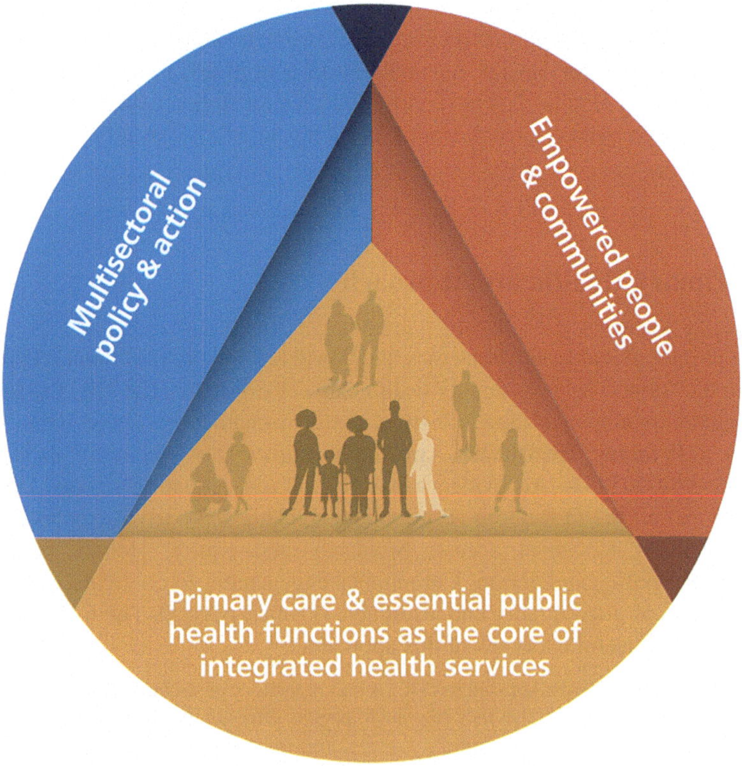

Fig. 5.2. Integrated elements in health services

Empowering Faculty: Primary Health Care Workforce

Research shows that accessible, affordable, high-quality, primary health care is a necessary component of any healthy community. Communities who do not have stable and accessible primary health care are vulnerable in many ways. There is also have strong evidence that tailored education and training methods can promote accessible, affordable, quality primary health care. The goals of SA share a striking resemblance to those of the Primary Healthcare Approach, in a way that can ground and justify the pursuit of faculty development that serves the aims of both SA and the Primary Healthcare Approach. Of particular relevance is Chap. 8 of the primer document which provides strategies to strengthen the health care workforce through education and workforce planning. Given the leadership roles of faculty within education systems, empowered faculty can make significant strides in this domain. Table 5.1 outlines the key areas most relevant for faculty empowerment.

Table 5.1 Key areas relevant to faculty empowerment illustrated in implementing the primary healthcare approach, the primer

Area of Interest	Chapter	Key Takeaways
Championing Interprofessionalism	8	– Optimizing task sharing can provide better and higher quality care
		– Learning interprofessionalism in medical education better prepares learners for professional practice
		– Collaborative practices expand services and provide greater stability to the health care system
Promoting primary care as a Speciality	8	– Promoting a culture where primary care is championed
Aligning medical school admissions with need	8	– Admission of students whose backgrounds support physician retention in needed areas
		– Providing supports for students who have lower socio-economic status
Adapting curriculum to enhance learning in primary care	8	– Earlier experiences in primary care support increased primary care providers
		– Integrating learners in communities supports primary care
		– Developing curriculum that utilizes the broad definition of PHC
Promoting community engaged curriculum strategies	7, 8	– Moving from a biomedical model to an holistic model of care
Advocate for publicly funded health care and health care education	8	– Physicians are respected community members and are important advocates for publicly funded health and education
Promoting integrated Technologies in Medical Education	11	– Health technologies can improve and support population health
		– Early learning and adoption of health technologies supports their use long term
Integrate digital health into medical education	13	– Greater access to health information strengthens health and connects rural and remote communities

But how can institutions practically and accountably transform and empower their faculty to work toward the shared goals of SA and the Primary Healthcare Approach? One effective way forward is through the use of the ISAT.

Empowering Faculty Using the ISAT

The Indicators for Social Accountability Tool (ISAT) [https://socialaccountability-health.org/] was recently updated to a 2.0 version, and it will soon incorporate interprofessional education and collaborative care standards as it is revised to reflect new realities in the field. In sum, the ISAT assists health training institutions in their journey to become more socially accountable to the public, the community, and the people who they serve. It addresses student recruitment, selection and support; faculty recruitment and development; what, how, and where students learn; research activities; governance and community engagement; school outcomes; and societal impact. The process of becoming socially accountable engages all of the key players at an institution in order to reflect on where the institution is in each domain and where there is room for improvement on their journey toward social accountability. As such, the ISAT assists in the process of institutional accountability, and the ISAT process provides institutions and their representatives with a vehicle to bridge primary care and social accountability, driving a global movement of people using social responsibility as a force for good.

Empowering faculty to uphold and advance SA is no easy task. In addition to change management techniques used by leaders to persuade faculty members to adopt SA as a key value, faculty must first understand what SA is in the context of medical education, then see a demonstrable need for its implementation, and then be empowered to uphold it through actionable strategies. To do this, faculty members require a clear starting point and frame of reference. Even if faculty members believe that SA is something that they ought to adopt as a professional value, instill in their students as a competency and virtue, and use to transform their institutions and policies for the sake of the public good, they still require a set of guidelines, standards, and self-assessment criteria for doing so.

The Institutional Self-Assessment Social Accountability Tool (ISAT) responds directly to this need by providing institutions and their decision-makers with a means to measure and evaluate their own journey toward greater Social Accountability.

The ISAT was developed in 2017 at a PAHO/WHO meeting that convened the developers (AMEE-ASPIRE, THEnet, and George Washington Institute for Health Workforce) of existing social accountability tools and global experts. Through a rating system that aspires to neutrality and objectivity, the ISAT provides health institutions across the globe with a means to track their progress, with a focus on the six core components mentioned above: (1) student recruitment, selection, and support; (2) faculty recruitment and development; (3) what, how, and where students learn; (3) research activities; (4) governance and stakeholder engagement; (5) school outcomes; and (6) societal impact.

Faculty Development components of the ISAT tool discuss the need for faculty to have training opportunities in response to the rapid changes in the world of medicine and health, including demographics, epidemiological transition, environmental challenges, emphasis on clinical quality and patient safety, financial challenges, and rapid advances in information technology, big data, and artificial intelligence. To increase the number and quality of the teaching faculty and to improve their skills in education and research, institutions should have an established Faculty Development program either as part of an education department or as a separate program. Such departmental development programs support continuous professional education using information technology and other communication tools. Faculty development programs may draw on various resources from the other departments at their university such as social and political sciences, engineering, other faculties of health sciences, and community-based organizations, all in order to shape a comprehensive curriculum on the social determinants of health and community development to prepare medical students for their community placements, and to support the community engaged service-learning education program. Faculty members can be instructed in pedagogical principles of interprofessional education and active student-centered and service learning during student community placements. Such programs can provide teaching and pedagogical resources to community practitioners recruited as adjunct faculty to improve their attributes/skills to be effective mentors, teachers, and preceptors.

For each component, there are suggested developmental phases, milestones, standards, and indicators that ground the ISAT verification process, which institutions can opt to engage in. The ISAT verification process involves third-party evaluation through the work of oversight committees, and inclusion in a global movement of other institutions and leaders. By evaluating institutional performance in relation to their (1) Developmental Phase according to Social Accountability Standards, (2) their Stakeholder Engagement, and (3) their Plans of Action to become more Socially Accountable and Transparent, the ISAT verification process provides a sort of peer review of institutional policies and practices, including the complexities of faculty development.

The role of faculty in advancing SA is essential. In the context of rapid global change and poly-crisis, the place of health and medicine is undergoing rapid transformation. To keep in step with large-scale social change, medical schools must respond to the shifting health needs of the societies they are tasked to serve, and they cannot do so unless faculty members are highly engaged in their professional service to the public. Despite the intensity of this task, in the context of environmental, epidemiological, political, and social change, faculty members do not often receive comprehensive training in education, pedagogy, communication, and the social and economic determinants of health. Beyond this, focused training is necessary for faculty members to remain connected to the communities they serve, and in response to this clear need, some institutions form faculty development programs to encourage continuous professional development and education.

It is in this context that the ISAT can contribute some measures and insights, including a call for more pluralistic forms of medical education that draw on the best of the Social Sciences and Humanities to enrich education and curriculum on the social political context of the social determinants of health. The ISAT encourages faculty development programs to broaden their reach from the health sciences, to community-based work, to forming partnership networks to encourage social connection and service learning. To track progress towards these goals, the ISAT institutional team composed of faculty, students, leadership, and community encourages institutions to situate themselves in one of four phases:

- Phase 1 describes an institution, program, or school where limited, or no attention is being paid to social accountability and where associated strategies are not currently being employed.
- Phase 2 describes a situation where leaders and faculty are early in the process of reflecting on or starting to implement strategies or policies associated with social accountability.
- Phase 3 suggests that the institution is intending to implement social accountability strategies, but it has not yet achieved the desired outcomes of these strategies.
- Phase 4 describes a situation where proactive processes and systems are in place to measure progress toward social accountability and where institutions can demonstrate the impact of strategies and policies associated with social accountability.

For faculty members who find themselves in Phase 2 where they are reflecting on the future implementation of Social Accountability principles, the task becomes turning these intentions to actions. It is important for faculty development programs to resource their surrounding institutional contexts to inform their pedagogical approach, ideally with the aim of becoming more invested in student-focused, community-driven, service-learning approaches that involve community members as adjunct faculty—for example, Indigenous Elders and Knowledge Keepers who can provide insights and grounding experiences that traditional physicians may not be able to provide.

But even before this stage, faculty recruitment plays a role in the social accountability of medical schools. As reflected in the ISAT guide, "Socially accountable institutions seek to attract faculty who have the competencies needed to address the health and health system needs of the region where the institution is located, and those who come from diverse socioeconomic and cultural backgrounds (ideally from the specific community it serves)." By recruiting faculty from the region that the school serves, the institution already shows its investment in its geographical and social situation—for example, consider the Northern Ontario School of Medicine University, and its efforts to recruit medical learners from northern, rural, remote, Indigenous, and Francophone populations.

ISAT 2.0: Revisions and Feedback Received

In early 2024, the ISAT was revised in light of feedback from content experts across the globe, with changes incorporated by Torres and Kennel. Below, the chapter details the updated faculty development criteria, and then highlights several pieces of feedback received.

The ISAT 2.0 provides a framework within which institutions can place themselves, from Phase 1, where there is no faculty development program, to Phase 2, where a faculty development program exists but only promotes conventional approaches (rather than prioritising Social Accountability), to Phase 3 where several milestones and indicators are met. In Phase 3 institutions have "a faculty development program that includes a focus on topics related to community needs (e.g. social determinants of health, community mobilization, etc.) as well as principles of student-centred and active learning, assessment of students, workplace-based learning, and community-based learning." This stage is indicated by the presence of faculty assessments and development programs that are meant to update and strengthen teaching competencies related to priority health needs, where educators are training in developing cultural competencies, humility, and skills.

Phase 4 represents an even more advanced stage of becoming a socially accountable institution where "The institution assesses faculty performance and community engagement; and provides faculty development programs aligned with the goals of socially accountable health professional education including active, student-centered and community-based learning." This stage is indicated by:

1. Proportion of faculty who completed clinical skills training relevant to identified priority **health care needs**.
2. Proportion of faculty who completed professional development in effective **community engagement**.
3. Proportion of faculty who are engaged in **social accountability aligned education, research, and service**.
4. Proportion of faculty members from the **local health workforce** (including practitioners and community members) who have completed courses on teaching methodologies including **inter-professional education and community service**.
5. Faculty, especially those from underserved groups, receive **personalized development and career enhancement**.
6. The institution has a program to **reward the quality of teaching and community engagement**.
7. Faculty are appraised of **best practices and strategies** to respond to society's health needs and are recognized and rewarded for doing so.
8. The institution includes Social Accountability Standards as part of **recruitment, hiring (contracts), orientation, and promotion**.
9. The institution provides a program to bring **awareness of and promote** Social Accountability.

Phase 4 is exemplified by having faculty development: to help them identify priority health needs, to undertake effective community engagement, to align education, research, and service, to draw from the local health workforce through interprofessional education and community service, to engage in career development, to reward high-quality teaching, to educate for best-practices and strategies, to embed Social Accountability in recruitment, hiring, orientation, and promotion, and to bring general awareness of Social Accountability.

The feedback received from global content experts on this part of the ISAT, which led to the revised list of recommendations above, can be summarised in several key themes.

The first key theme is acknowledging the **plurality of appointments** that fall under the category of "faculty." Content experts during the ISAT revisions process identified ambiguity in the first version of the ISAT where a narrow definition of the category of faculty could artificially limit the scope of reforming medical education toward greater Social Accountability. As such, in the ISAT 2.0 the term "Faculty members" refers to all members of the health care team within the institution. This broad and inclusive category is meant to expand the purview of Social Accountability, while acknowledging that this inclusiveness is not always reflected in more stratified institutions.

The second key theme of the ISAT revisions is moving beyond educating faculty in best practices of Social Accountability toward **embedding institutional incentives and rewards** for doing so. This requires dedicated programs within medical, public, health, and health sciences contexts that have real power to bring awareness and reward uptake of Social Accountability—for example, in the tenure review process, which might be reformed to incentivize socially accountable research (for more on this, see the other chapters in this volume). This effort toward embedding institutional incentives and rewards can involve orientation and education about the basics of Social Accountability, which can be extended to the building of accountability structures so that faculty members learn to balance the values of academic freedom with the obligations that they have to society and to educate medical professionals who will serve the public good.

The third key theme that arose from the general feedback on the ISAT is **global difference**, as exemplified by the fact that people cannot assume that faculty development will look the same across all institutions. In some contexts, faculty hiring and development will need to follow local and national laws and legislation that may stand in the way of forming local community connections. Across the board, the task of engaging in faculty development toward Social Accountability is challenged by the tension between the fact that Social Accountability is a normative and universal vision for medical education reform, and the reality that any universal vision will not apply in the same way to all specific social and geographical locations. This means that part of the task of engaging in faculty development toward greater Social Accountability is being both rigorous and flexible in the implementation of tools and resources like the ISAT 2.0. Rigid, punitive, and simplistic applications will not suffice. What is needed are flexible, contextual, and adaptable ways of developing faculty members as professionals who serve the public good through their medical education, research, and service activities, all according to the specificities of their contexts and its needs.

Conclusion

Faculty are a key component of successful Social Accountability implementation in health professions education, and the way toward faculty development and empowerment that advances Social Accountability is through the use of powerful paradigms like the Primary Healthcare Approach, and helpful tools like the ISAT. Schools should empower faculty members with appropriate faculty development activities in relation to Social Accountability, but true faculty empowerment also requires cultural shifts across and beyond the institutional level. Empowered faculty can drive innovation and champion the values of Social Accountability to inspire students and engage communities. In the long term, faculty members may become ambassadors of a school's Social Accountability mission, but this can only happen if they themselves are educated about the problems that confront healthcare systems in their contexts. Socially accountable medical education can only have a long-term sustainable impact if it is closely linked with other approaches to healthcare delivery like the Primary Healthcare Approach, and if the pursuit of Social Accountability is itself held accountable to flexible but rigorous standards like those set and revised in the ISAT.

Take-Home Message

To advance Social Accountability on a global scale through faculty activities and faculty development, the following five elements are required:

1. Developing enriching faculty development programs that educate for and prioritize Social Accountability.
2. Forging meaningful and long-term bonds of connection between faculty members and the communities they serve.
3. Broadening our vision of who faculty are and who faculty should be by investing in community members and scholars and professionals from disciplines beyond the sciences.
4. Embedding Social Accountability in ways that have integrity, so that Social Accountability is not another institutional check-box or buzz-word, but that it remains a critical principle that can move faculty and their institutions toward actions that improve health outcomes for all.
5. Including Social Accountability prioritization in faculty's tasks, evaluations, and responsibilities in the areas of education, research, and service.

References

1. DM I. Faculty development and academic vitality. Acad Med. 1993;68(10):760–3.
2. Burkle M, Rolfson D, Lang M. Designing an international faculty development program in medical education: capacity and partnership. Int Med Edu. 2023;2(1):26–34.
3. WHO_HSS_HRH_HEP2011.01_eng.pdf.
4. Mikkelsen JHH. Contextual learning to improve health care and patient safety. Educ Health (Abingdon). 2007;20(3):124.
5. McLean M, Cilliers F, Van Wyk JM. Faculty development: yesterday, today and tomorrow. Med Teach. 2008;30(6):555–84.
6. Pai NE, Young M, Danoff D, Plotnick LH, Cummings BA, Gomez-Garibello C, et al. Teachers' mindsets in medical education: a pilot survey of clinical supervisors. Med Teach. 2020;42(3):291–8.
7. Richardson D, Kinnear B, Hauer KE, Turner TL, Warm EJ, Hall AK, et al. Growth mindset in competency-based medical education. Med Teach. 2021;43(7):751–7.
8. Steinert Y, Mann K, Centeno A, Dolmans D, Spencer J, Gelula M, et al. A systematic review of faculty development initiatives designed to improve teaching effectiveness in medical education: BEME guide no. 8. Med Teach. 2006;28(6):497–526.
9. Elsanousi SEM, Khalafallah O, Habour A. Assessment of the social accountability of the faculty of medicine at University of Gezira. Sudan East Mediterr Health J. 2016;22(4):258–66.
10. Global strategy on HRH. Workforce 2030. Geneva: WHO; 2016.
11. Brian H. Demonstrating social accountability in medical education. Can Med Assoc J. 1997;156(3):365–7.
12. Pálsdóttir B, Neusy AJ, Reed G. Building the evidence base: networking innovative socially accountable medical education programs. Edu Health. 2008;21(2):177.
13. Taha MH, Abdalla ME, Saleh Wadi MM, Khalafalla HE, Akbarilakeh M. The implementation of social accountability in medical schools in eastern Mediterranean region: a scoping review. J Taibah Univ Med Sci. 2023;18(1):84–97.
14. Simpson D, Marcdante K, Souza KH, Anderson A, Holmboe E. Job roles of the 2025 medical educator. J Grad Med Educ. 2018;10(3):243–6.
15. Wood B, Fitzgerald M, Kendall C, Cameron E. Integrating socially accountable health professional education and learning health systems to transform community health and health systems. Learn Health Syst. 2021;5(3):e10277.
16. Shah AP, Cleland J, Ross S. Bringing social accountability education into hospital-based clinical practice. Med Educ. 2024;58:491–3.
17. Burdick WP, Morahan PS, Norcini JJ. Capacity building in medical education and health outcomes in developing countries: the missing link. Edu Health. 2007;20(3):65.
18. Wolcott MD, McLaughlin JE, Hann A, Miklavec A, Beck Dallaghan GL, Rhoney DH, et al. A review to characterise and map the growth mindset theory in health professions education. Med Educ. 2021;55(4):430–40.
19. ASPIRE. Recognition of excellence in social accountability of a medical school [internet]. AMEE.
20. Cheu HF, Sameshima P, Strasser R, Clithero-Eridon AR, Ross B, Cameron E, et al. Teaching compassion for social accountability: a parallaxic investigation. Med Teach. 2023;45(4):404–11.
21. Mashauri HL. Who should be a medical educator? Beyond knowledge and experience. Ann Med Surg (Lond). 2023;85(10):4650–2.
22. Abdalla ME, Khalafalla HE, Wadi M, Taha MH. Medical schools' efforts to build social accountability indicators and determinants in the eastern Mediterranean region: a scoping review. Edu Med J. 2022;14(4):1–12.
23. Berkhout JJ, Helmich E, Teunissen PW, van der Vleuten CPM, Jaarsma ADC. Context matters when striving to promote active and lifelong learning in medical education. Med Educ. 2018;52(1):34–44.

24. Leslie K, Baker L, Egan-Lee E, Esdaile M, Reeves S. Advancing faculty development in medical education: a systematic review. Acad Med. 2013;88(7):1038–45.
25. Abbasi MAN, ShafieeH PZ. Role of social Well-being and academic vitality in predicting the academic motivation in nursing students. Edu Strateg Med Sci. 2016;8(6):49–54.
26. Dash NR, Taha MH, Shorbagi S, Abdalla ME. Evaluation of the integration of social accountability values into medical education using a problem-based learning curriculum. BMC Med Educ. 2022;22(1):181.
27. Gonullu I, Artar M. Metacognition in medical education. Educ Health (Abingdon). 2014;27(2):225–6.
28. Schofield A, Bourgeois D. Socially responsible medical education: innovations and challenges in a minority setting. Med Educ. 2010;44(3):263–71.
29. Alborzkouh PNM, Zainali M, Abed Y, Shahgholy GF. A review of the effectiveness of stress management skills training on academic vitality and psychological Well-being of college students. J Med Life. 2015;8(4):39–44.
30. Gill AC, Singhal G, Schutze GE, Turner TL. Educational coaches: facilitating academic vitality and a pathway to promotion for clinician-educators. J Pediatr. 2021;235:3–5e3.
31. Fitzgerald M, Shoemaker E, Ponka D, Walker M, Kendall C. Global health and social accountability: an essential synergy for the 21(st) century medical school. J Glob Health. 2021;11:03045.
32. Cynthia, Larche Maxwell, Kennel Sean, Tackett David, Marsh Erin, Cameron (2025) Enhancing Social Accountability in Medical Education and Accreditation: A Meeting Report Advances in Medical Education and Practice Volume 16471–476 https://doi.org/10.2147/AMEP.S508928

Further Reading

Abdalla ME, Boelen C, Osman WN. Development and evaluation of an online course about the social accountability of medical schools. J Taibah Univ Med Sci. 2019;14(3):241–5. https://www.sciencedirect.com/science/article/pii/S1658361219300472

Part III
Community Engagement and the Voice of Society

Chapter 6
The Role of the Community in Medical Education

Lionel Green-Thompson, Tracey Naledi, Damaris Kiewiets, Bernhard Gaede, Tasleem Ras, and Dina-Ruth Lulua

Learning Outcomes

1. Define the concept of community and its distinction from society.
2. Analyze the role and amplification of community voice in medical education.
3. Examine power asymmetries in community-health professional relationships.
4. Evaluate strategies for empowering communities through education.
5. Gain insights from the Homestay Project case study.

Part 1: Framing the Community Voice

> …Community, it's not what you think a community is, community is what the community tells you it is, and you can't get that from teaching, you have to be there, and you have to see it and people have to come to you with that information.
> Final Year Medical Student.
> University of the Witwatersrand, 2012.

L. Green-Thompson (✉)
Faculty of Health Sciences, University of Cape Town, Cape Town, South Africa
e-mail: lionel.green-thompson@uct.ac.za

T. Naledi · T. Ras · D.-R. Lulua
University of Cape Town, Cape Town, South Africa

D. Kiewiets
University of Western Cape, Cape Town, South Africa

B. Gaede
University of KwaZulu-Natal, Durban, South Africa

M. E. Abdalla et al. (eds.), *Social Accountability of Medical Schools*,
https://doi.org/10.1007/978-3-031-94435-2_6

Defining Community

Green-Thompson et al. [1] quote a final year medical student who provokes a reframing of the role of the community in medical education. Simplistically, yet powerfully, it challenges our assumptions about how community is known, as well as the idea that community can be defined or understood solely through a pedagogical frame. When we read the student's words '*Community is what the community tells you it is*' we are alerted to the depth of authentic engagement required by the academy in order to fully comprehend the concept of community. Through the voice of the student, we hear that community is not an entity which is known, learned, or understood from a distance. There is a view that health professions education view of the community evolves from the notion that the community is a place where patients are or everything outside the tertiary teaching settings to the recognition that community is a vital and dynamic social construct [2]. In contrast, a meaningful understanding of community, this social construct, emerges from direct engagement and interaction with the community itself, in the words of the student "*...you have to be there, and you have to see it and people have to come to you with that information...*".

The student rounds up by calling us, within medical and health professionals' education, to *listen* to the community in order to truly engage it. Community identity and meaning cannot be imposed from our external perspective; instead, this meaning must be gleaned from the narratives, perspectives, and insights that community members share. The community voice should always be our starting point, because while medical institutions play a crucial role in educating healthcare professionals, society itself has an integral role in shaping this education. The *community voice* is integral during the design, implementation, and evaluation of medical curricula in order for healthcare professionals to genuinely meet the evolving health needs of society.

Strasser [2] describes that the presence of students in community-based settings such as within general practice is often experienced in a positive way by the visiting patients. In one such encounter, the patient tells their physician that doctors are better at communicating information with the patient in the presence of a student. The patient is quoted as saying: 'you're a better doctor when you have a student' [3] This patient (community member) perspective reflects the symbiotic [4] nature of the relationships which are nurtured between the students, the professionals, and the community in which they may be located for learning. Worley et al. [4] showed community had a positive impact on student community relationships which influenced the career choices of graduates. In addition, the community participated in selection of students, provided orientation to programmes as well as had local oversight when students were engaged in communities [4].

In considering the use of the word 'community' to encapsulate the voice in conversation with the health professions, we must also consider whether 'society' may be a more appropriate description. In describing an approach to global health, medical anthropologist Cecil Helman defines community as a "...small, intimately connected group, with a strong common feeling..." [5] as opposed to society that is "...a much larger, more impersonal group, with looser links between its members" [5]. In this sense, society could be said to comprise multiple communities with distinct identities, with loose interpersonal links, often held together by formalised membership of a legislated entity, such as nationhood. By seeking to engage with its multiple collaborative communities, the health professions community involves itself in society-building. We see ourselves as part of this broader society, and from this perspective our focus is on strengthening inter-community discourse, relationships, and accountability.

Ellaway et al. [6] offered a review of the literature and the multiple concepts of community: as a context and location, community in contrast to hospital settings, relationship-based engagement as opposed to context and often these are located within political and health systems which are not always nurturing of positive relationships. This BEME Guide No.35 goes on to define a community as follows: *discrete group of individuals bound together either by a) living in the same locality and b) sharing a common professional or personal interest* [6].

The Community Voice

Educating professionals (the academy) must seek the articulation of the community voice within health professionals' education through the diversity of its expressions from both local and global geographies. This voice comprises patients, citizens, families, communities, and the nation at large [7], voices that have often been historically silenced in the medical education conversation. The identity of the community voice is social, rooted in the context and their lived reality. We need greater appreciation of the overlapping dimensions that constitute this context: socio-cultural, linguistic, economic, and historical. The knowledge by which this social identity knows itself, its relations and its environment produces the speech that the community voice projects into its engagements with the health profession. The community identity knows itself and its world by through a legitimate system of producing knowledge, an episteme. Epistemology can be defined as "the theory of knowledge, its origins and nature, and the limits of knowledge" [8]. Knowledge, when conceptualised as a product of a particular episteme, facilitates three kinds of knowing: knowing what things are and their uses in the world, knowing how processes work, allowing us to uncover causal relationships between events and knowing who we are in relation to the world around us, both people and objects [9]. The community voice has evolved from within a particular epistemology that has a unique legacy, which in the case of Indigenous communities, may be several thousand years old. This may require deeper appreciation from teaching and academic environments.

Community voice is enabled through the deep human capital held within the community and facilitates this voice partnering with the voice of the health professions. The health professions education community also subscribes to a particular episteme, context, language, and aspirations which reflects our construct of how the world is and how it ought to be. When viewing the partnership with community from this perspective, we see that *engaging with the community voice is an issue of relationships*, with the nature and quality of this relationship defining whose voice echoes more clearly across space and time. The relationship itself is often manifest across multiple axes—often reflecting the axes of asymmetry.

The Current Axes of Relationship

It is no secret that the current status of this relationship is largely one wherein the health professions dominate the discourse, driven by a multitude of factors beyond the reach of broader society, one of which may be the tension between evidence-based practice and locally held culturally determined practice. Truly generative relationships need to be located in a socially just frame. In the pursuit of such relationships, we must appreciate that community voice is raised in the context of a generative relationship between society and the health profession.

Amplifying the community voice, broadens our perspective from a one-dimensional training regimen where the academy is dominant, to the point of harnessing firsthand community experiences and diverse perspectives to develop a holistic understanding of health, wellness and disease [10]. This amplification must take place within the context of a dynamic functional relationship between society on the one hand, and the health professional education community on the other. The synergistic meeting of the identities of profession and community is facilitated by areas of convergence (similarity or common ground) and threatened by areas of divergence (oppositional aspirations). The amplification of the community voice and an authentic integration into routine academic discourse may make it possible to identify these opportunities and risks. The question to ask now is: *How best do we frame relationships for amplification of community voice?*

Ubuntu, an ancient African indigenous philosophy, offers us a source of wisdom and direction to address this question. Ubuntu, commonly translated from its Nguni roots, refers to a collective humanity that animates a community without negating individuality—"I am because we are, and because we are, I am" [11], or in Desmond Tutu's words "I am a human because I belong" [12]. The community voice echoes in the place of the greater collective. If we were to adopt a set of organising principles from Ubuntu to think about the framing of the intergroup relationship that would facilitate the hearing of the community voice, we could start imagining a space where this voice took its rightful place in health professions education.

These principles would include embracing the inherent humanity of each voice, ensuring unqualified dignity to all, always undergirded by a firm adherence to respectful engagement. The interconnectedness that is so central to Ubuntu would mean that each party "is open and available to others, affirming of others, does not feel threatened that others are able or good; … is diminished when others are humiliated or diminished, when others are tortured or oppressed…" [12]. Affording dignity means that voices are heard, and opinions are valued. Ubuntu would induce us to act in the best interest of others, precisely because their best interests are inextricably interwoven with our own.

Ubuntu is a foundational humanist ethos, embracing the interaction between the reciprocal relationships within a community and the social determinants of a community's health [1]. The notion of a reciprocal community of relationships presupposes that the health professionals are themselves part of a community. This disrupts the idea of the community as an entity which exists outside of the health professional community. Figure 6.1 below, demonstrates the Ubuntu approach as an embracing philosophy in the South African national (potentially global) context, at the centre of which is this community of reciprocal relationships. These reciprocal relationships are centred on the relationship between health professional and patient. A microlevel demonstration of social accountability built under an anti-oppressive framework and allowing the entry of social determinants of health into the personal relationships [13]. Goel et al. [13] refer to this micro level as 'one patient at a time.' This level of reciprocal individual based relationship is linked to the global ubuntu framework by the interdependent systems of health care delivery and the attendant education system. This notion echoes the Lancet Commission of 2010 [14] which emphasised the interdependence of the health systems and their associated health professions education systems. These interdependent systems of education and health care are both community facing as well as in constant dialogue with the national context. When communities are properly engaged in relationship with their

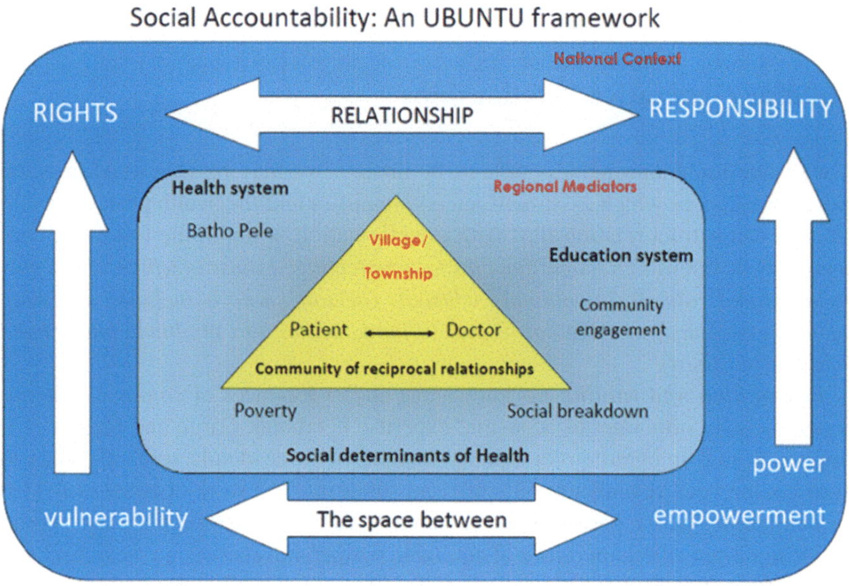

Fig. 6.1 Social Accountability- an Ubuntu framework demonstrating the relationship of local reciprocal relationships and national context [16]

healthcare workers, it has potential to advance them towards an attainment of their right to good health and their shared responsibility for maintaining the state of their health. The outer frame of ubuntu recognises the tensions between the vulnerability of community and their potential empowerment relationship with professionals in a bidirectional way. An essential dimension is that relationships dynamically occupy the space between these forces in tension.

Ubuntu is an African humanist philosophy which resonates globally in many Indigenous communities whose voices are making themselves heard in the global context. UbuntuWorks [15], as part of an organisational mission has curated reflections from multiple global communities on the connection to Ubuntu. The recurring themes of a values-based interdependence within community is echoed through global Indigenous communities which all reflect our shared stories. The people of Alaska (Yp'it) speak of a shared personhood which echoes in the Navajo (K'e) valuing this idea in the spirit of solidarity, love, and respect within a commitment to a community way of life. The Brazilian Kaxiwana tribe uses Txai saying: 'half of what's in you is also in me, and half of what's in me is also in you.' The Australian Aboriginals use the word 'anpernirrentye' to describe that we all belong to a single family connected through a web of relationships formed of a common life stream connecting us to all living things.

These shared expressions of the interrelatedness of all people and things lies at the heard of Ubuntu and is confirmed through the indigenous expressions from across the world. The need for relationships which value solidarity and love are integral to hearing the voices of community within our health professions education domain.

Building Generative Relationships

If we value the connectedness offered by ubuntu, we may be able to address the power imbalances which exist between communities and the health professions. In order to reconstruct relationships with transformation in mind, the following concepts may be relevant: *Recognition and valuing (changed sense of which voices may be heard and valued), Intentional inclusivity (deciding who is included and what inclusion is valued) and Mutual respect (a fundamental part of ubuntu and echoed in other traditions).*

Recognition and valuing the knowledge and experiences of community members as equally important as academic expertise is crucial. Cargo and Mercer [17] emphasize that integrating community insights with academic research leads to more comprehensive and culturally relevant solutions. The work of Israel et al. [18] on community-based participatory research (CBPR) further supports this point. CBPR highlights the importance of equitable partnerships between researchers and communities. CBPR principles advocate for involving community members in all phases of the research process, from defining the problem to disseminating the results. This collaborative approach not only enriches the research process but also ensures that the outcomes are more likely to be implemented and sustained within the community.

Intentional inclusivity of community members is essential to ensure diverse representation in decision-making processes [19]. This approach goes beyond merely inviting community members to participate; it involves actively seeking out and engaging a wide range of voices, especially those from marginalized or underrepresented groups. By doing so, decision-making processes become more democratic and reflective of the community's diverse perspectives, needs, and aspirations. Intentional inclusivity also requires deliberate efforts to identify and eliminate barriers that prevent certain groups from participating. This may include addressing language differences, ensuring accessible meeting locations, and creating an environment where all participants are heard.

Mutual respect, which involves a focus on building two-way relationships based on trust between medical institutions and the communities they serve, is foundational principle for effective and sustainable community engagement [20]. This respect must be demonstrated through genuine listening, acknowledging community concerns, and valuing the cultural, social, and experiential knowledge that community members bring to the table. Establishing mutual respect requires medical institutions to move beyond a top-down approach and embrace a more collaborative and participatory model of engagement [18]. This includes involving community members in the planning, implementation, and evaluation of health programs and policies.

It is in these processes and continued reflection that the voice of the community grows and is established as integral to medical education. Added to these are questions about control of resources needed to enact decisions. Mere inclusion of community voices in decision-making bodies but restricting their access to the means of implementing these decisions renders their involvement as a sort of tokenism [21]. A final manifestation of power lies in the ability to hold others accountable to the group's or intergroup's shared intentions. The amplification of the community voice in demanding socially accountable health professional education is a matter that could be transformative in its import and enacted through intentional community partnership.

Part 2: Community Partnerships

Community Partnership (CommPart) emphasizes the integration of community perspectives into the training and development of future healthcare professionals. By actively partnering with communities' medical schools ensure that their programs are not only academically rigorous but also relevant to local health needs [22]. It is the role of the health professions to empower people in community to engage with the social determinants of health [23]. There is need to educate the future health professional regarding the role of empowering communities. The professional should be taught not to act upon the community which is at risk because of the asymmetry of knowledge and power between themselves and the communities but rather collaborate with the said community. CommPart functions as the corner stone of social accountability in medical education, and there are strong links between community partnership and the attainment of health for all.

The people have the right and duty to participate individually and collectively in the planning and implementation of their health care.

This excerpt above from the Alma Ata declaration of 1978 [24] occupied the attentions of global health advocates in the decades which followed that declaration. The sentiments were echoed in the Ottawa Charter foe Health Promotion in 1986:

At the heart of this process is the empowerment of communities—their ownership and control of their own endeavours and destinies [25].

However, the Astana Declaration of 2019 [26] highlights the persistent unmet health needs of the global population, despite the significant advancements often celebrated over the past fifty years. This declaration asserts that the empowerment of individuals, families, communities, and civil society are fundamental pillars in effectively addressing health needs. Further it emphasizes the critical need to foster community participation in the planning, ownership, and accountability of both public and private health sectors. Highlighting that such participation is essential for developing health systems that are relevant and responsive to the specific needs of diverse communities [26].

The combination of Arnstein's Ladder of Citizen Participation [27] and McKnight's approach to community engagement [28], seen in Fig. 6.2 below,

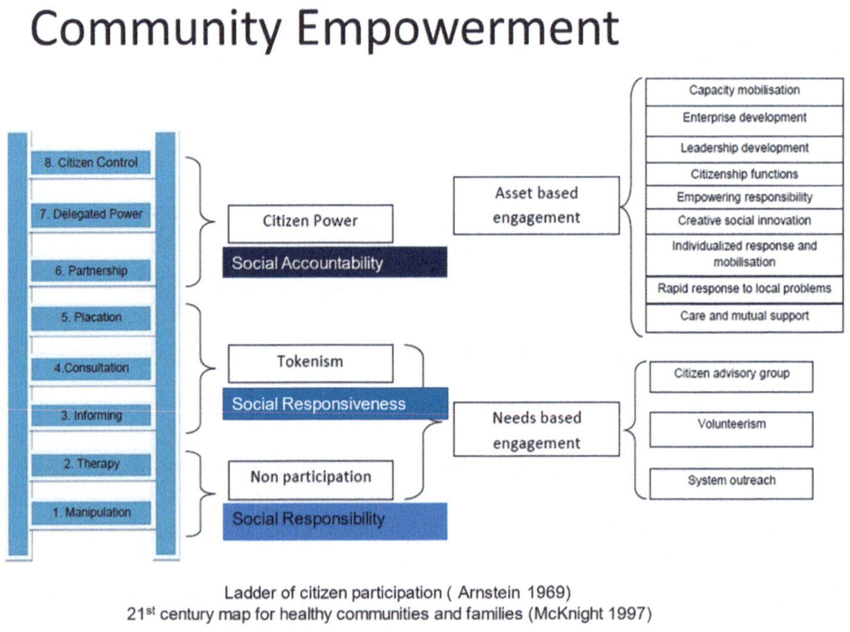

Fig. 6.2 The combination of Arnstein's Ladder of Citizen Participation and McKnight's approach to community engagement and Boelen's Scale of Social Obligation [7, 27, 28]

demonstrates the relationship between community partnership and community empowerment. By adding components from Boelens Scale of Social Obligation [7] to the illustration, namely *Social Responsibility, Social Responsiveness and Social Accountability* (see chaps. 1 and 9 for more details on the scale), we are able to graphically interpret the relationship between community partnership and community empowerment into the medical education conversation.

In the lowest two levels of the ladder health systems decide what the needs of a particular area are and make an intervention, in medical education [7] and colleagues refer to this non-participation of communities as *Social Responsibility*. At this level, faculties intuitively and implicitly consider the needs of society [7, 29]. With this approach the community is often left in the same position as it was before the intervention [27, 28]. Levels three, four and five offer more community engagement with efforts such as system outreach, volunteerism (community is co-opted to work for free) and citizen advisory group (a group chosen by the system to respond in a predetermined way). However, this engagement is considered tokenistic in nature as community engagement occurs, but impact and partnership of interventions are not measured. Boelen [7] describe this as *Social Responsiveness*, where there is an explicit response by medical schools to societal needs by directing the education, service, and research of the faculty to these community needs.

Laverack [23] argues that it is important that those who have power—often the medical communities—*work together with people in communities*. Adding that this power dispersal happens as much because people are looking to participate meaningfully as it happens because of a willingness to share vested power [23]. This community empowerment and partnership can be translated to what Boelen [7] describe as *Social Accountability*. In this instance, faculties not only explicitly identify community needs but go further to work collaboratively with communities, government, other sectors, health service organisations to ensure high quality, equitable and cost-effective health interventions which are measurable and produce change. Further the medical programmes produce graduates who are social change agents, who address social determinants of health and contribute to an adaptive health system.

Modelling Community Partnerships

Ratna and Rifkin [30] developed the CHOICE model for the empowerment of communities in order to facilitate the implementation of public health projects and programmes. The key elements of CHOICE are Capacity building, Human rights, Organizational sustainability, Institutional accountability, Contribution and Enabling environment [30]. The framework emphasises the continuum of actions and processes which lead to the effective empowerment of the communities especially in the achievement of improved health, see Table 6.1.

Having offered the CHOICE model as a lens for reflection of the Alma Ata declaration, Rifkin [31] later highlighted that power and control are often the reasons

Table 6.1 Ratna and Rifkin's CHOICE framework in tabular form [30]

C	Capacity building	People learning to do for themselves
H	Human rights	Participation in their own life decisions
O	Organisational sustainability	Allows programmes to continue for the long term
I	Institutional accountability	Building relationships of engagement with providers of services
C	Contribution	The contributions which active participants make
E	Enabling environment	Allowing partnerships between the professionals and lay people

that community participation has not had the desired or expected results [31].This power and control asymmetry directed the authors of this chapter to the creation of a community partnership model which speaks directly to the concept of power asymmetries, breaking boundaries, acknowledgement of the complexity of community engagement, the required negotiation between stakeholders, evaluation of impact and eventual unleashing potential.

Community Engaged Education

Abdalla et al. [32] posit that social accountability benefits communities through the education of graduates who are more attuned to the social determinants of health and the impact on treatment plans for their patients as well as within their communities [32]. This AMEE Guide No.175 [32] also lists possible learning approaches to support social accountability, three of which directly relate to communities (community-based education, service learning and community engagement as well as longitudinal integrated clerkships). The guide also offers six case studies all of which demonstrate various approaches to communities as stakeholders in the education enterprise ranging.

Community engaged education is seen as the final stage of a growing recognition of the role of the community. Evolving from the community-oriented thinking in which an institution may think about the importance of the community, through the idea of locating the education enterprise within communities to the final stage of communities becoming a part of the construction and determination of what needs to be a part of the learning endeavour. In order to ensure the role of community is fully realised, the relationships must be premised on trust. Chinekezi et al. [33] reporting on the AAMC Collaborative for Health Equity: Act, Research, Generate Evidence (CHARGE) project frame the principles of trustworthiness as essential for generative engagements. The principles they offer include recognition that communities already hold substantial education, the need to shift the definition of expertise away from the centre, that community engagement goes beyond a formal structure such as a community advisory board or an office. Their statement of principles emphasises that community engagement for the improvement of the community and its health outcome recognises that diversity is an essential part of the relationship and '*if you're going to do it, take your time, do it right*' [33] because the work is enduring beyond the scope of a possible project [33].

Longitudinal Integrated Clerkship (LIC)

The transformative nature [34] of longitudinal integrated clerkships is premised on the educational possibilities of continuity and relationships. The continuity of the relationships between the patients, the student and the teachers lies at the heart of this educational intervention which drives a different kind of learning in which the health outcomes for the community may be directly impacted. LIC offer the opportunity for community expression within the education enterprise across recognised symbiotic axes [4].

It takes a community to train a future physician [35]. This evocative title is from an article which describes the sources of social support for students during longitudinal integrated clerkships in rural Canada. Dube et al. describe social support as the perceived source of required assistance based on the relationships one has with people. The medical students in this study describe their relationship with the communities as essential to their sense of belonging. They offer three constructs for their integration: welcoming (their insertion into formal orientation activities), integration (awareness of students and willingness to let students be part of their clinical care) and farewell (an appreciation of the reciprocal relationships which benefit their learning) [35].

All of the above educational interventions have an essential sense of learning in new ways, relating in empowering ways and recognising the importance of context. See chap. 11 for more details on LIC.

The ABANTU Model: The People Model

Abantu is an Nguni word meaning *the people*.

The provocations in the twenty first century about the role of community in the education of health professionals continue to evoke images of the asymmetry of relationships. These asymmetries exist across a number of axes: **power** (the voice of the professional is privileged in the conversations of keeping communities healthy), **access** (all too often the social barriers and boundaries between professionals or their institutions preclude mutually respectful relationships), **cultural humility** (the inability to recognise the asset base within the complex social relationships in communities), **valued conversations** (the lack of recognition that communities have a view that needs to be respected as equally important in the

Table 6.2 ABANTU model

A	**Attention to Power**	Paying attention to the power dynamic inherited from a colonial frame of healing and wellness.
B	**Breaking boundaries**	The hierarchical nature of society means that professions may be seen as outside of and superior to communities
A	**Acknowledge**	Communities are a complex network of interactions of the multiple assets held within them. Harnessing the cultural, social, political, and economic capital held within communities benefits the education of their professionals
N	**Negotiate**	Conversations of dignity which respect diverse views. Compassionate listening for understanding
T	**Testing impact**	Creating spaces for co-creation with and amongst communities of innovative models of being and doing. Testing these in practice.
U	**Unleash the unique**	Unleashing the potential of each community through recognition of the unique spirit of each.

engagement on health and wellness), the **capacity to co-create** (the lack of openness to explore new ways of doing and being within relationship) and finally, the **assumption that all communities are the same** and can be engaged without recognition of their lived reality (unleashing unique spirit).

The following acronym offers a way to combine these emergent themes from this chapter and charter a course going forward about an ubuntu based framing of the ability of society to drive the agenda of institutions which educate professionals. At the heart of the ubuntu framing of community and its capacity for engagement are the people. A commonly used adage to capture the sense of ubuntu is: umuntu ngumuntu ngabantu (a person is a person through other people). Using the ubuntu frame, abantu (people) are a central space for the engagement within a reciprocal community of relationships as well the interaction of a community with other people (ABANTU). Abantu emphasizes community empowerment and collaboration (Table 6.2).

Part 3: Case Study the Homestay Project: Nelson R. Mandela School of Medicine (NRMSM) in Durban, KwaZulu-Natal Province, South Africa

Introduction

The "Homestay Project" was initiated in 2016 at the Nelson R. Mandela School of Medicine (NRMSM) in Durban, KwaZulu-Natal Province, South Africa. The project aimed to address various challenges faced by final-year medical students during their 7-week rural placement in KwaZulu-Natal, South Africa. The Homestay Project was conceptualized with three key objectives: exploring the viability of homestays as alternative accommodation, embedding students in the community for educational purposes, and fostering community development to align with the university's social accountability agenda.

Conceptualization and Objectives

The Homestay Project was driven by the need to provide final-year medical students with authentic, community-based learning experiences during their rural placements. The three main objectives were:

1. **Accommodation Alternative:** Investigate whether homestays could serve as a viable accommodation option for health sciences students placed in decentralized training platforms.
2. **Community-Embeddedness:** Assess the effectiveness of homestays in achieving community-embeddedness as part of community-based education.
3. **Community Development:** Explore opportunities for implementing community development activities to support social accountability within the decentralization of education.

The project aimed to position student learning within a real-life context, linking their education dynamically to the reality of the communities they served. The shortage of student accommodation in rural areas was seen as an opportunity rather than a limitation, with the homestay families envisioned as key agents in the process.

Setting up Homestays

Following a scoping review of homestays, the project team engaged with key stakeholders, including students, communities, and university administration, to ensure the project's success. This included sourcing local suppliers for furniture and setting up standards to address the unique challenges of deep-rural communities, such as the lack of piped water in homes.

Student Engagement The project team met with the Students Representative Council and final-year students to understand their expectations and concerns. This engagement helped shape the project to ensure that students' voices were heard throughout the process, particularly in developing standards for their stay.

Community Engagement Four rural sites in KwaZulu-Natal were selected for the project: Mseleni Hospital, Church of Scotland Hospital (COSH), St Andrews Hospital, and Bethesda Hospital. The project team engaged with the hospitals and communities at these sites to establish the homestays. In two of the sites, Mseleni Hospital and COSH, previous experience with international student homestays provided a foundation for the project. In the other two sites, the process was initiated from scratch, with significant engagement from local municipalities.

Experience of Homestays

The Homestay Project quickly gained popularity among medical students, with many actively choosing their host families in advance. Between 2016 and 2018, the number of students participating in homestays varied due to external funding constraints and accommodation challenges at hospitals.

Student Participation

- **2016:** 41 students were placed in homestays.
- **2017:** 108 students were placed in homestays.
- **2018:** 70 students were placed in homestays, with limited slots due to funding and accommodation issues.

Despite these challenges, the homestay experience was highly valued by students, contributing to the success of the program.

Community Member Feedback

Regular interviews with host families revealed that initial anxieties about hosting medical students quickly gave way to pride and a sense of accomplishment. Host families reported positive impacts, such as improved academic performance in their children and the development of social capital within the community. The relationships formed between students and host families often extended beyond the homestay period, with some students returning to celebrate their graduation with their host families.

Student Feedback

Focus group discussions with students highlighted the transformative impact of the homestay experience. Students reported that living in the community helped them contextualize their medical training and provided a supportive environment to manage the stresses of hospital work. The experience also fostered a sense of belonging, with students often feeling like members of their host families (Table 6.3).

Table 6.3 Reflecting on the Homestay Project within the ABANTU Model

A	**Attention to Power**: Paying attention to the power dynamic inherited from a colonial frame of healing and wellness.	The process of honouring both the students' perspectives and the community members' anxieties were critical to ensure full participation. The students, recognizing that they were the guests, and homestay families, recognizing their role as hosts, equalized the dynamics to a remarkable extent.
B	**Breaking boundaries:** The hierarchical nature of society means that professions may be seen as outside of and superior to communities	The project as a whole broke the hierarchical boundaries between rural households (perceived to be poor and unsophisticated) and medical students (perceived to be privileged and entitled).
A	**Acknowledge:** Harnessing the cultural, social, political, and economic capital held within communities benefits the education of their professionals.	The experience by the students was a profound process of discovering the human, social, cultural, and economic capital. Similarly, the community members experienced a similar, unexpected benefit of hosting the students, such as the status in the community or the impact on their children
N	**Negotiate:** Conversations of dignity which respect diverse views. Compassionate listening for understanding	The negotiations with the homestay families included a recognition of their inherent value to the project and an engaged process of finding to obstacles along the way. In the orientation of the students to the homestay project, the essence of respect, engagement and negotiation was emphasized. Solutions came out of the negotiations, rather than by decree.
T	**Testing impact:** Creating spaces for co-creation with and amongst communities of innovative models of being and doing. Testing these in practice.	In the iterative process of testing, improving, and re-testing of the placement of the students many lessons were learnt. A deep sense of adventure, and finding solutions made this project particularly exciting for students and homestay families.
U	**Unleash the unique:** Unleashing the potential of each community through recognition of the unique spirit of each.	The dynamic of each student with their homestay family was unique. The engagement, trust and depth of relationship that developed over just a few weeks for many of the homestay families and the visiting students was surprising.

Case Study Conclusion

The Homestay Project at UKZN successfully embedded medical students within rural communities, providing them with a deeper, more authentic learning experience. The project's success was driven by its focus on social accountability, community engagement, and the development of genuine relationships between students and host families. The experience not only shaped the students' perceptions of the communities they served but also contributed to the social cohesion and development of the rural areas involved.

Table 6.4 Role of Community in Medical Curriculum Development

Role of Community in Medical Curriculum Development	
Current Curriculum	
Providing cultural context	Community members offer insights into local cultural practices, beliefs, and social determinants of health, which can be integrated into the curriculum to improve cultural competence among medical students.
Identifying local health needs	Communities can help identify the most pressing health issues in their area, ensuring that the curriculum addresses these needs.
Feedback on curriculum content	Community representatives can review and provide feedback on curriculum content, helping to refine and enhance the relevance and applicability of the material being taught.
Future curriculum	
Participating in curriculum development committees	Involving community members in curriculum development committees ensures that the curriculum reflects the community's needs and values.
Co-create learning objectives	Communities can collaborate with educators to define learning objectives that are relevant to the community's health priorities, ensuring that students gain the necessary skills and knowledge to serve effectively.
Facilitating community-based learning opportunities	Communities can support the integration of community-based learning experiences into the curriculum, such as service-learning projects, internships, and fieldwork, which allow students to apply their knowledge in real-world settings.
Evaluation	Communities play a crucial role in the ongoing evaluation of medical education programs. Community members can be involved in evaluating the effectiveness of the curriculum, providing feedback on how well it prepares students to meet the community's health needs, as well as the quality and relevance of training for future healthcare professionals.

Further it facilitated community partnerships, community empowerment, and impressionable relationships between students and community families. Most strikingly it highlighted the profound benefits of community-integrated partnership models, ultimately demonstrating the significant impact of such initiatives on both medical education and community development (Table 6.4).

Eight Take Home Messages: The Role of Community in Medical Education in Practise (Table 6.5)

Table 6.5 Take Away Messages and Practical Implementation of Chapter

	Take Home Message	Role of Community in Medical Curriculum In Practise
1	**Authentic Community Understanding:** True comprehension of community in medical education requires direct, authentic engagement rather than a theoretical or distant approach.	**Formally embed regular, hands-on community engagement activities into the medical curriculum**. Design so students can gain a deeper understanding of the communities they will serve.
2	**Community-defined identity:** Community identity and meaning are determined by the community itself, not imposed by external perspectives, making community voice integral to medical curriculum design.	**Set up advisory panels with community members to provide input on the curriculum.** Ensure that the curriculum reflects the real identities and needs of the communities, making community voice a cornerstone of educational content and delivery.
3	**Society vs. community:** Distinguishing between 'community' and 'society' helps frame medical education within the broader context of multiple interconnected communities that impact society.	**Educate students to be able to differentiate between community and society**, use case studies to highlight how various communities contribute to broader societal health, helping students understand their roles within both contexts. Encourage students to reflect on these case studies and apply the lessons learned to their own practice.
4	**Community voice:** When community voice is heard at health education institutions, the nature of the graduate and healthcare is changed.	**Involve community representatives in key decision-making processes within health education institutions**. This could be through regular consultations, focus groups, or partnerships that directly influence the training and development of future healthcare professionals.
5	**Relational dynamics:** The relationship between the health profession and community must be socially just, focusing on mutual respect and valuing diverse community perspectives.	**Foster socially just relationships**: Implement mentorship programs where students learn from community leaders about the community they will serve. Train students and faculty on the importance of mutual respect, intentional inclusivity, and recognition.
6	**Power imbalances:** Addressing existing power imbalances between medical institutions and communities is crucial for fostering socially accountable and equitable healthcare education.	**Address power imbalances**: Include regular 'power' assessments in curriculum reviews to identify and address power imbalances between medical institutions and communities. Develop initiatives that redistribute power, such as community-led health programs or co-designed research projects.

(continued)

Table 6.5 (continued)

	Take Home Message	Role of Community in Medical Curriculum In Practise
7	**Community partnerships:** Active community partnerships in medical education enhance the relevance and effectiveness of health programs, aligning them with local needs and promoting social accountability.	**Build strong community partnerships**: Establish long-term partnerships with local communities and organizations. Engage in joint projects that address local health needs.
8	**Models for empowerment:** Frameworks like the ABANTU model provide actionable strategies for empowering communities and integrating their voices into medical education.	**Implement empowerment models**: Utilize frameworks like the ABANTU model to structure community engagement activities. Train students to use these models in their interactions with communities, ensuring that they approach their work with empowerment and collaboration in mind.

Concluding Thoughts

Community engagement models are essential for promoting social accountability in medical education. Each model lays a solid foundation for future healthcare professionals to be both skilled clinicians as well as accountable to the health needs of the communities they serve. By fostering a deep connection between medical schools and communities, these engagement models contribute to the development of a more equitable, effective, and socially accountable healthcare system.

The relationship between community and health practitioners is paramount in creating effective and sustainable health outcomes. Such a generative relationship is characterised by the sharing of power, mutual respect, trust, and fostering a collaborative environment where both parties work together to address health challenges. The African philosophy of Ubuntu, which emphasizes the interconnectedness and interdependence of all individuals, provides a valuable framework for understanding the importance of these relationships. Ubuntu, encapsulated in the phrase "I am because we are" [7] underscores the belief that the well-being of an individual is intrinsically linked to the well-being of the community.

The emergent idea in this chapter is seen in the ABANTU acronym, which places the people (abantu) at the centre of community engagement, highlights the need for reciprocal relationships and interactions within and beyond the community. By utilizing the framing of this model institutions can enhance the voice of the community and better align their educational strategies with the values and needs of the communities they serve.

In the context of healthcare, ABANTU translates into an approach where health practitioners recognize and dismantle power imbalances, break down barriers between health professions and community, acknowledge the complexity of communities, negotiate community nuance, test impact of co-creation and unleash solutions keeping in mind the unique context of the community. ABANTU highlights the significance of all of society involvement and the value of collective communal wisdom. By partnering with communities in the planning, implementation, and evaluation of health programs, practitioners can ensure that interventions are culturally appropriate, locally relevant, and more likely to be accepted and sustained.

When communities are valued for who they are and heard, they are more likely to engage actively with health initiatives, leading to improved health literacy and better health outcomes [10]. This collaborative dynamic also addresses power imbalances, empowering communities to take ownership of their health and hold health systems accountable.

Take Home Messages

Authentic engagement with communities is essential in medical education, offering deep insights into local health needs and cultural dynamics. Amplifying the community voice ensures curricula are relevant, responsive, and socially accountable. Addressing power imbalances between medical institutions and communities fosters collaboration, mutual respect, and equitable healthcare education. The African philosophy of Ubuntu provides a framework for building reciprocal relationships that emphasize interconnectedness and shared humanity. Case studies, such as the Homestay Project, demonstrate the transformative impact of embedding students in communities, enriching both their education and community development. Practical frameworks like CHOICE and ABANTU guide the integration of community voices into medical education, promoting socially accountable healthcare professionals who are prepared to address evolving societal health challenges.

References

1. Green-Thompson L, McInerney P, Woollard R. Envisioning a socially accountable doctor: a three-axis curriculum emerging from final-year medical student reflections. Scholarship Teach Learn South. 2018 Apr 24;2(1):76–94.
2. Strasser R, Worley P, Cristobal F, Marsh DC, Berry S, Strasser S, Ellaway R. Putting communities in the driver's seat: the realities of community-engaged medical education. Acad Med. 2015 Nov 1;90(11):1466–70.
3. Strasser R. Students learning medicine in general practice in Canada and Australia. Aust Fam Physician. 2016 Jan;45(1/2):22–5.
4. Worley P, Prideaux D, Strasser R, Magarey A, March R. Empirical evidence for symbiotic medical education: a comparative analysis of community and tertiary-based programmes. Med Educ. 2006 Feb;40(2):109–16.
5. Helman C. Culture, health, and illness. CRC Press; 2007 Jan 26. p. 426.
6. Ellaway RH, O'Gorman L, Strasser R, Marsh DC, Graves L, Fink P, Cervin C. A critical hybrid realist-outcomes systematic review of relationships between medical education programmes and communities: BEME Guide No. 35. Medical Teacher. 2016 Mar 3;38(3):229–45.
7. Boelen C, Woollard R. Social accountability: the extra leap to excellence for educational institutions. Med Teach. 2011 Aug 1;33(8):614–9.

8. Illing J. Thinking about research: theoretical perspectives, ethics, and scholarship. Understanding medical education: evidence, theory, and practice 2013 Oct 22:329–347.
9. Steup M, Neta R. Epistemology. Stanford Encycl Philos [Internet]. 2020;7(1):37–72. Available from: https://www.researchgate.net/publication/269107473_What_is_governance/link/548173090cf22525dcb61443/download%0Ahttp://www.econ.upf.edu/~reynal/Civilwars_12December2010.pdf%0Ahttps://think-asia.org/handle/11540/8282%0Ahttps://www.jstor.org/stable/41857625
10. Pálsdóttir B, Neusy AJ, Reed G. Building the evidence base: networking innovative socially accountable medical education programs. Edu Health. 2008 Jul 1;21(2):177.
11. Mbiti J. African religions and philosophy. New York: Praeger Publishers; 1969.
12. Tutu D. No future without forgiveness, vol. 16. New York: Doubleday; 1999. p. 34–6.
13. Goel R, Buchman S, Meili R, Woollard R. Social accountability at the micro level: one patient at a time. Can Fam Physician. 2016 Apr;62(4):287.
14. Frenk J, Chen L, Bhutta ZA, Cohen J, Crisp N, Evans T, et al. Health professionals for a new century: transforming education to strengthen health systems in an interdependent world. Lancet. 2010 Dec 4;376(9756):1923–58.
15. https://ubuntuworks.org/ubuntuworks-in-action/ubuntu-around-the-world/. Accessed 8 Sep 2024.
16. Green-Thompson LP. The nature of social accountability in south African medical practice and education—a qualitative reflection. [PhD thesis]. Johannesburg: University of the Witwatersrand; 2014.
17. Cargo M, Mercer SL. The value and challenges of participatory research: strengthening its practice. Annu Rev Public Health. 2008 Apr 21;29(1):325–50.
18. Israel BA, Parker EA, Rowe Z, Salvatore A, Minkler M, López J, Butz A, Mosley A, Coates L, Lambert G, Potito PA. Community-based participatory research: lessons learned from the centers for children's environmental health and disease prevention research. Environ Health Perspect. 2005 Oct;113(10):1463–71.
19. Minkler M, Wallerstein N. Part one: introduction to community-based participatory research. Community-based participatory research for health 2003:5–24.
20. Ahmed SM, Beck B, Maurana CA, Newton G. Overcoming barriers to effective community-based participatory research in US medical schools. Edu Health. 2004 May 1;17(2):141–51.
21. Majid U. The dimensions of tokenism in patient and family engagement: a concept analysis of the literature. J Patient Exp. 2020 Dec;7(6):1610–20.
22. Mahoney S, Boileau L, Floridis J, Abi-Abdallah C, Lee B. How social accountability can be incorporated into an urban community-based medical education program: an Australian initiative. Edu Health. 2014 May 1;27(2):148–51.
23. Laverack G. Improving health outcomes through community empowerment: a review of the literature. J Health Popul Nutr. 2006 Mar;1:113–20.
24. UNICEF. World Health Organization, & International Conference on Primary Health. Declaration of Alma-Ata International Conference on primary health care, Alma-Ata, USSR, 6–12 September 1978. Development, 1978:159–61.
25. World Health Organization. The Ottawa Charter for Health Promotion. 1986. Available from: http://www.who.int/healthpromotion/conferences/previous/ottawa/en/index1.html.
26. Declaration of Astana. Astana: global conference on primary health care. World Health Organization and the United Nations Children's Fund (UNICEF); 2018 [Accessed 18 Oct 2024]. Available from: https://www.who.int/docs/default-source/primaryhealth/declaration/gcphc-declaration.pdf.
27. Arnstein SR. A ladder of citizen participation. J Am Inst Plann. 1969 Jul 1;35(4):216–24.
28. McKnight JL. A 21st-century map for healthy communities and families. Fam Soc. 1997 Apr;78(2):117–27.
29. Boelen C. Building a socially accountable health professions school: towards unity for health. Edu Health. 2004 May 1;17(2):223–31.

30. Ratna J, Rifkin S. Equity, empowerment, and choice: from theory to practice in public health. J Health Psychol. 2007 May;12(3):517–30.
31. Rifkin SB. Alma Ata after 40 years: primary health care and health for all—from consensus to complexity. BMJ Glob Health. 2018;3:e001188.
32. Abdalla ME, Taha MH, Onchonga D, Preston R, Barber C, Green-Thompson L et al. Instilling social accountability into the health professions education curriculum with international case studies: AMEE Guide No. 175. Medical Teacher. 2024 Oct 11:1–4.
33. Chinekezi O, Andress L, Agonafer EP, Massick S, Piepenbrink S, Sutton KM, et al. From the national to the local: issues of trust and a model for community-academic-engagement. Front Public Health. 2023 Feb;24(11):1068425.
34. Worley P, Couper I, Strasser R, Graves L, Cummings BA, Woodman R, Consortium of Longitudinal Integrated Clerkships (CLIC) Research Collaborative, Banh KV, Barnard A. A typology of longitudinal integrated clerkships. Med Educ. 2016 Sep;50(9):922–32.
35. Dubé T, Schinke R, Strasser R. It takes a community to train a future physician: social support experienced by medical students during a community-engaged longitudinal integrated clerkship. Canadian Med Edu J. 2019 Jul;10(3):e5.

Further Reading

Boelen C, Woollard R. Social accountability: the extra leap to excellence for educational institutions. Med Teach. 2011;33:614–9.

Green-Thompson L, et al. Envisioning a socially accountable doctor: a three-axis curriculum emerging from final-year medical student reflections. Scholarship Teach Learn South. 2018;2:76–94.

Rifkin SB. Equity, empowerment, and choice: from theory to practice in public health. J Health Psychol. 2007;

Strasser R, et al. Putting communities in the driver's seat: the realities of community-engaged medical education. Acad Med. 2015;90:1466–70.

Chapter 7
Engaging with Underserved Communities in the Curriculum

Patrick O'Donnell, Bridget Kiely, David Blane, and Susan Smith

Learning Outcomes

1. Recognize how to engage with underserved communities to improve their health and enhance student learning.
2. Support students in becoming clinicians who can address social and structural determinants of health.
3. Recognize the importance of awareness about marginalization, its causes, and its effects on health for institutions, faculty, and students.
4. Develop knowledge of initiatives aimed at addressing health inequities and improving the health of underserved communities.

P. O'Donnell (✉)
School of Medicine, University of Limerick & Health Research Institute, University of Limerick, Limerick, Ireland
e-mail: patrick.e.odonnell@ul.ie

B. Kiely
RCSI University of Medicine and Health Sciences, Dublin, Ireland

D. Blane
School of Health and Wellbeing, University of Glasgow, Glasgow, UK

S. Smith
Discipline of Public Health and Primary Care, Trinity College Dublin, Dublin, Ireland

M. E. Abdalla et al. (eds.), *Social Accountability of Medical Schools*,
https://doi.org/10.1007/978-3-031-94435-2_7

Introduction

Opening Reflection

"I had known and adored Jeremy's family for several years. So when the sandy-haired, good-natured 8-year-old came to see me in my clinic with abdominal pain, I bent over backward to find out why his tummy hurt. I poked and prodded; did tests of his urine, stool and blood; and took X-rays, over the course of several months. When those tests came back normal, I did more. I had trained at a top medical school and gone on to one of the best residencies in my specialty; in Jeremy, I thought I had identified a real clinical mystery. But in the end, the mystery was not a best-seller: It turned out that Jeremy's family couldn't afford to buy food."

"It had never even occurred to me to ask his mother about how much food there was in the house. In Jeremy's case, I had diagnosed "abdominal pain" when the real problem was hunger; I confused social issues with medical problems in other patients, too. I mislabelled the hopelessness of long-term unemployment as depression and the poverty that causes patients to miss pills or appointments as noncompliance. In one older patient, I mistook the inability to read for dementia. My medical training had not prepared me for this ambush of social circumstance."

Gottlieb, L., 2010. Funding healthy society helps cure health care. *San Francisco Chronicle* [1].

This was written by a family doctor Professor Laura Gottlieb in the San Francisco Chronicle in 2010. She eloquently described blindly trying to care for her patients without adequately understanding their socioeconomic contexts. Shared decision making is a fundamental component of evidence based clinical practice, but it may not achieve best outcomes for patients unless shared solutions can be developed which take the patient's context into account.

The Importance of Focusing on Underserved Communities in the Era of Social Accountability

Social determinants of health (SDoH) have been defined as the life circumstances in which people are born, grow up, live, work and age, and the wider set of forces and systems shaping the conditions of daily life [2]. SDoH play a key role in shaping the health and well-being of individuals and communities. It is estimated that SDoH contribute to over 50% of **health inequities** [3]. For example, a report by the University College London Institute of Health Equity found that poverty was a risk factor for adverse childhood experiences, and these could subsequently lead to a multitude of chronic health issues such as respiratory problems, cancers, cardiovascular issues, mental health problems and others [4]. For this reason, the World Health Organization's commission on SDoH recommended re-orientation of health systems to emphasize health promotion and population health [5]. Despite progress on addressing health inequities worldwide, significant inequalities remain. The impacts of the COVID-19 pandemic have fallen so unequally that WHO Member States called for a World Report on the Social Determinants of Health Equity [6]. The vision of this initiative is "*A world where health equity is a shared value across society and where all social groups (categorized by income, occupation, education, ethnicity, gender, sexual identity or intersections of these factors) enjoy healthy living and working conditions*" [7]. Given the significant impact SDoH have on health and wellbeing, there has been a clarion call to prepare doctors and other allied healthcare professionals to address the SDoH at the patient and community level [8].

A **community** can be defined as "a group of people that interact and support each other, and are bounded by shared experiences or characteristics, a sense of belonging, and often by their physical proximity" [9], for discussion of the community definition, you can read chap. 6 While some communities may be defined by place, such as an inner-city community, others are defined by shared heritage and customs, such as the Roma or Irish Traveller communities. Communities, just like individuals, can be shaped by the social determinants of health. Communities that experience worse health and well-being outcomes because of their social determinants of health are often referred to as disadvantaged, deprived, marginalised, vulnerable or underserved as they cannot access the same economic, educational, social and cultural opportunities and services available to other groups. In the United States an Executive Order on Advancing Racial Equity and Support for Underserved Communities Through the Federal Government was signed in January 2021, and defined "**underserved communities**" as populations sharing a particular characteristic, as well as geographic communities, that have been systematically denied a full opportunity to participate in aspects of economic, social, and civic life [10]. In summary, there is no agreed terminology internationally, but the purposes of this chapter we are using the term 'underserved communities' as it reflects the structural inequalities underlying the inequitable distribution of the SDoH that lead to poor health outcomes.

Definitions and terminology differ in policy and practice relating to health inequities around the world. In the United Kingdom (UK) a National Health Service (NHS) initiative for addressing health inequalities is known as Core20PLUS5 and it focuses on the most deprived 20% of the national population as identified by the national Index of Multiple Deprivation (IMD) [11]. The IMD has seven domains with indicators accounting for a wide range of social determinants of health. 'PLUS' groups are defined as groups that may experience additional disadvantage such as minority communities, people with learning disabilities, people with multiple long-term health conditions and other groups that share protected characteristics defined in UK law. There are also some groups that experience extremes of social exclusion, and these are known as **inclusion health** groups. These include people experiencing homelessness, people with drug or alcohol dependence, vulnerable migrants, Gypsy, Roma and Traveller communities, sex workers, people in contact with the justice system, victims of modern slavery and others [12].

Communities usually experience disadvantage based on multiple social determinants as well as multiple sources of discrimination (for example gender, ethnicity, sexuality, disability). This is known as **intersectionality**, where multiple forms of discrimination and disadvantage are compounded and create unique obstacles that are difficult to address through a single-issue approach [13]. Intersectionality can apply at an individual level, related to membership of different communities, for example someone who identifies as queer and lives in a rural agricultural community, or at community level, for example a Roma community living in an economically deprived urban area.

Communities also exist within, and interact with, complex systems and power structures, such as health and educational institutions, government policies and legal structures. These systems and structures prohibit certain people and communities from accessing the necessary opportunities and services they require to optimise their health and wellbeing, a process referred to as structural inequality. The term **structural violence** refers to the resultant poor health and excess deaths, estimated at up to 20 million, that occur as a result of structural inequality [14]. With few exceptions, clinicians are not trained to understand such social forces or to alter them. The result of this failure is demonstrated in Dr. Gottlieb's article at the start of this Chapter [1]. To respond to the WHO vision for "*A world where health equity is a shared value across society*" doctors need to be trained to be able to recognise and respond appropriately to the causes of health inequities at an individual (micro), community (meso) and structural level (macro).

Virchow over 100 years ago observed that "physicians are the natural attorneys of the poor, and the social problems should largely be solved by them" when he was attending to patients during a cholera epidemic. He was encouraging doctors to be more active in attending to the structures affecting the communities they serve. Increasingly, there are calls for healthcare professional students to be trained in **structural competency**. Structural competency is defined as "the trained ability to discern how a host of issues defined clinically as symptoms, attitudes, or diseases (e.g., depression, hypertension, obesity, smoking, medication "non-compliance," trauma, psychosis) also represent the downstream implications of a number of upstream decisions about such matters as health care and food delivery systems, zoning laws, urban and rural infrastructures, medicalization, or even about the very definitions of illness and health" [15].

To support their students to become more structurally competent, medical schools need to consider their social accountability (SA). **SA** is the social contract that medicine has with society [16]. For care to be socially accountable, it must be equitably accessible to everyone and responsive to patient, community, and population health needs. It necessitates medical education and training that models and teaches advocacy, community responsiveness, and health care provision that addresses the priority health concerns of the population served [17].

Planning a Curriculum for Engaging with Underserved Communities

When developing a curriculum for engaging with underserved communities, it is worth remembering the many potential benefits of these endeavours if they are conducted in an appropriate and collaborative way. The following sections and the chapter on curriculum development inspired by social accountability will complment each other.

Rationale for Focusing Education on Engagement with Underserved Communities

In 1985 Julian Tudor Hart lamented that medical education was mainly concerned with "the production of specialist excellence, unsullied by prior contact with the society it serves. It is training the wrong people, at the wrong time, in the wrong skills, and in the wrong place" [18]. With the increased demand for healthcare professionals and the resulting expansion of clinical placement numbers, medical educational institutions have since needed to look beyond secondary-care settings for placements so that their numbers could increase, but also to enhance students understanding of the context and the needs of their patients [19]. Aretz [20] noted that if academic institutions are "creating healthcare professionals that match what societies need", then they "should become the catalyst for change, the hub for stakeholder interactions, and the breeding ground for the new healthcare workforce."

Student experience in primary care and general practice settlings provides exposure to lower-acuity health issues, chronic disease management and undifferentiated illnesses among other things [19]. Health services based in underserved communities, including those in rural areas and urban deprived settings, are now frequently being accessed for clinical placements, and as Perkins and Daly [21] wrote "there are good arguments for all medical students to have some experience of working in underserved areas because wherever they live and work in future they will treat patients from such communities and will benefit from their formative experiences." Consideration must also be given to the fact that most medical students tend to come from backgrounds of relative privilege despite efforts to widen participation in university education [22]. Students from underserved backgrounds and minority ethnic groups can also struggle when they have been successful in applying for medical degree courses, and this can be due to issues like being unfamiliar with the workings of universities or they can "find their identity conflicted" [23].

Student clinical placements are one important way that academic institutions can foster links with proximate underserved communities, but there are other possible activities such as health promotion initiatives, advocacy with and for communities on health and associated issues, the involvement of patients from underserved communities in the design and delivery of teaching and institutions taking strategic action to encourage students from underserved communities to enter the healthcare professions. One practical example of an academic institution taking time to discover the pressing needs of its surrounding community in Dublin has resulted in researchers from Trinity College publishing work with that community that found residents living in poor quality housing locally were 2.4 times more likely to have asthma compared to other residents [24, 25]. Another example is work by Dr. Kate Pitt who collaborated with people who were homeless and Brighton and Hove Common Ambition (a co-production and health service improvement project) to develop a comprehensive module on homelessness and health that comprised six sessions and was co delivered by experts by experience at Brighton and Sussex Medical School in 2023 [26]. Other examples of these types of activities are detailed in Table 7.1 below. We will explore how some of these types of initiatives may be utilised in the curriculum to improve student understanding of the context and needs of underserved communities.

Table 7.1 Examples of healthcare professional education initiatives that aim to improve the health of underserved communities

Category	Example projects	Reference
Health promotion/ information initiatives	American Medical Association medical student section's community service project idea book, which addresses the SDoH and is "designed to help your school organize community service events to encourage medical students to become more integrated with their communities"	[27]
Student led health initiatives	Student-run free clinics which can "act as primary care providers that bring health care to populations in need and are an important source of undergraduate medical education, guiding trainees through the art of history taking and physical examination." these clinics may have a particular role in communities that don't have current access to healthcare	[28]
Advocacy with/for communities on health and associated issues	Higher prevalence of asthma linked to unhealthy living conditions in Dublin south Inner-City community—research conducted in collaboration with a local deprived community found that residents of certain substandard apartments were 2.4 times more likely to have asthma compared to other local residents	[25 & 24]
Involvement of patients from underserved communities in curriculum design and delivery	Experts by experience of homelessness co-produced a medical student selected component on homelessness and health. Five workshops were held to co-design the curriculum, the course structure, content and teaching style. The experts were then involved in the delivery of the teaching.	[26]
Affirmative actions to support students from underserved communities to become healthcare students	Premedical honors college—From USA is an 8-year medical degree programme in Baylor College of Medicine and University of Texas designed to increase the number of physicians from underserved backgrounds who can then go on to address the health care needs of underserved populations in Texas	[29 & 30]

Potential Benefits of Engagement

Enhanced Learning Opportunities for Students

The potential for students to gain from placements in underserved areas is great [31]. Students themselves have described a feeling integrated with host communities, gaining an improved understanding of psychosocial matters, having positive experiences of teamwork and many other gains [31, 32]. Their placements also allowed them to develop close relationships with supervisors and colleagues [32].

It is important to highlight these positive experiences, as there is some evidence that interest in working with underserved communities among medical students declines over the course of their medical education [33]. Certain characteristics were associated with students being more keen to work with these groups in the future including students being of female gender, students identifying as being from an underserved or ethnic minority community themselves, students having exposure to marginalised groups during their medical education and students intending to practice in primary care [33]. This highlights the importance of creating positive and dynamic learning opportunities for students and how formative these experiences can be for career planning. This has been seen particularly with regard to rural practice, and Crampton et al. [32] found that all students in their review reported being more likely to seek to work in a rural post having completed a rural clinical placement as a student. There is also concern that universities may not utilise a variety of clinical placement settings such as areas of deprivation, and this may have knock-on effects on the future recruitment of clinical staff to work in these areas [34]. Ultimately these experiences and the enhanced understanding that students can gain from placements in underserved areas can help them to become socially accountable clinicians who have "'an obligation to denounce, to name and try to find mechanisms to address inequalities that they perceive' (PP_1–2) in their practice and in their sphere of influence" [35].

Service learning has been explored by universities globally to support healthcare professional students to learn about social and structural determinants of health and to give them some understanding of communities where they may end up working. It is considered a lever for transforming student attitudes and improving their knowledge in conjunction with community organisations [36]. As well as having a community service aspect to it, service learning should follow explicit learning objectives, with focused preparatory work and time allocated for facilitated reflection on student experiences [37]. These experiences can be beneficial to students and help link universities to the communities they are built to serve [36]. Without harnessing initiatives such as service learning, educators have asked "How do you teach a student to be community-based within the walls of the university? How do they learn to be a resource for a defined population they've never met? How do you teach them to be patient-centered clinicians without showing them this attitude in practice?" [38, 39]. Educators have acknowledged how difficult it is to teach about social and structural issues relating to health within the confines of traditional education settings [40, 41], and so service learning has a role as an effective bridge for these topics. Seifer [42] in her seminal work on service learning wrote that "balanced partnership between communities and health professions schools and a balance between serving the community and meeting defined learning objectives" was needed to be effective. One such project in Canada called the Making The Links (MTL) placed students in a variety of underserved settings including urban deprived communities, rural and remote areas and some international placements [38]. In those settings patients, community members and staff on the ground all worked to ensure that the placements met the goal of addressing community-identified need specific to each context [38].

Cultural and Structural Competency

Healthcare professional education has evolved in how it seeks to foster an understanding of the lived experience of marginalised and underserved groups. In the past the focus was on the development of cultural competency, described as "the trained ability to identify cross-cultural expressions of illness and health, and to thus counteract the marginalization of patients by race, ethnicity, social class, religion, sexual orientation, or other markers of difference" [15]. Now the aspiration is to give students an awareness of the concept of structural competency. This newer approach provides a lens for analysing and understanding health-related social justice issues by looking at the upstream structural causes of inequity such as the "economic and political conditions producing and racializing inequalities in health" [15, 43, 44]. Placements in and engagement with underserved communities provide the ideal setting for students and educators to see in real-life some of these structural impediments to equity in health, and also to see some of the levers and initiatives that may be useful to surmount those barriers [44]. Advocacy relating to housing and legal rights, and initiatives to support people to get their correct welfare benefits are some examples. Awareness of race as a determinant of health and the pernicious influence that racism can have on the health and wellbeing of individuals and minority ethnic groups is also key for students and educators to acknowledge and seek to address in their educational and clinical endeavours [15, 45].

Community Impact

Reeve et al. [31] conducted a review that found that medical and health professions schools which adopt socially accountable approaches to student placements in underserved communities were found to have some positive impacts on local health systems and the health of the communities. Another review reported positive feedback from communities themselves that had engaged with social accountability and student placement programmes [46], and one reported fostering a sense of empowerment among community members as a result of the activities [47]. There are limits to what can be attributed to these initiatives in terms of community benefits however, and Reeve et al. [31] said that "attributing health and workforce outcomes to medical school interventions is notoriously difficult due to the multiple complex factors involved in improving health outcomes, and the inability of descriptive studies to prove causality". Further discussion of the impact of socially accountable medical schools on community can be found in Chap. 10 of this book.

Widening Participation

One of the other potential benefits to engaging with underserved communities is the potential that the partnership may encourage students to consider applying for medicine and healthcare professional courses. Educators recognise that widening access to medicine and the healthcare professions will allow for the development of more diverse institutions which are representative of the communities they serve [48, 49], but it is unclear how institutions are actually operationalising this policy in many instances [49, 50]. There is some evidence from the American context that doctors who come from minority ethnic groups are more likely to work in "medically underserved areas" and "primary care health professional shortage areas" [51, 52], and this highlights another reason why targeted supports are needed to facilitate wider access to universities. Outreach programmes to pre-university students in underserved areas could seek to fill some of the gaps in understanding the potential of medical careers and the "deficits of social capital" that can act as a significant barrier to considering applying for healthcare courses [53].

Benefits for Educational Institutions

Academic institutions can have influence at local, regional and national levels in terms of trying to ensure health policies and practices are tailored to the needs of underserved communities [54]. Research that aims to do this needs to be conducted in a collaborative and sensitive way to be relevant and have the intended impact. Medical schools and other educational institutions should strive to meet "the pressing health care needs of society", and engagement with underserved communities can provide a great opportunity to do just that by adjusting institutional strategies to better align them with current health system challenges and community needs [55].

Developing a Curriculum

Designing an Appropriate Curriculum

Curriculum Integration

There have been many different approaches to integrating social accountability teaching relevant to working for underserved communities adopted in medical curricula worldwide [46]. Medical curricula are designed around Medical Graduate Profiles (MGPs), and meaningful and sustained integration of social accountability will mean incorporating these ideas and principles into the MGP. This would demonstrate commitment and then map the concept back into curricular content and related assessment. Abdalla et al [56]. described strategies for the integration of those relevant topics in a vertical and horizontal manner across a curriculum and they noted that a mixture of problem based learning and clinical presentations may be an efficient way of achieving the desired integration. Examples of existing curricular approaches have included community placements, advocacy initiatives, classroom-based teaching on relevant topics and others [46, 56]. Some authors describe initiatives to remodel their curriculum to provides relevant teaching that punctuates the educational journey of medical students before culminating in a community clerkship [35, 57]. It is unclear from many of the published reports what teaching in this area is mandatory for students, and what is optional. Fung and Ying [58] also highlighted the importance of multidisciplinary partnerships developed to deliver interprofessional education on social accountability, mirroring the way care is provided in the community. It has also been acknowledged that some of what is relevant for teaching students in preparation for placements in areas of deprivation may be different that other areas; for instance in the Scottish context general practitioners felt that supporting patients with addiction, multimorbidity, polypharmacy, psychosocial issues and child protection were key areas of relevance for their own learning [59], and these would then be witnessed by undergraduate students on placement. Important skills frequently employed in supporting patients included the engagement of 'hard-to-reach' patients who have competing priorities, striving to "promote and maintain therapeutic optimism" for both patients and clinicians in the face of challenges and the application of evidence-based medicine principles in these contexts [59, 60]. Clinical educators in underserved areas also need to be aware of how their teaching fits into the overall curriculum and what the universities and students expect from their time 'on the ground' [32]. Finally, the impact of the SDOH needs to be integrated into all clinical teaching, for example, ensuring socio-economic risk factors are considered across all conditions including, for example, cardiometabolic conditions, cancers and mental illness. Further discussion on this is in chap. 10.

Partnership and Curricular Co-design with Local Communities

Collaboration and effective communication with underserved communities is a fundamental consideration when developing social accountability initiatives [58]. The Partnership Pentagram developed by Boelen has identified that these communities are one of the five key stakeholders in initiatives focused on social accountability along with administrators, healthcare professionals, academics and policy-makers [61]. One example of the from Canada highlighted the work that was needed to begin and maintain these partnerships [57]. It described engagement with two Aboriginal communities in Canada and documented the process for integrating community perspectives and being open to revising and improving the programme as time went on. Other experts in the field have also highlighted the initial identification of priorities and shared goals for these programmes as crucial [41, 62]. The cultivation of strong relationships with communities is vital to the success of these plans, and can be difficult for institutions to grapple with, hence some authors have tried to simplify and describe how it might be done. One example is the Assess, Inquire, Deliver, Educate, Respond (AIDER) model created by Sandhu et al. [63] to help academics carry out this work in a collaborative way.

Delivering a Curriculum

Logistical Considerations and Preparing Students

Students attending placements in rural areas in particular have reported challenges relating to the costs of taking part and also the potential for being socially isolated while away [32, 64]. This highlights the importance of adequately preparing students and putting supports in place for them prior to going and throughout their placements. Meili et al. [38] described a project called 'Making the Links' that sought to teach students about caring for underserved groups and it began with a comprehensive orientation module of 20 h of teaching including language classes and cultural training. The participating students also had a supported reflection period at the end. Jarvis-Selinger, Ho [57] described a two-day orientation programme led by Aboriginal community Elders and clinician educators from the participating communities. This began to immerse the students in the culture and customs they would see, give them an understanding of the structure of the communities and the health issues they may encounter, while also fostering companionship between the students themselves who could support each other while away.

Student Assessment

The assessment of students who have taken part in social accountability initiatives with underserved communities is challenging [65]. Some authors discuss the use of student self-reported questionnaires on their attitudes as a way of examining whether teaching has been effective, while others feel that Objective Structured Clinical Examinations (OSCEs) are more appropriate [32, 33, 58]. While OSCEs are primarily designed to test clinical skills over a series of simulated patient encounters, Fung and Ying [58] felt that over years of clinical education they could be used to "engage with more complex sociocultural issues and become more intricate with expectations of diagnosis and management", and that student should eventually be able to "consider social factors in their assessments and management". The use of tools such as the self-reported 'Medical Student Attitudes Toward the Underserved' (MS-ATU) questionnaire and the 'Medical Student future Intention to Work with the Underserved' (MS-IWU) questionnaire is notable for this purpose. The combination of OSCEs and these types of questionaries together may provide a comprehensive indication of whether an institution is meeting the goal of providing socially accountable education [33]. As Leinster [65] also pointed out, there is considerable overlap between the concepts of professionalism and social accountability, and there are similar challenges and debates on how best to assess them. Fung and Ying [58] in a paper written to encourage educators to address social accountability teaching wrote that examining of social accountability learning needs to happen as part of routine assessments of core medical subjects and the devising of management plans. Other educators have developed novel approaches to assessment, with Metzl and Petty [43] creating the 'Structural Foundations of Health' (SFH) evaluation instrument for their work at Vanderbilt University which tested the core structural competency skills of students as well as gathering their demographic information. Gholar, Palokas [66] reviewed the breath of structural competency teaching and assessment and found that it was being taught to medical, nursing, social work, pharmacy, and other students. They also found that there were a variety of qualitative, quantitative and mixed methods assessments in use [66].

Evaluating a Curriculum and Potential Challenges

Evaluation of Programmes

The evaluation of any programmes implemented is important in order to keep them focused on the needs of the communities involved and the challenges that students may be facing while taking part. Continuous improvement based on feedback from all stakeholders is necessary, but also evaluation reports can form an important tool for advocacy on some of the wider needs of underserved communities. For example,

Noya et al. [67] interviewed graduates from their rural track of training and found that one of major impediments to delivering high quality education in the remote settings was inadequate infrastructure and poor practice conditions. They concluded that policy makers needed to understand these issues and rectify them for educators and communities to be able to work toward the shared goal of training and recruiting more healthcare workers to rural underserved areas.

Challenges

Resource Constraints

Perkins and Daly [21] wrote that "underserved communities are by definition low in skills that are relatively abundant in teaching hospitals and often face problems in the recruitment and retention of (general) medical staff", highlighting that the very fact that these areas are underserved means that there can be great challenges in placing healthcare students there when clinicians are often overstretched and have limited capacity to facilitate teaching. This bears out what Julian Tutor Hart wrote in the 1970s that "the availability of good medical care tends to vary inversely with the need for it in the population served" [68]. The provision of care to patients in underserved and deprived areas can be personally and professionally challenging for clinicians, and the pressure on their time can mean that they may be less likely to engage in the training of students [60]. Butler et al. [34] examined data from Northern Ireland and found that practices in areas of high deprivation were less involved in teaching undergraduates than those in more affluent areas. One potential consequence of this uneven distribution of placements and lack of exposure is that students may feel less confident about working in areas of deprivation in the future [32]. Providing diverse educational experiences in a variety of contexts is key to the delivery of social accountability teaching, and as Fung and Ying [58] wrote on this topic—"the status quo of medical education focuses on understanding the "average" patient. However, social accountability requires active efforts to consider marginalized communities who are often medically underserved with unique social and medical needs. Medical schools have the responsibility to support diverse learning environments for medical students to be able to identify and intervene on these needs." This is particularly important given the general lack of diversity in medical student cohorts.

Reluctance of Stakeholders

There can be reluctance on the part of students, educators and institutions to fully pursue socially accountable initiatives with underserved communities. Linked to the aforementioned resource constraints and challenges for clinicians in these areas, this can manifest as a poor experience for students and they can give feedback that supervisory and clinical arrangements are less satisfactory than expected [32, 64]. As well as that, students have expressed concern at the limited range of medical conditions seen, not being comfortable living in a community so close to their patients, having a perceived lack of structure of the placement and having difficulties with accommodation and logistical issues [21, 32, 64]. These experiences and perceptions can make subsequent students less likely to consider applying for these types of social accountability initiatives.

Faculty leadership and finding academic 'champions' who are keen to drive social accountability agendas in educational institutions are key to the success and comprehensiveness of these initiatives [69, 70]. It can be difficult to start on the path of changing how an institution engages with these topics, and as Boelen, Pearson [69] wrote "faculty often denigrates concepts like "social accountability" as "soft", not true bio-medical science, whilst discouraging students to take the concept seriously. Working in the "social accountability" space moves people out of the comfort zone, a zone they control, into an arena where they have to learn from others and share credit." Showing the value of social accountability to all stakeholders is a challenging but vital step in terms of resource allocation and the potential sustainability of any programmes.

Sustainability

Maintaining and enhancing engagement with underserved communities takes time and funding [57]. There is an ethical imperative to ensure careful sustained engagement as there have been communities who have been 'let-down' by short-lived initiatives in the past. Acquiring sustainable funding can be a challenge, quite often it is conditional and for a short duration and there may be requirements to quickly show tangible benefits from these programmes. As well as funding, social accountability concepts needs to be embedded within the curriculum, with clear linkage to the medical graduate profile, as there is potential for relevant initiatives to cease when 'champions' move on [70] In order to build trust and truly engage with underserved communities in an ethical and sustainable way, these initiatives need full commitment from all stakeholders involved.

Case Studies

Case Study 1—University of Glasgow Medical School

Glasgow is home to some of the most stark health inequalities in the UK, with a 17-year gap in male life expectancy at birth across Glasgow's neighbourhoods and an equivalent 13-year gap in female life expectancy [71]. Glasgow has the lowest healthy life expectancy (HLE) in Scotland; men are estimated to live for 54.6 years in good health and women for 57.6 years [71]. In the context of these sobering statistics, the University of Glasgow's medical school has introduced several initiatives over the past 10 years to increase its social accountability, aiming to both widen access to the medical profession for those from more disadvantaged backgrounds and to improve students' understanding of socioeconomic disadvantage across the curriculum. This case study will present examples of initiatives in both these areas.

Initiatives to Widen Participation

Widening Participation (WP) for medical school entry has been encouraged to ensure access and participation for underrepresented groups (e.g. those living in the 20% most deprived postcodes in Scotland; SIMD20, Scottish Index of Multiple Deprivation) that are less likely to apply for medical school entry and even less likely to be successful [72]. Glasgow medical school is involved in two main WP initiatives.

- *REACH Scotland*—this is a national programme, established through support from the Scottish Funding Council, with the overall aim of widening participation to high demand professions, including medicine. Pupils from any secondary school in the west of Scotland (who meet certain eligibility criteria) can take part in the programme over the final 3 years of school (S4 to S6). The programme introduces pupils to medicine and supports their applications [73]. More than 500 pupils have been supported since the programme began in 2010.
- *Gateway to Medical Studies Programme*—this initiative, formerly called the Glasgow Access Programme (GAP), was set up in 2017 with funding from the Scottish Government as part of the national widening participation directive [74]. It is a pre-medical year which is targeted to students from certain underrepresented or disadvantaged backgrounds (e.g. resident in a SIMD20 postcode; refugee or asylum seeker; care experienced) and provides automatic progression to the MBChB programme for students who satisfactorily complete the programme. The programme includes teaching on basic sciences and communication skills and has tailored content from GPs working in the most socioeconomically disadvantaged and underserved communities in Scotland who are linked to the Scottish Deep End Project [75].). More than 100 students have taken part in this programme so far.

On a less formal basis, staff and students at the medical school have recently set up the Widening Access to Medicine Student Society (WAMS) and are actively promoting various initiatives (e-mentoring, social networking events etc) designed to raise awareness of WP among the student population.

Initiatives to Improve Student Understanding

There is teaching on the social determinants of health across the medical school curriculum at the University of Glasgow, with a plan to add 'Tackling health inequalities' as a vertical theme. Examples of current teaching which all students experience includes a "Community Diagnosis" project in Year 1, a block called "Keeping People Healthy" in Year 2 which teaches mental health and problem substance use issues, a session in Year 3 on inclusion health focussed on the experience of homelessness and trauma informed care, and a cross-cultural communication skills session in Year 4. Specific initiatives that students can choose include:

- *Community Orientated Medical Experience Track (COMET)*—in recognition of the fundamental role of General Practice within health systems, this innovative scheme, launched in 2019 with Scottish Government funding, provides selected medical students with an enhanced experience of General Practice [76]. Central to the COMET programme is increased patient contact in primary care settings, including a longitudinal placement in the same GP practice (roughly one day per month) covering a 2-year period. There are places for 30 COMET students each year and they all start in Year 2 with a 5-week Student Selected Component (SSC) about the SDOH and Tacking Health Inequalities. This involves placements in a range of health and community settings (including time within a Deep End practice). Other SSC options (in Year 3 or 4) include topics such as Gender based violence and LGBTQIA+ health inequalities. The first cohort of COMET students graduated in summer 2024.
- *Student Selected Components (SSCs)*—SSC options (in Year 3 and 4) open to any medical student include topics such as Gender based violence and LGBTQIA+ health inequalities. There are also SSCs in Deep End GP practices. These are practices with the highest percentages of registered patients who live in the 15% most socioeconomically disadvantaged SIMD postcodes [75]. The Scottish Deep End Project is a collaboration between Deep End and academic GPs with the aim of ensuring the NHS is at its best where needs are greatest [77]. Activities include advocacy, research and teaching and students undertaking these SSCs will get a taste of the challenges faced by primary care teams delivering care to underserved communities. All SSCs are based around a set of specific learning outcomes and online resources that students and tutors can utilise. There have also been four Deep End student conferences since 2017.

Case Study 2—The Latin American Social Medicine and Collective Health Movement

The Latin American Social Medicine and Collective Health movement (LASMCH) has played a crucial role in shaping medical education in that region since the 1970s. Rooted in principles of social justice, equity, and a deep understanding of the social determinants of health, the movement has influenced the training of healthcare professionals, especially in medical schools, by embedding these values in undergraduate and postgraduate "Collective Health" initiatives across Latin America [78].

Collective health involves understanding health as a shared social responsibility and addressing systemic inequalities through policy and structural change. Brazilian and Argentine medical schools have pioneered this approach, training doctors to not only serve individual patients but to advocate for public health reforms that address the root causes of health inequities, such as wealth inequality and access to healthcare.

The LASMCH movement is organised under the Latin American Social Medicine Association (*Asociación Latinoamericana de Medicina Social* [ALAMES]), which was founded in 1984 [79], its country-level chapters, as well as by prominent country-specific organisations, like the Brazilian Association of Collective Health (Associação Brasileira de Saúde Coletiva [ABRASCO]).

Though not as well known in the Anglophone world, important contributions made by Latin American social medicine scholars and activists pre-date more recent work such as the World Health Organization's commission on social determinants of health and Metzl and Hansen's 'structural competency' [80]. Several generations of health professionals in Brazil and Mexico have, for instance, been trained in a social medicine framework that trains them to recognise how poverty, housing, education, and labour conditions influence health outcomes.

There is clear recognition in Latin America of the importance of health care systems based on strong primary care [81]. However, the reality on the ground is that there is considerable scope for enhancing the social accountability of medical schools in Latin America, with a need for more robust policies to increase the volume and quality of training in primary care in particular [82].

Take-Home Message

In this chapter we have examined the continuum of curricular planning, development, delivery and evaluation while sensitively engaging with underserved communities. We have explained that institutions and educators need to understand how to engage with humility when interacting with underserved communities to work to improve their health and to foster student learning. We have also highlighted that educators need to support students to become clinicians who can understand and begin to address the social and structural determinants of health. To do this effectively, we need to understand why it is important for institutions training healthcare professionals, faculty members and students to be aware of disadvantage and marginalisation, and their causes and effects on health. We have also described some exemplars of good practice where initiatives have been developed to seek to address these issues.

References

1. Gottlieb L. Funding healthy society helps cure health care. San Francisco Chronicle; 2010.
2. Dahlgren G, Whitehead M. The Dahlgren-Whitehead model of health determinants: 30 years on and still chasing rainbows. Public Health. 2021;199:20–4.
3. Marmot M, Allen JJ. Social determinants of health equity. Am J Public Health. 2014;104(S4):S517–S9.
4. Allen M, Donkin A. The impact of adverse experiences in the home on children and young people. London: Institute of Health Equity; 2015.
5. Lewis JH, Lage OG, Grant BK, Rajasekaran SK, Gemeda M, Like RC, et al. Addressing the social determinants of health in undergraduate medical education curricula: a survey report. Adv Med Educ Pract. 2020;Volume 11:369–77.
6. World Health Assembly. Social determinants of health–Seventy-fourth World Health Assembly WHA74.16 Agenda item 22.1 Geneva: World Health Assembly; 2021. Available from: https://apps.who.int/gb/ebwha/pdf_files/WHA74/A74_R16-en.pdf. Accessed 09 Jan 2024.
7. World Health Organization. Special initiative for action on the social determinants of health for advancing health equity [internet]. Geneva: WHO; 2024. Cited 2024 Aug 11th. Available from: www.who.int/initiatives/action-on-the-social-determinants-of-health-for-advancing-equity
8. Lewis JH, Whelihan K, Roy D. Teaching students to identify and document social determinants of health. Adv Med Educ Pract. 2019;10:653–65.
9. Cobigo V, Martin L, McHeimech R. Understanding community. Canadian J Disab Stud. 2016;5(4):181–203.
10. The White House. Executive order on advancing racial equity and support for underserved communities through the Federal Government [internet]. Washington DC: The White House; 2021. [Cited 2024 Aug 8th]. Available from: www.whitehouse.gov/briefing-room/presidential-actions/2021/01/20/executive-order-advancing-racial-equity-and-support-for-underserved-communities-through-the-federal-government/
11. Government of the UK. Accredited official statistics–English indices of deprivation 2019. London: Ministry of Housing, Communities & Local Government; 2019. [Cited 2024 Aug 6th]. Available from: www.gov.uk/government/statistics/english-indices-of-deprivation-2019
12. Public Health England. Inclusion Health: applying all our health London: Government of the UK; 2021 [Cited 2024 Jul 9th]. Available from: www.gov.uk/government/publications/inclusion-health-applying-all-our-health/inclusion-health-applying-all-our-health
13. Scottish Government. Using intersectionality to understand structural inequality in Scotland: evidence synthesis Edinburgh: Scottish Government; 2022 [Cited 2024 Jul 5th]. Available from: www.gov.scot/publications/using-intersectionality-understand-structural-inequality-scotland-evidence-synthesis/documents/
14. Farmer PE, Nizeye B, Stulac S, Keshavjee S. Structural violence and clinical medicine. PLoS Med. 2006;3(10):e449.
15. Metzl JM, Hansen H. Structural competency: theorizing a new medical engagement with stigma and inequality. Soc Sci Med. 2014;103:126–33.
16. Dharamsi S, Ho A, Spadafora SM, Woollard R. The physician as health advocate: translating the quest for social responsibility into medical education and practice. Acad Med. 2011;86(9):1108–13.
17. Boelen C, Heck JE, Organization WH. Defining and measuring the social accountability of medical schools. World Health Organization; 1995.
18. George HJ. The world turned upside down: proposals for community-based undergraduate medical education. J R Coll Gen Pract. 1985;35(271):63.
19. Thistlethwaite JE, Kidd MR, Hudson JN. General practice: a leading provider of medical student education in the 21st century? Med J Aust. 2007;187(2):124–8.
20. Aretz HT. Some thoughts about creating healthcare professionals that match what societies need. Med Teach. 2011;33(8):608–13.

21. Perkins D, Daly M. What is the evidence for clinical placements in underserved areas? Med Educ. 2013;47(10):958–60.
22. Steven K, Dowell J, Jackson C, Guthrie B. Fair access to medicine? Retrospective analysis of UK medical schools application data 2009-2012 using three measures of socioeconomic status. BMC Med Educ. 2016;16(1):11.
23. Krstić C, Krstić L, Tulloch A, Agius S, Warren A, Doody GA. The experience of widening participation students in undergraduate medical education in the UK: a qualitative systematic review. Med Teach. 2021;43(9):1044–53.
24. Trinity College Dublin. Higher prevalence of asthma linked to unhealthy living conditions in Dublin south Inner City community Dublin: Trinity College Dublin; 2024 [Cited 2024 Aug 16th]. Available from: www.tcd.ie/news_events/articles/2024/higher-prevalence-of-asthma-linked-to-unhealthy-living-conditions-in-dublin-south-inner-city-community/
25. Mc Carthy N, Hayes C, Creane D, O'Ciardha D, Smith SM, Campbell A. Health data to support local communities Dublin: Trinity College Dublin; 2024 [Cited 2024 Aug 16th]. Available from: www.tara.tcd.ie/handle/2262/104420
26. Brighton & Hove Common Ambition. Coproducing medical student training Brighton: Brighton & Hove Common Ambition; 2023 [Cited 2024 Jul 12th]. Available from: www.bhcommonambition.org/2023/08/22/coproducing-medical-student-training/
27. American Medical Association. AMA-MSS COMMUNITY service project IDEA book Chicago: American Medical Association; 2021 [Cited 2024 Jul 20th]. Available from: www.ama-assn.org/system/files/mss-csc-idea-book.pdf
28. Rupert DD, Alvarez GV, Burdge EJ, Nahvi RJ, Schell SM, Faustino FL. Student-run free clinics stand at a critical junction between undergraduate medical education, clinical care, and advocacy. Acad Med. 2022;97(6):824–31.
29. Thomson WA, Ferry PG, King JE, Martinez-Wedig C, Michael LH. Increasing access to medical education for students from medically underserved communities: one program's success. Acad Med. 2003;78(5):454–9.
30. Center for Educational Outreach. Houston Premedical Academy Houston: Baylor College of Medicine; 2024 [Cited 2024 Jul 20th]. Available from: www.bcm.edu/departments/huffington-department-of-education-innovation-technology/center-for-educational-outreach/career-pathways/b-s-m-d-programs/houston-premedical-academy
31. Reeve C, Woolley T, Ross SJ, Mohammadi L, Halili SB Jr, Cristobal F, et al. The impact of socially-accountable health professional education: a systematic review of the literature. Med Teach. 2017;39(1):67–73.
32. Crampton PES, McLachlan JC, Illing JC. A systematic literature review of undergraduate clinical placements in underserved areas. Med Educ. 2013;47(10):969–78.
33. Leaune E, Rey-Cadilhac V, Oufker S, Grot S, Strowd R, Rode G, et al. Medical students attitudes toward and intention to work with the underserved: a systematic review and meta-analysis. BMC Med Educ. 2021;21(1):129.
34. Butler D, O'Donovan D, McClung A, Hart N. Do undergraduate general practice placements propagate the 'inverse care law'? Educ Prim Care. 2022;33(5):280–7.
35. Dubé TV, Cumyn A, Fourati M, Chamberland M, Hatcher S, Landry M. Pathways, journeys and experiences: integrating curricular activities related to social accountability within an undergraduate medical curriculum. Med Educ. 2024;58(5):556–65.
36. Playford D, Bailey S, Fisher C, Stasinska A, Marshall L, Gawlinski M, et al. Twelve tips for implementing effective service learning. Med Teach. 2019;41(1):24–7.
37. O'Neil EH. Health professions education for the future: schools in service to the nation. San Francisco: Pew Health Professions Commission; 1993. p. 2.
38. Meili R, Fuller D, Lydiate J. Teaching social accountability by making the links: qualitative evaluation of student experiences in a service-learning project. Med Teach. 2011;33(8):659–66.
39. Rosser W. Sustaining the 4 principles of family medicine in Canada. Can Fam Physician. 2006;52(10):1191.
40. Stephenson A, Higgs R, Sugarman J. Teaching professional development in medical schools. Lancet. 2001;357(9259):867–70.

41. Faulkner LR, McCurdy RL. Teaching medical students social responsibility: the right thing to do. Acad Med. 2000;75(4):346–50.
42. Seifer SD. Service-learning: community-campus partnerships for health professions education. Acad Med. 1998;73(3):273–7.
43. Metzl JM, Petty J. Integrating and assessing structural competency in an innovative Prehealth curriculum at Vanderbilt University. Acad Med. 2017;92(3):354–9.
44. Neff J, Holmes SM, Knight KR, Strong S, Thompson-Lastad A, McGuinness C, et al. Structural competency: curriculum for medical students, residents, and Interprofessional teams on the structural factors that produce health disparities. MedEdPORTAL. 2020;16:10888.
45. Rivara FP, Bradley SM, Catenacci DV, Desai AN, Ganguli I, Haneuse SJPA, et al. Structural racism and JAMA network open. JAMA Netw Open. 2021;4(6):e2120269-e.
46. Mihan A, Muldoon L, Leider H, Tehfe H, Fitzgerald M, Fournier K, et al. Social accountability in undergraduate medical education a narrative review. Education for Health. 2022;35(1):3–8.
47. Strasser R, Hogenbirk JC, Minore B, Marsh DC, Berry S, McCready WG, et al. Transforming health professional education through social accountability: Canada's northern Ontario School of Medicine. Med Teach. 2013;35(6):490–6.
48. Alexander K, Fahey Palma T, Nicholson S, Cleland J. 'Why not you?' Discourses of widening access on UK medical school websites. Med Educ. 2017;51(6):598–611.
49. Cleland J, Buxton J, Hughes E, Patterson F. Translating government policy into practice: how new UK medical schools enact widening participation. Med Educ. 2024;n/a(n/a):1247–56.
50. Ellaway RH, Malhi R, Bajaj S, Walker I, Myhre D. A critical scoping review of the connections between social mission and medical school admissions: BEME guide no. 47. Med Teach. 2018;40(3):219–26.
51. Walker KO, Moreno G, Grumbach K. The association among specialty, race, ethnicity, and practice location among California physicians in diverse specialties. J Natl Med Assoc. 2012;104(1):46–52.
52. Xierali IM, Nivet MA. The racial and ethnic composition and distribution of primary care physicians. J Health Care Poor Underserved. 2018;29(1):556–70.
53. Martin AJ, Beska BJ, Wood G, Wyatt N, Codd A, Vance G, et al. Widening interest, widening participation: factors influencing school students' aspirations to study medicine. BMC Med Educ. 2018;18(1):117.
54. Boydell V, McMullen H, Cordero J, Steyn P, Kiare J. Studying social accountability in the context of health system strengthening: innovations and considerations for future work. Health Research Policy and Systems. 2019;17(1):34.
55. Boelen C, Woollard B. Social accountability and accreditation: a new frontier for educational institutions. Med Educ. 2009;43(9):887–94.
56. Abdalla ME, Taha MH, Onchonga D, Magzoub ME, Au H, O'Donnell P, et al. Integrating the social determinants of health into curriculum: AMEE guide no. 162. Med Teach. 2024;46(3):304–16.
57. Jarvis-Selinger S, Ho K, Novak Lauscher H, Liman Y, Stacy E, Woollard R, et al. Social accountability in action: university-community collaboration in the development of an interprofessional aboriginal health elective. J Interprof Care. 2008;22(sup1):61–72.
58. Fung OW, Ying Y. Twelve tips to center social accountability in undergraduate medical education. Med Teach. 2022;44(11):1214–20.
59. MacVicar R, Williamson A, Cunningham DE, Watt G. What are the CPD needs of GPs working in areas of high deprivation? Report of a focus group meeting of 'GPs at the deep end'. Educ Prim Care. 2015;26(3):139–45.
60. Blane DN. Medical education in (and for) areas of socio-economic deprivation in the UK. Educ Prim Care. 2018;29(5):255–8.
61. World Health Organization. Towards unity for health: challenges and opportunities for partnership in health development. 2000.

62. Woollard RF. Caring for a common future: medical schools' social accountability. Med Educ. 2006;40(4):301–13.
63. Sandhu G, Garcha I, Sleeth J, Yeates K, Walker GR. AIDER: a model for social accountability in medical education and practice. Med Teach. 2013;35(8):e1403–e8.
64. Roberts C, Daly M, Kumar K, Perkins D, Richards D, Garne D. A longitudinal integrated placement and medical students' intentions to practise rurally. Med Educ. 2012;46(2):179–91.
65. Leinster S. Evaluation and assessment of social accountability in medical schools. Med Teach. 2011;33(8):673–6.
66. Gholar VM, Palokas M, Tacy J. Structural competency curriculum in health sciences education: a scoping review. JBI Evidence Synthesis. 2023;21(7):1408–52.
67. Noya F, Carr S, Thompson S. Social accountability in a medical school: is it sufficient? A regional medical school curriculum and approaches to equip graduates for rural and remote medical services. BMC Med Educ. 2024;24(1):526.
68. Tudor HJ. The inverse care law. Lancet. 1971;297(7696):405–12.
69. Boelen C, Pearson D, Kaufman A, Rourke J, Woollard R, Marsh DC, et al. Producing a socially accountable medical school: AMEE guide no. 109. Med Teach. 2016;38(11):1078–91.
70. Preston R, Larkins S, Taylor J, Judd J. Building blocks for social accountability: a conceptual framework to guide medical schools. BMC Med Educ. 2016;16(1):227.
71. Glasgow Centre for Population Health. Understanding Glasgow–the Glasgow indicators project. Glasgow: University of Glasgow; 2022. [Cited 2024 Jul 10th]. Available from: www.understandingglasgow.com/indicators/health/overview
72. Sartania N, Haddock G, Underwood M. The challenges of widening access to the medical profession: how to facilitate medical careers for those at a genuine disadvantage [version 2]. MedEdPublish. 2019;7(277):277.
73. University of Glasgow. Reach Scotland Glasgow: University of Glasgow; 2024 [Cited 2024 Jul 10th]. Available from: www.gla.ac.uk/study/wp/reach/
74. University of Glasgow. Gateway to medical studies Programme. Glasgow: University of Glasgow; 2024. [Cited 2024 Jul 20th]. Available from: www.gla.ac.uk/schools/medicine/mus/admissions/gateway-to-medical-studies-programme/
75. Scottish Deep End Group. The Scottish deep end project. Glasgow: University of Glasgow; 2024. [Cited 2024 Jul 12th]. Available from: www.gla.ac.uk/schools/healthwellbeing/research/generalpractice/deepend/
76. University of Glasgow. Community orientated medical experience track (COMET). Glasgow: University of Glasgow; 2024. [Cited 2024 Jul 18th]. Available from: www.gla.ac.uk/schools/medicine/mus/communityorientatedmedicalexperiencetrackcomet/
77. Watt G, Brown G, Budd J, Cawston P, Craig M, Jamieson R, et al. General practitioners at the deep end: the experience and views of general practitioners working in the most severely deprived areas of Scotland. Occasional Paper (Royal College of General Practitioners). 2012;89:i.
78. Harvey M, Piñones-Rivera C, Holmes SM. Structural competency, Latin American social medicine, and collective health: exploring shared lessons through the work of Jaime Breilh. Glob Public Health. 2023;18(1):2220023.
79. Breilh J. Critical epidemiology and the people's health. USA: Oxford University Press; 2021.
80. Sesia PM. Global voices for global (epistemic) justice: bringing to the forefront Latin American theoretical and activist contributions to the pursuit of the right to health. Health Hum Rights. 2023;25(1):137–47.
81. Macinko J, Montenegro H, Nebot Adell C, Etienne C. Renewing primary health care in the Americas. Rev Panam Salud Publica. https://www3pahoorg/hq/dmdocuments/2010/Renewing_Primary_Health_Care_Americas-PAHOpdf. 2007;21(2-3):73–84.
82. Puschel K, Rojas P, Erazo A, Thompson B, Lopez J, Barros J. Social accountability of medical schools and academic primary care training in Latin America: principles but not practice. Fam Pract. 2014;31(4):399–408.

Further Reading

Abdalla ME, Taha MH, Onchonga D, Magzoub ME, Au H, O'Donnell P, et al. Integrating the social determinants of health into curriculum: AMEE guide no. 162. Med Teach. 2024;46(3):304–16. https://doi.org/10.1080/0142159X.2023.2254920.

Deep End REPORT 33 Increasing undergraduate education in primary care in areas of socio-economic deprivation (the Deep End) https://www.gla.ac.uk/media/Media_608446_smxx.pdf

PLOS Collection on Social Medicine in the twenty-first Century https://collections.plos.org/collection/social-medicine/

Chapter 8
From Community-Oriented Medical Education to Social Accountability

Rukhsana W. Zuberi and Mohi Eldin Magzoub

Learning Outcomes

1. Trace the historical perspectives of community-oriented medical education (COME).
2. Identify why COME was conceptualized and implemented.
3. Recognize the challenges associated with implementing COME and Community-based Education (CBE).
4. Recognize the rationale for transitioning to social accountability in medical education.
5. Differentiate between COME and socially accountable medical schools.

Evolution of Medical Education: From Community-Oriented to Socially Accountable Practices

In the post Flexner era, nearly all medical education was based within universities and hospitals, where acute care drove the agenda of curative medicine, leaving little time for preventive and promotive medicine: how to keep the people healthy. The social determinants of health were not given due importance.

Consequently, medical students who graduated from these institutions possessed limited knowledge or experience about existing community issues and lacked the necessary skills to work outside the hospitals [1].

R. W. Zuberi (✉)
Aga Khan University, Karachi, Pakistan
e-mail: rukhsana.zuberi@aku.edu

M. E. Magzoub
United Arab Emirates University, Al Ain, UAE

M. E. Abdalla et al. (eds.), *Social Accountability of Medical Schools*,
https://doi.org/10.1007/978-3-031-94435-2_8

Many medical colleges recognized this inequity of health services distribution and, as a counterbalance, initiated community-oriented medical education (COME) programmes, but unfortunately, without clear goals and explicit strategies. The Network of Community-Oriented Educational Institutions for Health Sciences (now Network-TUFH) united the health professions education institutions with the common goal of promoting relevance in health professions education, research and services. It defined COME and conceptualized community-based education.

Community-oriented medical education focuses on both population groups and individuals, and emphasizes the health needs of the community concerned [2]. Community-Based Education is a means of achieving educational relevance to community health needs. It consists of learning activities within a community, where the community is the learning environment in which not only students, but also teachers, members of the community, and representatives of other sectors are actively involved in the educational experience.

When faculty teach students in the community, they not only contribute to services in the community increasing access, but also equip the students with experiential learning, competencies to engage with communities, and management skills and leadership. It also leads to interprofessional education and increased community-based research.

Implementation of COME and CBE was challenging. Initially the lack of common well-defined goals and strategies, and later establishing partnerships, variability in educational experiences, issues with student assessment, monitoring and programme evaluation, and the high cost made it unfeasible. Usually, CBE was left to a single department to implement. In addition, community expectations from the programme were enormous and could not be fulfilled.

Alas, the people's health needs remained unmet. Given the hindrances of COME and the globalisation of medicine and health care a new approach was needed.

As per the World Health Organization's (WHO) definition of Social Accountability of Medical Schools 1995, (see chap. 1 for the definition) [3] medical schools must work with all stakeholders to increase efficiency and effectiveness. The Global Consensus for Social Accountability of Medical Schools (GCSA)," [4] emphasizes ten main areas: Anticipating society's health needs; forming partnerships; adapting to the changing roles of doctors and other health professionals; outcome-based education; creating responsive and responsible governance; refining the scope of standards and continuous quality improvement in education, research and service delivery; establishing mandated mechanisms for accreditation; global principles relevant to the local context; and defining the role of society. This approach transcends geographical boundaries and addresses broader societal challenges. See chap. 1 for more details on the GCSA.

Historical Perspectives of the Evolution of Community-Oriented Medical Education

The Flexner report, published in 1910, convinced the medical community in the United States that the prevalent approach to medical education, which relied on apprenticeship, was inadequate in producing physicians of high quality. The report emphasized the necessity of enhancing the scientific foundation of medical knowledge and medical practice [5]. Medical education should be academic and should be located in universities. As a result, Universities in both developing and developed countries have widely followed Flexner's model. The paradigm has resulted in an increased emphasis on factual biomedical knowledge as well as disciplines and departments of basic medical sciences. Consequently, the volume of information that medical students need to learn, and the number of content-experts required to teach this information have also grown [5]. The majority of instructions is teacher centered with a passive role of students. Teaching takes place within classrooms, laboratories, and specialized university hospitals with little exposure to community sites. Consequently, medical students who graduate from these institutions possess limited knowledge about the existing community issues and lack the necessary skills to work outside the hospitals, leave alone in rural and under-served areas [1].

The discipline of medical education began to emerge in the late 1950s with the formation of the first Department of Medical Education at the University of Illinois in Chicago, USA, as well as the establishment of Departments of Preventive Medicine and Public Health in several universities worldwide [6]. Simultaneously, inside the community, the human rights movement advocated for equal opportunities across all aspects of human life, including healthcare [7]. Governments recognized the disparity in access to services among their population and established social security and welfare agencies to provide equitable health services to individuals, irrespective of their socio-economic, age, or ethnic origins. The recognition of public health's significance in tackling the socioeconomic determinants of health, such as education, housing, water sanitation, and others, has become evident. In 1978, the global recognition of the significance of primary health care in providing services attained a significant milestone. This was due to the Alma Ata declaration on primary health care and the widespread endorsement of the "Health for all by the year 2000" goals [8]. All these movements have contributed to the development of community-oriented medical education in the late 1970s.

Prior to the establishment of the Network of Community-Oriented Educational Institutions for Health Sciences (later the name has changed to Towards Unity for Health (TUFH) in 1987, several health professions education institutions had already embraced the community-oriented education (COME) approach, even without clear definitions, goals, and strategies being explicitly formulated. TUFH was a consortium of predominantly health professions institutions united by the common goal of promoting relevance in health professions education, research and services. It had a significant impact in spreading the concept of COME extensively. It also exerted remarkable efforts in conceptualizing and defining COME and community-based education (CBE).

In 1995, the World Health Organization (WHO) developed the concept of social accountability [9]. As a result the Network opened its doors to health systems and community organizations to enjoy memberships and the name was changed to TUFH.

What is COME and CBE

Community-oriented medical education is defined as a type of teaching of health personnel that focuses on both population groups and individuals, and that takes into account the health needs of the community concerned [2]. CBE is defined as a means of achieving educational relevance to community needs and, consequently, as a way of implementing a community-oriented educational programme. It consists of learning activities that are based extensively in the community which a learning environment in which not only students, but also teachers, members of the community, and representatives of other sectors are actively involved throughout the educational experience [10]. Community-based education activities take place within a community or in any of a variety of health services settings at the primary and secondary care level. As the definitions explain, COME is an educational philosophy where the objectives of the institution are based on the relevant national or local priority health problems, while CBE as one of the instructional methods with community-based learning activities to operationalize COME [10]. As such there may be a medical school which can be described as community-oriented but not community-based with minimal exposure of students to community sites.

Rationale of Community-Oriented Education and Community-Based Education

Contribution to Resolving Inequity in Health Services Provision

COME is expected to contribute to the solution of inequity of health services distribution by graduating physicians who are willing and able to work in rural and underserved areas. Many countries such as Norway, decided to establish medical schools in underserved and rural areas to provide opportunities for students to be well-versed in working competently in the community health facilities [11]. Australia encouraged medical schools to establish rural branches in remote areas. In fact, empirical research has demonstrated that graduates of community-oriented health professions instutions are more likely to opt for working in rural areas [12]. Longitudinal studies have shown that the impact of rural ducation is sustained over time, with a higher proportion of graduates from these programmes eventually practicing in rural or underserved areas compared to those who did not have similar educational experiences [12, 13].

Enhanced Student Learning

COME/CBE both enhanced students' learning by providing an authentic learning relevance/environment that closely resembled the students' future working environment. Learning in community-based education was supported by educational theories, mainly the constructivist (CT) and experiential learning theories (ELT). ELT emphasizes learning though experience and CBE provided opportunities for students to learn through concrete experience during interactions of students with real patients and community members [14]. Students had the opportunities to reflect on these experiences and develop deeper understanding of health disparities, cultural competencies and health care delivery challenges. This allowed students to develop the gained knowledge and skills in subsequent interactions or future clinical practice. Key aspects of COME/CBE that are supported by CT include active learning, social interaction, contextual learning and scaffolding. Through these theories, CBE encourages students to develop critical thinking, adaptability, and a deep understanding of the practical aspects of healthcare, which are essential for their future roles as healthcare professionals. Evidence from empirical studies support the workplace experiences including community-based education of enhancing learning of students [15].

Contribution to Provision of Services in the Community

In fact, many community-based programmes fall under the category of services programme on the taxonomy proposed by Magzoub and Schmidt 2000, that make health services available to the community as soon as students begin to learn in that community [13]. The taxonomy is based on the nature of activities carried out by the students in the community, in addition to the level of community and faculty involvement in these programs. These services range from curative services to community-development activities, and three categories have been suggested. It distinguishes between programs that are mainly focusing on services to the community around them. The services may range from restricted curative services in primary care facilities (first category) to broader full-fledged community development. The second category include programs that are primarily research-oriented. In this category, students and staff are mainly involved in studying the problems at community-based health facilities level or in the community at large. The third category includes an education-focused programme, be it a primary care unit, a defined community or a working environment including some aspects of community development [10].

In this regard, communities are not used as other laboratories for students to learn. Services enhance partnerships with communities and give the collaborating instutions political and moral support. These programmes may serve as models to be replicated by local governments, nongovernmental organizations (NGOs) or the international community.

Equip Students with Unique Competencies

With the recent development of competency-based medical education, community-based education provides students with the essential skills and abilities that they would not acquire through other means, such as leadership skills, teamwork capabilities, and the capacity to engage with the community. During their field work, students have an exceptional chance to utilize these abilities, which are crucial for their future careers. In addition, CBE offers a chance to integrate and reinforce skills acquired in other areas of the curriculum, including problem-solving, clinical expertise, and management abilities [13].

Improvement of Student Assessment and Programme Evaluation

Community-based education may provide opportunities for improving student assessment and programme evaluation. As the community dispenses a site for learning, it also provides a chance for assessing important student competencies in context, eg., communication, management and leadership skills [16, 17]. Also, the community is a source of independent assessors for both students and the programme, such as community leaders or health personnel working in primary health care units [18].

Enhanced Interprofessional Education and Collaboration

Medical students were provided with opportunities to learn with other students from various health professions including nursing, pharmacy, physiotherapy, and others, in order to and prepare student to work better together in the future.

Some medical schools provided opportunities to work with other students out of the health field such as students studying education, agriculture and economics, thus enhancing multidisciplinary collaboration [19].

Enhanced Research Production

Community-based education provided opportunities for enhancing research among though students, faculty and other stakeholders. Gaffar et al. demonstrated that community-based medical schools produce more research compared to noncommunity-based medical schools [20].

Implementation of Community-Oriented & Community-Based Education

Establishing concrete guidelines for implementing community-oriented and community-based education programmes was challenging due to the diverse nature of communities involved. Communities within the same country or region can vary significantly in terms of development, health status, socioeconomic conditions, and cultural practices. Furthermore, the resources available for CBE programmes also differ across institutions within the same region. Consequently, country-specific, regional, community, and institutional factors collectively shape the identity of a CBE programme, making it difficult to establish universal guidelines. However, a general framework was formed to guide the effective implementation of these programmes [21].

Establishing Partnerships

The first step was to create strong partnerships between the community, healthcare services, and health professions educational institutions. These partnerships should define specific roles for each stakeholder involved in the programme. It is crucial that all partners are engaged in every phase of the programme, from planning through implementation to evaluation [22].

Defining Shared Goals and Objectives

Shared, feasible, and implementable goals and objectives were to be established, reflecting the interests of all partners. For instance, communities should benefit from improved healthcare services, while educational institutions should achieve their educational and research goals.

Developing Educational Objectives

Educational objectives should be specific, attainable, measurable, time-bound and relevant to the community's health priorities. The development of these objectives should involve active participation from all stakeholders, ensuring alignment with the institution's learning outcomes, programme delivery, instructional methods, and assessment strategies [23].

Implementation

The responsibility for implementing CBE should be shared among all faculty members within the medical school, rather than being confined to a single department. How that was to be achieved was not well understood. A reasonable proportion of credit hours, ideally not less than 20% of the curriculum duration, should be allocated to CBE. The programme should start early in the curriculum and continue throughout all phases of study. Resources and costs should be shared among all stakeholders, and faculty development programmes should enroll and include adjunct faculty from community sites [24].

Student Assessment

Assessment strategies and methods for students were to be identified, ensuring they were valid, reliable, and relevant to the nature of the CBE programmes. All stakeholders, including community members, were to participate in student assessments. Student portfolios could provide unique opportunities for collecting data from various activities, offering a comprehensive evaluation of student performance [25].

Monitoring and Evaluation

The programme was to be closely monitored and evaluated using sensitive and measurable key performance indicators. Continuous feedback and improvement processes were to be in place to ensure the programme met its objectives and adapted to changing community needs.

Following these steps provided a structured approach to implementing community-oriented CBE programmes, ensuring they were effective, sustainable, and responsive to the unique needs of each community [10].

Case Study [1]

This vignette may demonstrate how CBE programmes are implemented.

We are a group of four students in the third year from the Faculty of Medicine, Sudan. Abbara village was selected for us during the summer field training course which ran three consecutive summers. Our first task was to identify problems in this village. We decided to collect the data through a structured questionnaire, interviews with community leaders, and an observation checklist. These tools were developed with the help of our tutors, senior colleagues and colleagues from the

Faculties of Agriculture and Economics. When we reached the village we had a warm welcome from the Sheikh, he asked his son and one of the few educated ladies to be our guide during our 1 week stay in the village. We lived in the Sheikh's house for 1 week which was a wonderful experience. We accomplished the task of data collection successfully. We returned to the University main campus for data analysis and listed all health and health related problems of the village. The findings were discussed with our tutors, colleagues and the community leaders. With the criteria for prioritizing problems, we selected childhood diarrhea as our priority problem.

In the second phase of our community-based education in the following year, we chose a latrine construction programme as an intervention to address this priority problem. The objective was to increase the availability of latrines by 30% in 1 year. We submitted a joint project with the village health committee to the Blue Nile Health Project. They agreed to provide slabs for any completed four-meter depth latrine. Our role was to encourage families to dig their four-meter pit. It was difficult to convince families to change their behaviour, i.e. not to get rid of their excreta in the open air. Through time and personal contact, we convinced the Sheikh to make a start. In far less time than we had expected our target was achieved.

The programme was evaluated in the last phase, in the third year. There was a significant reduction in the incidence of diarrhea when compared with the base line data. During the presentation of our work, we were criticized, as the reduction of diarrhea incidence might not have been due to our intervention. It might have been the result of other factors which we had not controlled, including improved socio-economic status and water supply. At first this was a disappointing comment, but it has stimulated us to read more about the community-based quasi experimental study design and the control of confounding variables. We concluded that we could not be sure the reduction was due to our intervention. What we can be sure about is that the community and we ourselves were satisfied with our input, and we learned a lot from this experience.

Challenges of Community-Based Programs

Community-oriented Medical Education (COME) and Community-based education (CBE) offer numerous benefits, but they also present several challenges that institutions must address to ensure successful implementation and sustainability. Here are some of the main challenges:

Resource Limitations and High Cost Community sites in community settings, including rural hospitals, primary care facilities, and community organizations, did not have the required facilities, healthcare infrastructure, and resources to provide comprehensive and effective hands-on education for students, as compared to urban health facilities. This potentially restricted the breadth and depth of acquired experiences and outcomes. Furthermore, the implementation of COME/CBE typically necessitates substantial financial commitment towards transportation, accommodation, faculty development, and resources for community locations. This can place a huge strain on finances and can result in compromising the quality of training [26].

Variability in Educational Experiences Students were posted in various community settings, and they were requested to attain unified learning objectives which led to inconsistent educational experiences. For instance, the types of patients and conditions and population health problems encountered can differ significantly between urban and rural settings. Ensuring a standardized curriculum across diverse community sites can be very challenging.

Student Adaptation Students faced challenges adjusting to different cultural, social, and linguistic contexts in community settings, and in the amount of welcome they attained from the communities. This hindered interaction with community members and negatively impacted student learning and comfort levels. Additionally, safety concerns in some community settings, particularly in conflict-prone or resource-limited areas, posed risks to students.

Community Engagement and High Expectations Community leaders had high expectations of services provided by the students and the participating institutions, which created mistrust and hindered community engagement—something that was crucial for student learning achievements.

Logistical Issues Transporting students to and from community sites, especially in remote areas, was logistically challenging and costly. Additionally, coordinating schedules between the educational institutions, community sites, and students can be complex, particularly when balancing academic requirements and community services [27].

Programme Evaluation and Student Assessment Assessing the impact of CBE on community health outcomes was challenging due to several confounding factors that influenced outcomes. Quasi experimental designs that control these confounding factors may be very difficult and expensive to implement. Student assessment , though authentic, is also very challenging as many raters from various stakeholders are involved and creating reliable and valid instruments for assessing performance of students in community setting is difficult to design.

Sustainability Ensuring the sustainability of CBE programmes requires long-term commitment from all stakeholders, including continuous funding, faculty involvement, and community engagement. Additionally, community-based programmes must be adaptable to fast changing community needs and expectations. Moreover, the shortage in faculty and their rapid turnover was another challenge affecting sustainability.

Addressing these challenges requires careful planning, ongoing support, and a collaborative approach involving educational institutions, healthcare providers, students, and community members, and other organizations.

The hindrances given above and faculty non-compliance because of the misconception of low quality of medical education in COME, came to be serious issues in its implementation. Community oriented medical education was largely faculty driven and not all COME programmes had CBE; which is an essential element for experiential learning. Additionally, COME is an internal intervention within the walls of the participating academic institutions. A new approach emphasizing the responsibilities of a medical school that addressed broader and global societal challenges was needed, where the global precepts could be adapted for local relevance.

The Rationale for Social Accountability

In 1948, as part of its constitution, the WHO defined health as a state of complete physical, mental and social well-being and not merely the absence of disease or infirmity [28].

However, many derogatory labels were appended to Community-Oriented Medical Education (COME), as if COME produced bare-foot doctors and unskilled primary care health workers, and was it costly in the bargain (see above). Unfortunately, the word ‘community’ [29] may have been the trigger, as the specialty of Community Health or Community Medicine did not become very popular, as it supposedly ignored the basic sciences. The word “community” often seems to bring out the connotation that this kind of medicine is just for the poor and the have nots—as if COME was only for the benefit of those in the lower socioeconomic strata of society. This is particularly strange as each one of us is a part of many communities: the community of students, the community of doctors, the community of the rich and the powerful, to cite a few examples. When COME fell into disrepute, primarily because of a lack of understanding of what it implied and what power it wielded for improving the health of nations, a new approach was needed, and Social Accountability came into being.

The concept is nothing new. Traditionally, medical schools have always been significantly important players in being responsible for and for improving the health of our nations. In addition to all humane and health for all benefits of COME, Social Accountability highlights and emphasizes the institutional responsibilities. Social Accountability is not an option, it is an integral responsibility of every medical school.

The world is a global village. The globalisation of medicine and health care demanded an approach that would transcend geographical boundaries and address broader societal challenges. Social Accountability is not a replacement for COME, it is a much broader, more holistic mega-concept. It not only targets the immediate and future needs of the community but also takes into consideration the broader responsibilities of medical professionals in our interdependent global societies.

The World Health Organization (1995) definition of Social Accountability of Medical Schools [3] holds the medical school responsible to integrate its precepts into all three areas of health care delivery, education and research. Medical schools must work with all stakeholders to increase efficiency and effectiveness. It emphasizes the importance of all specialties and how each specialty must contribute to improve the health of the nation in their own spheres spheres, in their own disciplines, in their own specialties—thus making the medical schools, in partnership with the Government agencies and other health professionals, accountable for the health of the nation and its people. Lastly, it deals not only what the problems people face today, but the medical school through its collective wisdom must anticipate the health issues of tomorrow and start addressing them today through their education, service and research programmes—to be well prepared for the health issues of tomorrow.

After much discussion, a consensus document, "Global Consensus for Social Accountability of Medical Schools," was published by [4] with more than 130 signatories from universities and organizations from all over the world including THEnet, WHO, World Federation of Medical education (WFME), Foundation for Advancement of International Medical Education and Research (FAIMER), and others.

Obligations of a Medical School

As medical schools are responsible for the health issues of the individuals, families, and people of the nation, they need to align their efforts to produce the appropriate workforce needed. In order to do that, the standards delineating the quality of medical education have to be reviewed and revised to ensure that social accountability is suitably incorporated and embedded into the fabric of the standards. International and national accreditation systems must reflect and pursue this. The GCSA (2010) has made it easier for medical schools to enhance their Social Accountability paradigm. Goals for education, research and service all need to be aligned to the priority health needs and challenges. This is the responsibility of not only the leadership but of every faculty member of the medical school [30].

Global Movement

The global move towards social accountability became very apparent in its historical progression. The next step was to identify what a socially accountable medical school would look like [31]. The medical school would target current, and anticipate and prepare for future priority health needs, redirect its service, education and service towards these challenges, specifically targeting the social determinants of health. It would graduate "fit for purpose" high quality doctors with the most appropriate competencies to deliver equitable and excellent health care. The medical school would build and enhance sustainable partnerships with all stakeholders in the area or region, and use external evaluation and accreditation to measure its performance and effectiveness [31]. Programme evaluation and accreditation must measure and show the effectiveness of programmes in improving not only the health system but actually the health of the people and their explicit needs.

Gathering Momentum

Canada was one of the first countries to adopt social accountability as an essential precept for medical schools. In 2001, Canada's federal department of health and all Canadian medical schools, jointly declared a commitment to Social Accountability [32].

In the meantime, the Association of Medical Education in Europe initiated awards to acknowledge excellence in medical education and the first three **Aspire-to-Excellence Awards** were chosen and announced in 2012 to recognize medical schools with Excellence in Student Assessment, Excellence in Student Engagement in the Curriculum and Excellence in Social Accountability [33, 34]. The first awards were bestowed at the AMEE Conference in Prague in 2013. The main themes extracted from the award winning institutions were: SA clearly depicted in the school's mission; diversity of student body; curriculum relevant to the social, cultural and priority health needs; student learning in clinical and service areas reflecting the social and cultural diversity and health needs; community-based education; research based on priority health needs; and a positive impact on the health of the community, region and country, especially on the health of the vulnerable and the underserved [35].

In Tunis in 2017, [36] the World Summit on Social Accountability endorsed social accountability precepts and produced a practical action plan for the way forward for increasing information, committing to the knowledge and skills essential for socially accountable health education institutions, working towards building accreditation systems which provided due importance to social accountability in its content, and enhancing social justice [37].

Student Declaration on Social Accountability in Health Professions Education (2017)

Student Declaration on Social Accountability in Health Professions Education was endorsed by the International Federation of Medical Student Association (IFMSA), The Student Network Organisation (ISNO) of the Network Towards Unity for Health (TUFH), the International Pharmaceutical Students' Federation (IPSF), the International Association of Dental Students (IADS), the International Veterinary

Students' Association (IVSA), the Tunisian Medical Students' Association (Associa-MED), and World Rural Doctors in Training (Rural Seeds) [38].

The Student Declaration strongly recommended that the action plan cited in the Tunis Declaration at the World Summit for Social Accountability should be actively followed: stakeholder partnerships; emphasis on key competencies for socially accountable health professionals; the medical school's impact on the health of the people must be a part of the accreditation; and lastly, that medical schools must build governance structures and leadership skills to enhance their socially accountability mandate.

Several medical schools in the East and the West have tried to re-orient their curricula to align it to the precepts of social accountability, and have done a great job [39, 40]. Several themes have been identified which are based on the ten main tenets of the GCSA: student selection, mission and governance, communication with stakeholders, community-oriented and community-based medical education, provision of health services, responding to emerging community health needs, impactful faculty and student research, and involvement in health policies.

However, there were still some gaps to be addressed, for example, addressing regional health issues, social determinants of health issues and cost–effectiveness in both education and research, and planning for quality services. A lack of SA accreditation in SA has been identified as a serious barrier [39, 40].

Take-Home Messages

- Community-oriented medical education was conceptualized to promote the health of the people by taking student learning outside the ivory towers of universities and hospitals.
- It fell into disrepute because of local variabilities, lack of clarity regarding its goals, high cost, faculty resistance due to misperceptions. The enormous challenges made it difficult to implement and sustain.
- Social accountability is a wide concept which addresses broader and global societal challenges in our interdependent global society. SA is a responsibility of medical schools, who must work with all stakeholders. to increase efficiency and effectiveness.
- The spectrum of social accountability in increasing order consists of social responsibility, social responsiveness and social accountability.
- The vision, mission and governance mist support the equity, relevance, quality and effectiveness in its education, service and research missions. The graduates must have all required competencies and should be employable where most needed.

References

1. Magzoub MMA, Ahmed BO, Salih ST. Eleven steps of community-based education as applied at Gezira medical school. Anna Comm-Orient Edu. 1992;5:11–7.
2. WHO Study Group. Community-based education of health personnel–Technical Report Series No. 746, Geneva; 1987.
3. Boelen C, Heck JE, Organization WH, others. Defining and measuring the social accountability of medical schools 1995.
4. Boelen C, Woolard B. Global consensus for social accountability of medical schools. http://healthsocialaccountability.org/. 2010;
5. Bannerman. Community-based education programmes; a literature survey. Centre for Educational Development University of Illinois; 1985.
6. Swanwick T, Forrest K, O'Brien BC. Understanding medical education: evidence, theory, and practice. 3rd ed. Wiley-Blackwell; 2019.
7. White K. Life and death and medicine. Sci Am. 1983;229(3):23–33.
8. First Meeting. Alma-Ata 1978–Primary Health Care [Internet]. 1978 [cited 2024 Jul 31]. Available from: https://www.unicef.org/media/85611/file/Alma-Ata-conference-1978-report.pdf
9. Boelen C, Heck JE, of Development of Human Resources for Health WHO Organization. Defining and measuring the social accountability of medical schools/Charles Boelen and Jeffery E. Heck. World Health Organization; 1995. p. WHO/HRH/95.7. Unpublished.
10. Magzoub MEMA, Schmidt HG. A taxonomy of community-based medical education. Acad Med. 2000;75(7):699–707.
11. Strasser R, Couper I, Wynn-Jones J, Rourke J, Chater AB, Reid S. Education for rural practice in rural practice. Educ Prim Care. 2016 Jan 2;27(1):10–4.
12. Worley P, Martin A, Prideaux D, Woodman R, Worley E, Lowe M. Vocational career paths of graduate entry medical students at Flinders University: a comparison of rural, remote and tertiary tracks. Med J Aust. 2008 Feb 4;188(3):177–8.
13. Rabinowitz HK, Diamond JJ, Markham FW, Hazelwood CE. A program to increase the number of family physicians in rural and underserved areas: impact after 22 years. JAMA. 1999;281(3):255–60.
14. Latessa R, Beaty N, Royal K, Colvin G, Pathman DE, Heck J. Academic outcomes of a community-based longitudinal integrated clerkships program. Med Teach. 2015 Sep 2;37(9):862–7.
15. Worley P, Strasser R, Prideaux D. Can medical students learn specialist disciplines based in rural practice: lessons from students' self reported experience and competence. Rural Remote Health. 2004;4(4):338.
16. Magzoub MEMA, Schmidt HG, Abdel-Hameed AA, Dolmans D. Student assessment in community settings: a comprehensive approach. Med Educ. 1998 Jan;32(1):50–9.
17. Magzoub ME. Studies in community-based education: programme implementation and student assessment at the Faculty of Medicine. Sudan: University of Gezira; 1994.
18. Schmidt H, Feletti G, Magzoub M, Nooman Z, Vluggen P. Assessment by community members. In: Handbook of community-based education: theory and practices. Network Publications; 2000.
19. Reeves S, Fletcher S, Barr H, Birch I, Boet S, Davies N, et al. A BEME systematic review of the effects of interprofessional education: BEME guide no. 39. Med Teach. 2016 Jul 2;38(7):656–68.
20. Gaffar AM, Magzoub MEMA, Mahmoud I. Do community-based medical schools produce more community-based research? A review of four medical schools in Sudan and Saudi Arabia. Health Prof Edu. 2020 Mar;6(1):19–30.
21. Fleishon HB, Itri JN, Boland GW, Duszak R. Academic medical centers and community hospitals integration: trends and strategies. J Am Coll Radiol. 2017 Jan;14(1):45–51.

22. Riley K, Myers W. Partnerships between academic medical centers and health systems: essential collaboration for improved health outcomes. Acad Med. 2011;86(7):829–34. https://doi.org/10.1097/ACM.0b013e31821dbe7f.
23. Pálsdóttir B, Neusy AJ, Reed G. Building the evidence base: networking innovative socially accountable medical education programs. Educ Health (Abingdon). 2008 Jul;21(2):177.
24. Mlambo M, Dreyer A, Dube R, Mapukata N, Couper I, Cooke R. Transformation of medical education through decentralised training platforms: a scoping review. Rural Remote Health. 2018;
25. Magzoub MEMA, Abdelhameed AA, Schmidt HG, Dolmans DHJM. Assessing students in community settings: the role of peer evaluation. Adv Health Sci Educ. 1998;3(1):3–13.
26. Ali SK, Baig LA. Problems and issues in implementing innovative curriculum in the developing countries: the Pakistani experience. BMC Med Educ. 2012 Dec 16;12(1):31.
27. Baig LA, Akram DS, Ali SK. Development of the community-oriented medical education curriculum of Pakistan: a case report on the National Initiative on curriculum development. Edu Health [Internet]. 2006;19(2) Available from: https://journals.lww.com/edhe/fulltext/2006/19020/development_of_the_community_oriented_medical.9.aspx
28. World Health Organization. https://apps.who.int/gb/bd/PDF/bd47/EN/constitution-en.pdf. Constitution of the World health Organization.
29. Hamad B. Community-oriented medical education: what is it? Med Educ. 1991;25(1):16–22.
30. Boelen C, Woollard R. Social accountability: the extra leap to excellence for educational institutions. Med Teach. 2011 Aug 20;33(8):614–9.
31. Boelen C, Woollard B. Social accountability and accreditation: a new frontier for educational institutions. Med Educ. 2009 Aug 20;43(9):887–94.
32. Cappon P, MacDonald N, McMurtry R, Mickael N, Parboosingh J, Rowe W, et al. Social accountability: a vision for Canadian medical schools. Ottawa: Institute for International Medical Education; 2001.
33. Aspire Recognition Of Excellence In Social Accountability Of A Medical School.
34. Boelen C. Why should social accountability be a benchmark for excellence in medical education? Educación Médica. 2016 Jul;17(3):101–5.
35. Rourke J. Social accountability: a framework for medical schools to improve the health of the populations they serve. Acad Med. 2018;93:1120–4. https://doi.org/10.1097/ACM.0000000000002239.
36. The Network. World summit on social accountability. In: Towards Unity for Health (TUFH). Tunisia; 2017.
37. Kherigi I, Chirchi T. Social accountability in Tunisia: processes of learning in civic innovation between 2011 and 2021. In: Social accountability initiatives in Morocco, Tunisia, and Lebanon: civic innovation in the Arab world after 2011. Switzerland Cham: Springer Nature; 2024. p. 83–137.
38. World Summit on Social Accountability. Student declaration on social accountability in health professions education. Tunisia: Hammamet; 2017.
39. Abdalla M, Taha M, Wadi M, Khalafalla H. What makes a medical school socially accountable? A qualitative thematic review of the evaluation of social accountability of medical schools in the eastern Mediterranean region. East Mediterr Health J. 2022 May 29;28(5):381–9. https://doi.org/10.26719/emhj.22.016.
40. Püschel K, Riquelme A, Moore P, Rojas V, Perry A, Sapag JC. What makes a medical school socially accountable in Latin America? A report from a Latin American panel based on a qualitative approach. Med Teach. 2017;39(4):415–21. https://doi.org/10.1080/0142159X.2017.1296119. https://pubmed.ncbi.nlm.nih.gov/28285565/

Part IV
Curriculum Development & Reform for Social Accountability

Chapter 9
The Role of Social Accountability in Re-envisioning Medical Education for the Twenty-First Century

Amy Clithero, Marlene P. Ballejos, Erin Bouquin, Natasha Dark, Anthony Fleg, Hannah Herring, Pearl Huynh, Debra Klamen, Tom Limanovich, Samantha Longley, Kristin Markle, Tom Markle, Sarah Nickolich, Natalie Reid, Heidi Honegger Rogers, Arindam Sarkar, Kevin M. Schroeder, Sookyun Suh, Melissa Torbey, William Ventres, Lindsey Yelton, Tegan Whitney, and Arthur Kaufman

Learning Outcomes

1. Recognize the role of Social Accountability in shaping medical education and its societal impact.
2. Identify key elements of Social Accountability that can be adapted to various institutional or regional contexts.
3. Recognize Social Accountability as a foundational pillar in improving community health through medical education.

A. Clithero (✉) · M. P. Ballejos · E. Bouquin · N. Dark · A. Fleg · H. Herring · P. Huynh · T. Limanovich · S. Longley · K. Markle · T. Markle · N. Reid · M. Torbey · L. Yelton · T. Whitney · A. Kaufman
University of New Mexico School of Medicine, Albuquerque, NM, USA
e-mail: aclithero@salud.unm.edu

D. Klamen · S. Suh
Southern Illinois School of Medicine, Springfield, IL, USA

S. Nickolich
Pennsylvania State Health, Hershey, PA, USA

H. H. Rogers
University of New Mexico, College of Nursing, Albuquerque, NM, USA

A. Sarkar
Baylor College of Medicine, Houston, TX, USA

K. M. Schroeder
Department of Health, Exercise, and Sports Sciences, University of New Mexico, Albuquerque, NM, USA

W. Ventres
University of Arkansas for Medical Sciences, Little Rock, AR, USA

M. E. Abdalla et al. (eds.), *Social Accountability of Medical Schools*,
https://doi.org/10.1007/978-3-031-94435-2_9

The Twentieth Century will be chiefly remembered by future generations not as an era of political conflicts or technical inventions, but as an age in which human society dared to think of the welfare of the whole human race as a practical objective. Arnold J. Toynbee.

History of Medical Education

Although we can trace medical education back from early civilization to the Renaissance and Enlightenment period, where the importance of understanding the whole patient, we will begin our history with the late 19th-early twentieth century, when the social medicine movement emphasized the importance of addressing social determinants of health and promoting community health and well-being which laid the foundation for community-oriented approaches to medical education. This period also saw the advent of general practitioners who provided primary care services to their communities. The rise of formal medical education is often said to have occurred in 1910, at least in the United States, with the publication of the Flexner Report, which standardized medical education and shifted towards classroom- and hospital-based instruction, which some educators recognized as detrimental to preparing students for the realities of practicing medicine in different communities.

While the Flexner Report ushered in a new era of medical education that improved the process of training and ensuring the scientific biomedical model of disease was routinely taught, it also negatively impacted the education of minorities, in particular African Americans. The Flexner Report called for separate medical education. Still, it held these distinct medical schools to the same standards as medical schools for white students, which forced the closure of all but two African American schools, Howard and Meharry. This has led to health disparities and a long history of structural racism, inequality, and lack of diversity [1]. Overall, however, the history of medical education reflects a continuous quest for excellence and adaptation to meet the changing needs of society and healthcare. This quest continues with today's challenges, including increasing patient demand, workforce shortages, and a growing understanding of the profound effect social, political, and structural determinants have on health. It is time to revisit the early nineteenth century and refocus on community health by emphasizing primary care, equity, and relevance to communities while incorporating new technologies, such as artificial intelligence, to improve access and the cost-effectiveness of education and service delivery.

Introduction to Social Accountability in Medical Education

In the 1970s, the World Health Organization (WHO) was publicly dissatisfied with the large investment, but poor society benefits from most medical schools worldwide. This was exacerbated by physician migration from poor to rich countries. One study showed that for every physician graduate in a low-income country who migrated to Western Europe or North America, that low-income country lost ~$150,000 it invested in that physician's training but would never receive the benefit of that investment. The high-income country receiving that graduate saved ~$400,000 for the physician it didn't have to train. This was a massive subsidy of the richer by the poorer countries [2]. In response, the WHO subsidized the creation of The Network for Community-Oriented Medical Education and invited many medical schools from across the globe to create a new kind of medical education geared to their populations' needs. This initiative was evolved until we reach the era of social accountability (SA), more details on this evelovement is written in chapter No.1.

The WHO identified SA as The responsibility of medicals schools to align their activities with the health needs of the local community, region, or nation it serves. These priorities are collaboratively determined by the government, health service organizations, and the public [3]. The WHO was not alone in recognizing social accountability as a critical mandate. The Global Consensus on Social Accountability for Medical Schools is a landmark document created in 2010 by 130 organizations and individuals delineating four components for medical schools to address, highlighting the need for schools "to reorient their education, research, and service priorities." [4].

Medical schools that aspire to SA strive to train a "fit-for-purpose" health workforce. It produces 'the right doctors to practice the right medicine with the right partners at the right time and place.' [5] This requires embedding the curriculum with socially accountable values and shifting from traditional training focusing on the individual biomedical disease model to broader social accountability.

What exactly are socially accountable medical schools? Schools must work collaboratively and in partnership with local communities to effectively respond to community health priorities and eliminate health inequities. They recognize the historical health disparities that occur in populations from colonization, structural racism, and environmental damage and pollution that put populations at risk of accelerated disease from exposure. It entails a commitment to addressing health's social/structural and ecological/environmental determinants and promoting health equity. Working with communities leads to a shared understanding and mutual goals. This collaboration moves schools from intentions to address health priorities to adding a layer of accountability through demonstrating impact [6].

SA in healthcare emphasizes responsiveness to society's needs, particularly marginalized or underserved populations. It is a step beyond responsibility and responsiveness. The social obligation scale is a visualization of this progression in meeting society's needs:

Social Obligation Scale [6]

	Responsibility	Responsiveness	Accountability
Social needs identified	Implicitly	Explicitly	Anticipatively
Institutional objectives	Defined by faculty	Inspired by data	Defined with society
Educational programs	Community-oriented	Community-based	Contextualized
Quality of graduates	Good practitioners	Meeting professionalism criteria	Health system change agents
Focus of evaluation	Process	Outcome	Impact
Assessors	Internal	External	Health partners

Education cannot be disconnected from health systems. SA is about changing the status quo through transformative learning. The emphasis is on the importance of interdependence between communities and education to build a health system focused on health equity. This begins with the medical student admissions process to select the students who mirror the populations they will serve and embedding the curriculum with foundational themes and curricular components.

Admissions: Selecting the "Right" Medical Student

There is a significant healthcare access gap internationally, partly related to the current medical school access gap [7, 8]. The WHO has recognized this gap as a priority for action since it impacts the quality of life and well-being of the population and contributes to the economic burden of societies. Furthermore, improving populations' health contributes to decreasing the discrepancies and inequalities in societies. The world is vast and very diverse, and students should be holistically chosen to reflect the communities they will serve. This, of course, is not our current reality, as students from poor, underserved, and rural backgrounds, as well as minoritized individuals, have less access to medical schools, which tend to be made up of individuals from majority-status, wealthy, and urban backgrounds who attend schools in major urban centers. Minimizing the gap between medical education access and global healthcare needs may significantly improve healthcare overall, so we are committed to re-imagining medical (school) education in this area. We need to increase the penetration of medical education training without building numerous new medical schools worldwide, which is cost-restrictive and relies on a limited pool of faculty, which is logistically not feasible.

Integrating SA into the medical school admissions process is paramount in ensuring the alignment of medical education with the needs and values of society and the medical school mission. Medical schools can cultivate a more inclusive and representative student body by considering factors such as socioeconomic background, first-generation college students, rural and underserved backgrounds, cultural diversity, and community engagement in the selection criteria. This approach not only addresses disparities in healthcare access and outcomes but also enriches the learning environment by fostering a diverse array of perspectives and experiences. Furthermore, emphasizing SA encourages aspiring physicians to recognize their responsibility to serve marginalized and underserved populations, promoting equity and social justice in healthcare delivery. Ultimately, by prioritizing social accountability in admissions, medical schools can play a pivotal role in shaping future healthcare professionals equipped to address society's complex and evolving needs.

By carefully considering applicants' demonstrated commitment to SA through their experiences, commitment to serving diverse populations, achievements, and personal attributes, medical schools can select candidates who are not only academically qualified but also possess the compassion and dedication necessary to address the healthcare needs of diverse and underserved populations.

It is critical to remember that it is our privilege and responsibility to open access to students from poor, underserved, and/or rural backgrounds, as well as minoritized individuals, to build the next generation of physicians. If we are to improve healthcare in our world, building a cadre of physicians passionate and large enough to do so is imperative.

Success story- Walter Sisulu University in Mthatha, South Africa
This school was established to address inequities in their community by ensuring rural and black medical school candidates have an opportunity to succeed. Their admission process selects candidates that reflect the community they serve. Walter Sisulu participated in a multischool longitudinal study. They found their matriculating students intended to practice primary care and, upon graduation, remained in underserved areas, reflecting their success [9].

Foundational Medical School Themes

Theme 1: Primary Care

A curriculum that reinforces primary care principles is foundational [10]. These principles emphasize communities' health and social needs by addressing the social determinants of health and providing community-based care [11]. Principles include care that is person & family-centered, continuous, comprehensive & equitable, team-based & collaborative, coordinated & integrated, accessible, and high-value.

The primary healthcare system emphasizes comprehensive care, disease prevention, and health promotion. It also envisions action on social determinants, individual and community input on health policy and planning, and cost-effective use of resources. It embodies the spirit of SA by utilizing workers trained both "socially and technically." Family medicine, in particular, has an ecological approach to care by partnering with families and communities for optimal health. Family physicians are taught to educate, treat, and prevent disease at both an individual and a community level, which is a central goal of SA—meeting the community's needs. In addition, persons with access to this specialty have better health outcomes with lower costs to the healthcare system and downstream costs to patients [12, 13].

Medical school curriculums and programs focusing on rural, underserved, primary care, and family medicine are robust contributors to physicians practicing in areas of need [14, 15]. Given the evidence that this improves outcomes, reduces costs, and promotes equity, SA demands advocacy for healthcare systems built on robust primary care services.

Theme 2: Competency-Based Medical Education

(CBME) is a model that focuses on learners' attainment of specific skills and abilities rather than completing them in a set amount of time. When it comes to SA in medical education, CBME offers several advantages:

1. Targeted Learning Objectives: CBME allows educators to identify and prioritize the competencies most relevant to the needs of the communities they serve. By aligning education with community health priorities, medical graduates are better equipped to address the population's healthcare needs, thus enhancing SA.
2. Outcome-Based Assessment: CBME emphasizes the assessment of learners based on demonstrated competencies rather than traditional metrics like time spent in training. This approach ensures that graduates are proficient in the skills necessary to address the health challenges faced by their communities. Without traditional time-bound advancement from one stage of training to the next, Artificial Intelligence (AI) could play an essential role in operationalizing CBME.
3. Flexibility and Adaptability: CBME offers flexibility in curriculum design, allowing medical education programs to adapt to changing healthcare needs and societal demands. This adaptability enables medical schools to respond effectively to emerging health issues and disparities within their communities, thereby improving SA. For example, a student who has demonstrated on their workplace-based assessments that they can perform all the expected clinical activities without supervision should graduate early or have additional flexible months of residency interview preparation, research, or elective coursework time.
4. Continuous Quality Improvement: CBME promotes a growth mindset with learners and a culture of continuous improvement. By regularly assessing and refining the curriculum based on feedback from stakeholders and performance data from learners, institutions can ensure that their graduates are well-prepared to meet the healthcare needs of their communities.

CBME improves SA by aligning educational outcomes with community health priorities, emphasizing outcome-based assessment, fostering flexibility and adaptability, promoting community engagement, and encouraging continuous quality improvement in medical education programs, as well as fostering success amongst student populations who have historically struggled in a more "traditional" teaching/evaluating format. Although CBME is most widely incorporated into undergraduate medical education in places like the Netherlands, Canada, and Australia, the United States and other countries recognize its benefits to learner well-being and the effectiveness of the clinical learning environment.

Theme 3: Resilience and Wellness

A 2022 survey on burnout conducted by the American Medical Association, Mayo Clinic, and Stanford Medicine found that 62.8% of physicians experience burnout, which is markedly increased from prior levels (38.2% in 2020 and 43.9% in 2017) [16]. Other current surveys found that nearly one in five physicians intends to leave their practice within 2 years [17]. While these studies are based in the U.S. and were conducted during the COVID-19 pandemic, it is reasonable to assume that despair and burnout are experienced worldwide. We placed resilience and wellness as a theme rather than a curricular topic. A compassionate healthcare system is vital to maintaining compassionate physicians who extend that care to patients and the community. Curricula across the globe have sought to address the skills needed to thrive in the medical field. For example, teaching faculty skills can assist learners in identifying their strengths and ways to cope with daily stressors [18]. Medical schools also seek to address financial, spiritual, and social wellness. However, equipping practicing physicians and learners with more resilience and approaching the topic as an individual issue is not the solution for systemic system-wide burnout. Thus, we recommend an institutional approach. One way this can be achieved is by including compassion training in medical curricula, role modeling compassion, taking a policy approach, and integrating it into the culture [19].

This theme should be addressed at the start of medical school. Students must be informed, encouraged, and allowed to make time for themselves. Reinforce self-care and ensure there is no negative professional impact for doing so. Linking with the theme of CBME, which reduces the burden time-based education places on students, ensuring that when a student or physician is experiencing burnout, a family crisis, or another major life event, they have not only the resources to care for themselves, their families, and their patients healthily, but they also have the option. Anecdotally, there is a reason why, when flying, you are instructed to put on your oxygen mask before assisting anyone else with theirs.

Success story—the University of new Mexico School of Medicine
The UNM SOM offers free services to students and faculty to combat burnout. There are licensed psychologists and therapists. Exercise is an essential component of the approach in addition to mental health services. The student wellness group provides classes focusing on movement or sets up games that require movement. A community coalition called "running for medicine" meets weekly near the university to encourage people of all ages and abilities to move for a few hours daily and foster a sense of community. Also, one of the more accessible courses is "writing for wellness." there are scheduled meetings where people are encouraged to journal about their experiences. This workshop is helpful because it allows people to work through their emotions and trauma safely [20].

While physicians are extremely resilient, there must be more grace around caring for yourself. It's okay to ask for help. It's ok to take time off. If this mentality were built into the medical school system, everyone would be better for it. Patients would have well-rested doctors who are at 100% when they are being seen. There may be less burnout in a field many went into for their love of helping others. A policy approach to ensure a holistic approach is warranted. This will assist in identifying where burnout may occur within the learning environment. "*Social accountability without compassion is not SA; compassion humanizes institutional policy by engaging sympathy and care*." [19].

It is imperative that the role of SA be applied institutionally, both intrinsically and extrinsically, with respect to policies affecting medical students. The debunked abridgment of the English jurist and politician John Selden, in his 1654 book *table talk,* produced the famous quote, "do as I say, not as I do," which applies keenly to what not to do as a medical institution. Social accountability requires an approach where medical institutions recognize students as members of the communities we seek to serve. This holistic approach is rooted in a growth mindset that doesn't neglect that medical students are people too. Therefore, institutions are in a prestigious position to lead and grow social accountability, whereby future doctors benefit and then apply the same principles to the communities they serve. Thus, this sets the stage for reducing upstream problems and producing downstream benefits. Neglecting this facet of medical education directly opposes the mission statement of any self-proclaimed socially accountable institution.
L.Y.—student voice

Socially Accountable Curricular Components

While there is a whole chapter in this book devoted to discuss the details of how to build a sociallay accountble curriculum, the below section will discuss the general components and charetristics for such a curriculum.

The curricular components we selected are not exhaustive, as there are many topics that physicians need to know about to care for patients effectively. Rather, we selected topics that the literature has shown to be effective in keeping graduates in the community, those that make a difference in population health and assist in reducing health inequities. Finally, the topics we include empower physicians to work with communities. It is one thing to know that issues exist; it is socially accountable to do something about them. Finally, we recognize that contexts are different. There is an urgent need for funding, additional faculty, disruptions such as war, and other issues that can make progress toward SA challenging. Remember—SA is an aspiration to progress toward, and implementation will differ in your context.

The chronic underinvestment in the education and training of physicians in some countries and the mismatch between educational strategies, health systems, and population needs often result in health inequities. Health inequities extend to the ability of people to access timely, cost-effective, and quality healthcare services delivered by skilled practitioners. Albeit more pronounced in rural and remote areas, health inequities are a global concern and are driving transformations in healthcare. As part of these transformations, education for physicians should focus on SA, i.e., educating students with the skills to address local health priorities. Health professionals need to be both person and community-oriented to improve population health. In order for health profession educators to create socially accountable physicians, they must move learners from awareness of accountability as an expectation to action by incorporating it as an aspect of professional identity that informs medical practice [21].

Community Engagement and Service Learning

Service learning in medical education is a powerful tool that allows students to engage with communities and apply their knowledge in real-world settings. By incorporating SA into this approach, students not only gain valuable hands-on experience but also learn to reflect on the impact of their actions on society. This intersection between service learning and SA fosters a sense of responsibility and empathy in future healthcare professionals, equipping them with the skills needed to address the diverse needs of patients and communities. Through this integrated approach, medical schools can produce socially conscious and culturally competent physicians committed to serving the greater good. Providing this training within communities helps students build a connection to the community, making it more likely they will return after graduation. Community can be defined in many ways, but for authentic, socially accountable engagement, community engagement and service learning must include collaborative delivery, design, and evaluation. Students must have a deep understanding and appreciation of the communities they serve [22].

Community experiences help build confidence in clinical skills and develop empathy for patients as persons, not just patients, by connecting classroom learning. Service-learning experiences in underserved areas can help students understand the social determinants of health and develop a sense of social responsibility. Immersion in a rural setting during undergraduate training is a crucial component, with at least 1 year in a mix of regional hospitals and general practice having the most substantial positive effect on future practice in rural areas [23]. There is also emerging evidence that community placements positively impact student competencies, with rurally-based students doing at least as well as or better in improving their clinical skills than students studying in urban hospital-based settings [24, 25].

Success Stories

Canada—the northern Ontario School of Medicine: All students undertake the whole third year living and learning in a large rural or small urban community outside the medical school training sites. Students are based in family practice, where they meet patients and follow them, including into specialist and/or hospital care. Community members actively host students and contribute to their educative experience [26–28].

Australia—Flinders University: All Flinders students are exposed to at least nine weeks of teaching in a rural environment. Some students (approx. 50%) may opt to spend their entire third year in a rural site [29].

The Philippines: Ateneo de Zamboanga School of Medicine: Students do ten months during their fourth year of study in a rural environment.

These schools have had extraordinary success in students selecting primary care and family medicine as their specialty and practicing in rural/remote areas [27, 30, 31].

Social Determinants of Health

> Medical education does not exist to provide students with a way of making a living, but to ensure the health of the community. ~ Rudolf Virchow.

Good healthcare does not mean good health. Where people live, work, play, and accumulate life experiences more significantly affect health than biology and genetics. To improve health, learners need to think beyond the four walls of a clinic or hospital and address the determinants of health, including the social and structural determinants. Each community is unique in its social determinants; thus, identifying them is the first step in creating solutions.

Poverty and social inequity are two critical determinants of ill health worldwide [32, 33]. Many, if not all, intractable health problems have as their root cause social determinants, including health inequities between economic and ethnic groups and poor access to healthcare. SA is not the exclusive responsibility of physicians and academic institutions. Physicians, however, have a social contract with society and the professional power to enact societal change related to health. Medical schools, primarily publicly funded ones, have an ethical responsibility to their communities to produce practitioners who can address the public's broad interests, specifically social issues relating to the public's health and well-being. Inherent within this responsibility is for the schools to identify societal needs and demonstrate results [34].

The current approach to Social Determinants of Health (SDoH) training within medical education too often celebrates cultural humility without exposing learners to the harsh realities that there is an entirely different target vocabulary, medication formulary, and approach to healthcare depending on where patients live, work, and eat. Exposing equity deficiencies within one's institution requires vulnerability to admit that patient-centered, community-centered care can be unsettling work.

The philosophy of care to impart to learners is that helping individual patients and communities is arduous and can be thankless. Even a student who overcame numerous SDoH barriers themselves to become physicians will need to continuously re-evaluate the undeniable forms of prejudice, bias, and privilege that inevitably arise in their patient-physician relationships.

Socioeconomically Disadvantaged Populations Poverty is not only a lack of income—it is also poverty of the mind due to a lack of stimulation and educational opportunities, poverty of the spirit as a result of neglect and positive role models, and poverty of choice and options that allow for hope and optimism. Exposing physicians early in their medical school training to the complex healthcare needs of the underserved has positively impacted their attitudes and abilities toward addressing these inequities [35]. Furthermore, long-term education programs designed to train medical students to meet the needs of the impoverished have been found to influence their intentions to practice in underserved communities [36, 37]. Educating future physicians to effectively address health care disparities through patient care and health policy advocacy is a proactive approach to bringing about systemic change in the health care systems.

Education to address SDoH—Cultural and Structural Competency to achieve health equity: Vulnerable and disadvantaged populations worldwide experience health disparities and worse health outcomes [38]. Their health needs require understanding the challenges in accessing and receiving appropriate care [39]. Training in cultural and structural competency helps graduates respond to the needs of patients from diverse backgrounds who contend with systemic inequities. This training includes addressing implicit bias, promoting anti-racist practices, and restructuring the healthcare system toward robust, community-embedded, person- and people-centered primary care.

To address the critical issues of underserved populations, foundational courses in cultural and structural competency can be created, or existing courses can be reviewed and revised [40–42]. Cultural elements to consider include various factors, including age, language, socio-economic status, and ethnicity; structural elements are multiple, as well, spanning from the dynamics of how power is expressed in clinical interactions regarding the politics of universal health care. Providing quality community-centric care to eliminate health disparities requires a cultural and structural understanding of the local and global communities in which health professionals practice.

During my outpatient pediatrics rotation, I encountered a young mother of three children who had just arrived as a refugee from a another country. We used a telephone translator to conduct the encounter for a rash on her son's arm. Slowly, through the static of the phone, I learned that she was living in temporary public housing and had walked several miles to the clinic that day–two children slung across her back–due to the complexity of the bus system and no other transportation. At the end of the encounter, I recalled the "teach back" technique we had been taught in medical school, and I asked the patient to explain the simple instructions regarding the prescribed cream. To my surprise, she had entirely misunderstood the directions and thought that her son would be taking oral medication instead. At this moment, I reflected on how powerful communication can be and how easily an already existing inequity can lead to worse care simply via poor communication. Between my use of medical jargon, the telephone interpreter, and the mother's understandable exhaustion and disorientation in a new country's medical system, it made sense that we weren't on the same page. Meeting this patient where she was was not enough; when we approach inequity, we must approach it with even more care. This experience highlights how essential a thorough education in cultural competence is in order to successfully bridge the gap between the medical world and marginalized populations.

T.W.—student voice

More than just receiving education on cultural and structural determinants is required. Physicians must practice cultural humility, which means including the social context of the patient's life in patient care and acknowledging cultural unknowns as a clinical practitioner. Practicing structural humility means recognizing the unique expertise of community members and partnering with them to support equitable systemic changes in providing clinical and non-clinical services. Both can revolutionize healthcare [43–45]. This transformative potential is further amplified as it improves patient satisfaction and quality of care and strengthens the patient-provider relationship [46, 47]. Advancing humility in medical practice to address implicit bias and foster a socially accountable healthcare system is a shared responsibility. Each stakeholder, from educators to policymakers, plays a vital role in ensuring that cultural and structural competency becomes a fundamental part of medical education and practice.

Global Health

> The physicians are the natural attorneys of the poor, and the social problems should largely be solved by them. ~ Rudolf Virchow.

Within this dialogue of SA and its importance to medical education is the argument for integrating global health education into this framework. This argument stems from the longstanding adage of "local is global'', wherein the practice of medicine involves working with increasingly global patient populations, including (but not limited to) immigrants, migrants, refugees, and first-generation citizens from immigrant families. With this increase in patient diversity comes the need to tackle social inequalities, the historical marginalization of vulnerable minority populations, and the lack of healthcare access in rural and urban areas, thus reflecting an overall need to address healthcare inequalities [48]. Learning opportunities can take many forms, including student exchanges, short-term engagements in global health, observation of clinical practice in under-resourced settings, teaching, and research. Experiential education is vital through formal curricula, elective tracks, or pre- and post-experience reflective courses. Although students from well-resourced countries often travel to other countries with the altruistic motive of "helping" the people who live there, this intention must be balanced to ensure that students and the host institutions benefit from each other equitably.

Global health education links to SA because medical education that trains future physicians to address the needs of vulnerable populations improves student attitudes toward the underserved and increases interest in primary care professions. Specifically, medical students participating in global health experiences are more likely to care for immigrants and marginalized minorities, change their career interests from subspecialty to primary care medicine, report better diagnostic skills, and have increased interest in public health and volunteerism [49]. While global health education is broad in spectrum and can be designed from a local or global approach, it comes with challenges and ethical considerations. Global health has problematic roots in colonialism, and much has been written about the importance of decolonizing global health education. While this topic is outside the scope of this chapter, it is crucial to consider this perspective and move towards reexamining problematic assumptions and practices underpinning the bedrock of past global health partnerships [50]. Should firsthand global health educational experiences occur, partnerships should be bi-directional, sustainable, and, above all else, prioritize the needs of the focus community [51].

Overall, incorporating global health into a social accountability framework within medical schools is not so much a paradigm shift as a "reconceptualization of boundaries." Regions, borders, or countries do not bind medical professionals in our increasingly globalized society. It doesn't matter where the patient arrives from; all that matters is that a doctor can provide quality health compassionately to whoever walks through the door.

Interprofessional Collaboration

Intersectionality between SA and interprofessional education (IPE) and collaborative practice is grounded in shared values and ethics that prioritize equitable access to healthcare and promotion of the well-being of communities. IPE complements SA by fostering collaboration and mutual respect among healthcare professionals from diverse disciplines. The Interprofessional Education Collaborative (IPEC) competencies outline essential skills for effective teamwork, communication, and shared decision-making [52]. The (IPEC) guides health professionals on the behaviors of interprofessional collaboration, including the values and ethics for working together across disciplines to fully engage in our responsibilities for SA. The first sub-competency (VE1) is to *"promote the values and interests of persons and populations in health care delivery, One Health and population health initiatives."* [52] Health professionals must take responsibility for designing and delivering the health systems and services necessary to ensure that everyone has equal access to the environments supporting health and well-being and essential health care services.

Integrating SA and IPE collaboration into their daily practice is a core duty for medical professionals. Medical professionals are responsible for showing up and participating in collaborative systems change, health care promotion, prevention, care delivery models, and advocacy for individuals and communities experiencing adverse health outcomes because of social, structural, and environmental disparities. Interprofessional professionalism emphasizes the importance of behaviors that build relationships as the foundation before entering partnerships to address health and well-being with individuals or communities. Grounded in the understanding of the interconnectedness of health and the ecological and social environments, healthcare professionals are uniquely responsible for collaborating across disciplines to address complex local and global challenges comprehensively. By aligning values, ethics, and competencies within a social accountability framework and interprofessional collaboration, healthcare professionals can drive meaningful change at individual and systemic levels, ultimately advancing health equity and improving community outcomes.

Leadership

Advocacy and Policy Engagement

> Medicine is a social science, and politics is nothing more than medicine on a grand scale. ~ *Rudolf Virchow.*

Values and ethics form the foundation of SA, guiding healthcare professionals to prioritize justice, fairness, and inclusivity in their practice. This commitment extends beyond individual actions to encompass systemic changes that address underlying social, political, and environmental factors influencing health outcomes. While physicians can make a difference one patient at a time, they can change the lives of hundreds of thousands of patients via health policy. This might involve engaging in grassroots advocacy efforts, partnering with policymakers, or joining professional organizations dedicated to health equity and SA. However, the evidence and research amassed that supports the educational change envisioned above may not be sufficient to bring about needed change. Innovators can face fierce headwinds when authority and traditional power bases in medical schools feel threatened. It takes great patience, wisdom, and skill among education reformers to overcome arrogance, accept criticism, and invite critics to build upon and improve reform plans [53].

Advocacy of health policy for physicians may feel outside the scope of medical practice and external to clinical learning. Engaging in advocacy as a medical student can feel daunting due to a lack of experience in the political and legal realms. For example, a patient with severe depression and anxiety, unaware of their legal rights, may miss their referred appointment with the psychiatrist for fear of losing their job; performance at the job and in the patient's personal life continues to decline in the setting of untreated psychiatric illness [54]. Physicians and lawyers can advocate for patients' rights and well-being through medical-legal collaboration. Advocacy within legal parameters affects social determinants of health, such as employment, thus creating the opportunity to advance health equity in the community. This bridges IPE and SDoH education for action.

With the demanding schedule that medical students face in their required curriculum, incorporating education on advocacy, especially interprofessionally, may be challenging to coordinate. Solutions include skills-based workshops such as "A Letter Writing Lunch," where students call local and state representatives to pitch health policy via pre-written scripts. This activity demonstrates how future physicians can participate in civic responsibility [55]. Although fragmented health policy education activities are pertinent to increasing awareness of the physician's role in advocacy, longitudinal advocacy education, beginning in medical school and extending to post-graduate education, may have the greatest potential to create the next generation of socially accountable physicians [56].

Leadership Development Although diversity, equity, and inclusion in the workplace have been emphasized recently, healthcare leadership is largely defined by ranks and titles, and physicians are often perceived as leaders in interprofessional settings. According to a scoping review of 114 interprofessional articles related to leadership, desired leadership capabilities and characteristics are vaguely defined [57]. Brewer et al. suggest the need for a sophisticated and shared understanding of leadership that includes broader inclusion of interprofessional representation in healthcare.

A national survey in academic medicine revealed that most leadership development programs (97% of respondents) were aimed at physician faculty [58]. In contrast, less than 26% of Academic Medical Centers that offer leadership development opportunities include non-faculty staff. It also needs to be clarified whether these programs were offered in an interprofessional setting. The lack of interprofessional or other leadership professional development programs represents missed opportunities to teach leadership as healthcare leaders lead people from multidisciplinary and professional backgrounds. There is a lack of interprofessional education opportunities for leadership development and a significant gap in diversity among senior leadership [57]. Selecting and supporting diverse leaders with a strong commitment to addressing health disparities and equity will be crucial for navigating healthcare challenges stemming from those disparities.

Success Case: Interprofessional Leadership Development Program
The Southern Illinois University School of Medicine (SIU SOM) launched a leadership development program called accelerate, which follows an internal needs assessment to cultivate the next generation of leaders. The program is specifically designed to empower emerging leaders who have supervised in the past 5 years at SIU SOM, primarily focusing on practical application. Unlike most leadership programs in academic medicine, this initiative extended enrollment beyond faculty, with approximately 70% of participants being non-clinical administrative staff. This 1-year program emphasized practical skill-building, strength-based character development, and individualized goal-setting.

The Future: Artificial Intelligence

The utopian possibilities of leveraging artificial intelligence and adaptive learning within medical education open the door to solving multiple issues at the heart of SA for students and institutions. We can envision a future in which students are empowered, through free and open access to a learning management system, to join the medical profession based on their own merits rather than the limitations placed upon them by the happenstance of their birth. In striving to live up to the potential and promise of SA, artificial agents can assist institutions in creating custom instructional content based on the unique local needs of their communities. While the development of such a system may sound like pure science fiction, we make the case that the reality is much closer at hand. More so, there is a moral obligation to strive towards such a paradigm shift to remove barriers to student access for greater equity and match the critical healthcare challenges of the next century.

A prudent and fundamental reaction to such a bold assertion is asking both, "Why and how?" Why would we suggest that the future of medical education may well pivot on bold new technologies rather than remain as it always has been? And how would such a feat even be accomplished in the first place? There is a critical need to train more future physicians as access to healthcare in many parts of the world can be difficult or delayed due to the mismatched ratio of doctors to patients. Even after receiving primary care, a referral to a specialist can lead to a months-long wait for additional diagnostic testing and treatment, if one can be found at all. In parallel, local medical services can be limited, requiring long travel to see a physician. Yet, despite these persistent shortfalls in healthcare personnel, there is little that medical training institutions are able to do to meet the demand of training physicians in adequate numbers. We lack the educational bandwidth in faculty, clinical exposure, and residency programs to increase the number of medical degrees conferred each year dramatically. While more medical schools are opening, the process is slow and methodical. However, developing adaptive learning curriculums and content for medical schools enables basic science medical education to exist entirely online. In shifting the earlier preclinical phases of education towards adaptive learning supported by AI, we can open pathways for students who might otherwise be excluded and free up resources for our faculty to expand clinical education to increase our overall output of future doctors. This envisioned model fits splendidly with the Competency-Based Medical Education model and has the potential to decrease disparities in access to not only geographically and socioeconomically disadvantaged students but also students with learning disabilities.

There are multiple benefits of adaptive learning systems. One of the most profound is that they allow for a student's proper scaffolding and support throughout a curriculum. With a complete ontological map of the domain of knowledge, assessments can be created that provide practice and evaluation but also give insight into exactly what concepts students understand and which they struggle with. The system can also see what lower-order concepts a student might be missing, causing confusion or mistakes. Therefore, in gaining the picture of what a student understands of the ontology, each student can be provided with customized lessons, assessments, and assignments focusing on what they most need to know, with little wasted time or effort. This level of academic customization isn't possible for modern medical school programs that often educate a hundred or more students simultaneously. Students are forced to adapt to the instructors' pace, pedagogy, and teaching style rather than the curriculum adjusting to their needs. Therefore, an adaptive learning AI fundamentally flips the model of how students can engage with and learn complex information, creating a learning environment customized to their needs rather than a generalized instruction often aimed toward the "average" student. When done well, the student has a near-perfect educator who can assist in helping them build their understanding effectively, with the right concepts, and at the right speed.

Additionally, since adaptive learning ontologies can be run by an AI through a learning management system and connected to the Internet, these courses can function perpetually any day and at any time. Adaptive learning systems lack the encumbrances of traditional medical school classrooms. There would be no limit to the number of students who could enroll, where they could access the information, or what speed they would be gated at to progress through the material. In effect, medical adaptive learning systems would remove one of the great gatekeepers from the profession: the limited number of spots offered by a physical brick-and-mortar school. The cost of such a program could be free, removing another of the classic gatekeepers from medical schooling, as Open MIT and other educational institutions have provided free online educational courses to anyone interested.

Beyond the enhanced equity, inclusion, and access that an adaptive learning AI would provide for medical education, it would also result in a seismic shift for students with disabilities. Content could be automatically generated to follow the universal design standards and even augment the presentation of educational materials to customize it to improve comprehension for individuals with specific disabilities.

One of the most exciting possibilities, and one of the clear benefits of adaptive learning systems, is the automatic support they can provide to learners with disabilities. These AI systems can automatically close caption speakers or lectures and provide descriptions of images or read-aloud text to adjust for color blindness or text size, just to list a few possibilities. Not only can there be a future where educational content is created and customized for each learner's specific conceptual needs, but the materials presented can also be adjusted to help offset disabilities. Such a dramatic shift in the accessibility of content would lead to greater equity and would hopefully encourage more individuals who have the potential to become physicians but may be hesitant to join the profession due to their disability to try."
K.M—student voice

If moving away from traditional assessment modalities and toward AI as a potential evaluation system of student knowledge seems far-fetched, that future is already here. The U.S. National Board of Medical Examiners is openly exploring using natural language processing (NLP) as an alternative assessment model in which written text or spoken words can be evaluated and scored by AI, and it is looking to generate test questions from AI. Therefore, the future of medical education is one in which artificial intelligence plays a central role. One where AI can assist with student learning is as a constant tutor who knows exactly how to support the needs of the medical student and can even work as a collaborator throughout the learning process. Yet, we strive to push toward open social equity. In that case, we must also build up online learning management systems supported by AI, which can help break down the historical barriers that often limit who is capable of joining the medical profession. Yet, our vision of the future does not mean we cannot begin achieving greater health equity today with already available technologies.

Conclusion

SA is an aspiration and can be a strategy to achieve optimal community health. It is both an institutional and personal responsibility. It is not solely academic learning, nor does it replace technical skills. Think of it as continuous quality improvement see the Fig. 9.1 below [59]. CQI skills are a continuous improvement method beyond assuring technical competence. Part of a continuous quality improvement (CQI) process is ensuring learners are selected, trained, sustained, and followed up on to meet social accountability.

Consideration of a student's characteristics at admission and sustaining initial motivation through community immersion with mentors who reinforce the values of primary care and community involvement throughout the curriculum can assist students in "becoming" socially accountable as part of their professional identity formation. Social accountability is a competency-based value best demonstrated by physicians acting as change agents in partnership with their communities [60]. The primary challenge of a socially accountable curriculum is changing existing curriculum content or context where it is delivered without significant resources and support. However, it is worth doing, as graduates of socially accountable medical schools perform just as well or better than graduates of traditional medical schools

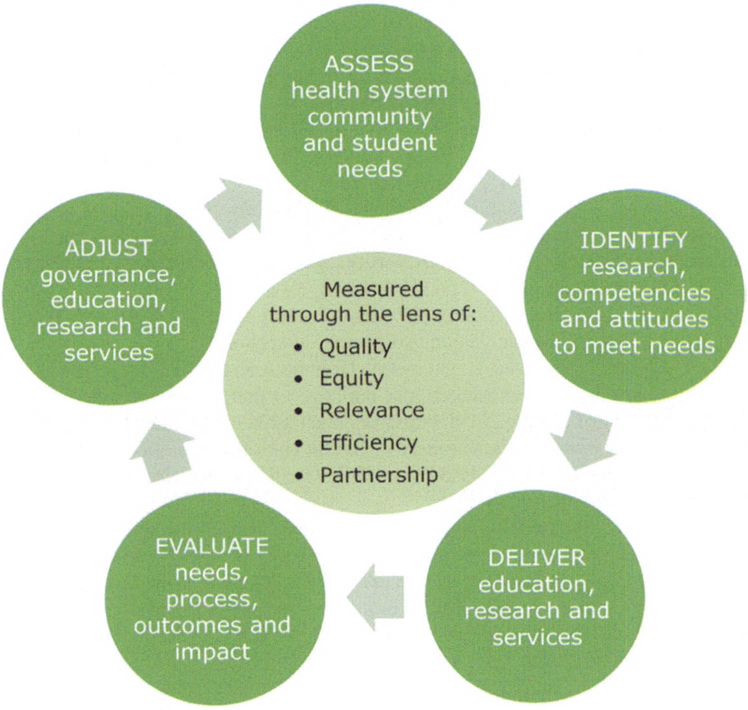

Fig. 9.1 SA with CQI understanding

[61]. Is it realistic to expect that all physicians will "become" socially accountable? Probably not. However, as academic training facilities, we owe it to learners and the communities they train to give them the tools to try.

> Never doubt that a small group of thoughtful, committed citizens can change the world. Indeed, it is the only thing that ever has. —Margaret Mead.

References

1. Steinecke A, Terrell C. Progress for whose future? The impact of the Flexner report on medical education for racial and ethnic minority physicians in the United States. Acad Med. 2010;85:236. https://doi.org/10.1097/ACM.0b013e3181c885be.
2. Saluja S, Rudolfson N, Massenburg BB, Meara JG, Shrime MG. The impact of physician migration on mortality in low and middle-income countries: an economic modelling study. BMJ Glob Health. 2020;5:e001535. https://doi.org/10.1136/bmjgh-2019-001535.
3. Boelen C, Heck JE, Health WHOD of D of HR for. Defining and measuring the social accountability of medical schools. 1995 [cited 23 May 2017]. Available: https://apps.who.int/iris/handle/10665/59441
4. Boelen C. Global consensus on social accountability of medical schools. Sante Publique. 2011;23:247–50.
5. Boelen C, Woollard R. Social accountability: the extra leap to excellence for educational institutions. Med Teach. 2011;33:614–9. https://doi.org/10.3109/0142159X.2011.590248.
6. Boelen C, Dharamsi S, Gibbs T. The social accountability of medical schools and its indicators. Edu Health. 2012;25:180. https://doi.org/10.4103/1357-6283.109785.
7. Health and care workforce in Europe: time to act. [cited 14 Apr 2024]. Available: https://www.who.int/europe/publications/i/item/9789289058339
8. WHO | Global Strategy on Human Resources for Health–Synthesis paper development. In: WHO [Internet]. [cited 10 Nov 2016]. Available: http://www.who.int/workforcealliance/media/news/2014/consultation_globstrat_hrh/en/
9. Larkins S, Johnston K, Hogenbirk JC, Willems S, Elsanousi S, Mammen M, et al. Practice intentions at entry to and exit from medical schools aspiring to social accountability: findings from the training for Health equity network graduate outcome study. BMC Med Educ. 2018;18:261. https://doi.org/10.1186/s12909-018-1360-6.
10. THEnet—Training for Health Equity Network—Section 3: What Do We Do? [cited 9 Nov 2016]. Available: http://thenetcommunity.org/social-af-section-3/
11. Epperly T, Bechtel C, Sweeney R, Greiner A, Grumbach K, Schilz J, et al. The shared principles of primary care: a Multistakeholder initiative to find a common voice. Family Med [Internet]. 2019 [cited 17 Nov 2019]. https://doi.org/10.22454/FamMed.2019.925587.
12. Starfield B. Primary care: an increasingly important contributor to effectiveness, equity, and efficiency of health services. SESPAS report 2012. Gac Sanit. 2012;26(Suppl 1):20–6. https://doi.org/10.1016/j.gaceta.2011.10.009.
13. Starfield B, Shi L, Macinko J. Contribution of primary care to health systems and Health. Milbank Q. 2005;83:457–502. https://doi.org/10.1111/j.1468-0009.2005.00409.x.
14. Goodfellow A, Ulloa JG, Dowling PT, Talamantes E, Chheda S, Bone C, et al. Predictors of primary care physician practice location in underserved urban or rural areas in the United States: a systematic literature review. Acad Med. 2016;91:1313–21. https://doi.org/10.1097/ACM.0000000000001203.
15. Reid SJ, Couper ID, Volmink J. Educational factors that influence the urban-rural distribution of health professionals in South Africa: a case-control study. S Afr Med J. 2011;101:29–33.

16. Shanafelt TD, Hasan O, Dyrbye LN, Sinsky C, Satele D, Sloan J, et al. Changes in burnout and satisfaction with work-life balance in physicians and the general US working population between 2011 and 2014. Mayo Clin Proc. 2015;90:1600–13. https://doi.org/10.1016/j.mayocp.2015.08.023.
17. Sinsky CA, Brown RL, Stillman MJ, Linzer M. COVID-related stress and work intentions in a sample of US Health care workers. Mayo Clinic Proceedings: Innovations, Quality & Outcomes. 2021;5:1165–73. https://doi.org/10.1016/j.mayocpiqo.2021.08.007.
18. Gheihman G, Singh TA, Cooper CA, McKeon BA, Hirsh DA, Simpkin AL. Everyday resilience: equipping faculty with practical exercises to promote resilience among medical students. MedEdPORTAL. 2021. [cited 6 Jun 2024];17 https://doi.org/10.15766/mep_2374-8265.11076.
19. Cheu HF, Sameshima P, Strasser R, Clithero-Eridon AR, Ross B, Cameron E, et al. Teaching compassion for social accountability: a parallaxic investigation. Med Teach. 2023;45:404–11. https://doi.org/10.1080/0142159X.2022.2136516.
20. Ninham BD. Running medicine provides 'healing journey' in Albuquerque. The Journal [Internet]. [cited 6 Jun 2024]. Available: https://www.the-journal.com/articles/running-medicine-provides-healing-journey-in-albuquerque/
21. Clithero-Eridon A, Albright D, Ross A. Conceptualising social accountability as an attribute of medical education. African J Primary Health Care Family Med. 2020:12. https://doi.org/10.4102/phcfm.v12i1.2213.
22. Talib Z, Palsdottir B, Briggs M, Clithero A, Cobb NM, Marjadi B, et al. Defining community-engaged health professional education: a step toward building the evidence. NAM. Perspectives. 2017. [cited 2 Feb 2022];7 https://doi.org/10.31478/201701a.
23. O'Sullivan B, McGrail M, Russell D, Walker J, Chambers H, Major L, et al. Duration and setting of rural immersion during the medical degree relates to rural work outcomes. Med Educ. 2018;52:803–15. https://doi.org/10.1111/medu.13578.
24. Satran L, Harris IB, Allen S, Anderson DC, Poland GA, Miller WL. Hospital-based versus community-based clinical education: comparing performances and course evaluations by students in their second-year pediatrics rotation. Acad Med. 1993;68:380–2.
25. Worley P, Esterman A, Prideaux D. Cohort study of examination performance of undergraduate medical students learning in community settings. BMJ. 2004;328:207–9. https://doi.org/10.1136/bmj.328.7433.207.
26. Halili S'B' Jr, Cristobal F, Woolley T, Ross SJ, Reeve C, Neusy A-J. Addressing health workforce inequities in the Mindanao regions of The Philippines: tracer study of graduates from a socially-accountable, community-engaged medical school and graduates from a conventional medical school. Med Teach. 2017;39:859–65. https://doi.org/10.1080/0142159X.2017.1331035.
27. Hogenbirk JC, Strasser RP, French MG. Ten years of graduates: a cross-sectional study of the practice location of doctors trained at a socially accountable medical school. PLoS One. 2022;17:e0274499. https://doi.org/10.1371/journal.pone.0274499.
28. Walker L, Isaac V, Walters L, Craig J. Flinders University rural medical school student program outcomes. Aust J Gen Pract. 2021;50:319–21. https://doi.org/10.31128/AJGP-06-20-5492.
29. Tesson G, Curran V, Pong R, Strasser R. Advances in rural medical education in three countries: Canada, the United States and Australia. Edu Health. 2012;18:405–15.
30. Halili S'B', Cristobal F, Woolley T, Ross SJ, Reeve C, Neusy A-J. Addressing health workforce inequities in the Mindanao regions of The Philippines: tracer study of graduates from a socially-accountable, community-engaged medical school and graduates from a conventional medical school. Med Teach. 2017;39:1–7. https://doi.org/10.1080/0142159X.2017.1331035.
31. Walker L, Isaac V, Walters L, Craig J. Flinders university rural medical school student program outcomes. Aust J Gen Pract. 2021;50:319–21. https://doi.org/10.31128/AJGP-06-20-5492.
32. WHO Commission on Social Determinants of Health, World Health Organization. Closing the gap in a generation: health equity through action on the social determinants of health: Commission on Social Determinants of Health final report. Geneva, Switzerland: World Health Organization, Commission on Social Determinants of Health; 2008.

33. Braveman PA, Egerter SA, Mockenhaupt RE. Broadening the FocusThe need to address the social determinants of health. Am J Prev Med. 2011;40:S4–S18. https://doi.org/10.1016/j.amepre.2010.10.002.
34. Gibbs T. Sexy words but impotent curricula: can social accountability be the change agent of the future? Med Teach. 2011;33:605–7. https://doi.org/10.3109/0142159X.2011.590251.
35. Furin J, Farmer P, Wolf M, Levy B, Judd A, Paternek M, et al. A novel training model to address health problems in poor and underserved populations. J Health Care Poor Underserved. 2006;17:17–24. https://doi.org/10.1353/hpu.2006.0023.
36. Ko M, Edelstein RA, Heslin KC, Rajagopalan S, Wilkerson L, Colburn L, et al. Impact of the University of California, Los Angeles/Charles R. Drew University medical education program on medical students' intentions to practice in underserved areas. Acad Med. 2005;80:803–8. https://doi.org/10.1097/00001888-200509000-00004.
37. McDougle L. Matching community need with physician training: the OSU urban family medicine program. J Natl Med Assoc. 2006;98:687–9.
38. Starfield B, Gérvas J, Mangin D. Clinical care and Health disparities. Annu Rev Public Health. 2012;33:89–106. https://doi.org/10.1146/annurev-publhealth-031811-124528.
39. Jensen N, Kelly AH, Avendano M. Health equity and health system strengthening–time for a WHO re-think. Glob Public Health. 2022;17:377–90. https://doi.org/10.1080/17441692.2020.1867881.
40. Neff J, Holmes SM, Knight KR, Strong S, Ariana T-L, McGuinness C, et al. Structural competency: curriculum for medical students, residents, and interprofessional teams on the structural factors that produce health disparities. MedEdPORTAL. 16:10888. https://doi.org/10.15766/mep_2374-8265.10888.
41. Kripalani S, Bussey-Jones J, Katz MG, Genao I. A prescription for cultural competence in medical education. J Gen Intern Med. 2006;21:1116–20. https://doi.org/10.1111/j.1525-1497.2006.00557.x.
42. Goss E, Iyer S, Arnsten J, Wang L, Smith CL. Liberation medicine: a community partnership and health advocacy curriculum for internal medicine residents. J Gen Intern Med. 2020;35:3102–4. https://doi.org/10.1007/s11606-019-05518-1.
43. Kirmayer LJ. Rethinking cultural competence. Transcult Psychiatry. 2012;49:149–64. https://doi.org/10.1177/1363461512444673.
44. Shepherd SM. Cultural awareness workshops: limitations and practical consequences. BMC Med Educ. 2019;19:1–10. https://doi.org/10.1186/s12909-018-1450-5.
45. Tervalon M, Murray-García J. Cultural humility versus cultural competence: a critical distinction in defining physician training outcomes in multicultural education. J Health Care Poor Underserved. 1998;9:117–25. https://doi.org/10.1353/hpu.2010.0233.
46. Hook JN, Davis DE, Owen J, Worthington EL, Utsey SO. Cultural humility: measuring openness to culturally diverse clients. J Couns Psychol. 2013;60:353–66. https://doi.org/10.1037/a0032595.
47. Botelho MJ, Lima CA. From cultural competence to cultural respect: a critical review of six models. J Nurs Educ. 2020;59:311–8. https://doi.org/10.3928/01484834-20200520-03.
48. Ventres W, Page T. Bring global health and global medicine home. Acad Med. 2013;88:907–8. https://doi.org/10.1097/ACM.0b013e3182952940.
49. Crump JA, Sugarman J. Working group on ethics guidelines for global health training (WEIGHT). Ethics and best practice guidelines for training experiences in global health. Am J Trop Med Hyg. 2010;83:1178–82. https://doi.org/10.4269/ajtmh.2010.10-0527.
50. Eichbaum QG, Adams LV, Evert J, Ho M-J, Semali IA, van Schalkwyk SC. Decolonizing global health education: rethinking institutional partnerships and approaches. Acad Med. 2021;96:329–35. https://doi.org/10.1097/ACM.0000000000003473.
51. Yarmoshuk AN, Guantai AN, Mwangu M, Cole DC, Zarowsky C. What makes international Global Health University partnerships higher-value? An examination of partnership types and activities Favoured at four east African universities. Ann Glob Health. 2018;84:139–50. https://doi.org/10.29024/aogh.20.

52. IPEC Core competencies for interprofessional collaborative practice: version 3.
53. Kaufman A. Leadership and governance. Acad Med. 1998;73:S11–5. https://doi.org/10.1097/00001888-199809001-00004.
54. Girard VW, Cannon Y, Bhatnagar P, Coleman S. How medical-legal partnerships help address the social determinants of mental health. Arch Psychiatr Nurs. 2021;35:123–6. https://doi.org/10.1016/j.apnu.2020.10.014.
55. Robinson R, Mishori R. The efficacy of short, skills-based workshops in teaching advocacy to medical students: a pilot study. PRiMER. 2023;7:7. https://doi.org/10.22454/PRiMER.2023.427789.
56. Oandasan IF, Barker KK. Educating for advocacy: exploring the source and substance of community-responsive physicians. Acad Med. 2003;78:S16–9.
57. Nguyen J, Sen-Crowe B, Sutherland M, McKenney M, Elkbuli A. Gender distribution of deans among US medical schools: towards equity in academic medicine. J Surg Res. 2022;271:41–51. https://doi.org/10.1016/j.jss.2021.10.018.
58. Lucas R, Goldman EF, Scott AR, Dandar V. Leadership development programs at academic health centers: results of a national survey. Acad Med. 2018;93:229–36. https://doi.org/10.1097/ACM.0000000000001813.
59. Clithero A, Ross SJ, Middleton L, Reeve C, Neusy A-J. Improving community Health using an outcome-oriented CQI approach to community-engaged Health professions education. Front Public Health. 2017;5:26. https://doi.org/10.3389/fpubh.2017.00026.
60. Frenk J, Chen L, Bhutta ZA, Cohen J, Crisp N, Evans T, et al. Health professionals for a new century: transforming education to strengthen health systems in an interdependent world. Lancet. 2010;376:1923–58.
61. Woolley T, Clithero-Eridon A, Elsanousi S, Othman A-B. Does a socially-accountable curriculum transform health professional students into competent, work-ready graduates? A cross-sectional study of three medical schools across three countries. Med Teach. 2019;41:1–7. https://doi.org/10.1080/0142159X.2019.1646417.

Further Readings

Boelen C. Prospects for change in medical education in the twenty-first century. Acad Med. 1995;70(7):S21–8. https://journals.lww.com/academicmedicine/abstract/1995/07000/prospects_for_change_in_medical_education_in_the.17.aspx

Jacobs C. Advancing a social justice agenda in health professions education. Critical Studies in Teaching and Learning. 2020;8(2) https://www.ajol.info/index.php/cristal/article/view/203981

Mullan F, Chen C, Petterson S, Kolsky G, Spagnola M. The social mission of medical education: ranking the schools. Ann Intern Med. 2010;152(12):804-811.https://www.acpjournals.org/doi/full/10.7326/0003-4819-152-12-201006150-00009.

Chapter 10
Embedding Social Accountability into the Medical Curriculum: Strategies, Insights, and Real-World Applications

Dervla Kelly, Siobhán Neville, and Mohamed Elhassan Abdalla

Learning Outcomes

1. Recognize the importance of orienting health professions curricula toward social accountability.
2. Review the relationship between societal needs, healthcare systems, and curriculum design.
3. Discuss strategies for planning a socially accountable curriculum.
4. Explore teaching, learning, and assessment methods that foster social accountability.
5. Analyze case studies of successful integration of SA into health professions education.

Introduction

The curriculum is a sophisticated blend of educational strategies, course content, learning outcomes, educational experiences, assessment, the educational environment and plan of work that enables learner growth [1]. Orienting health professions curricula towards social accountability means that the institution, faculty, and students have an outward-looking population focus aimed at producing graduates who can better serve societies and improve health systems. Rather than the curriculum

D. Kelly · M. E. Abdalla (✉)
School of Medicine, University of Limerick, Limerick, Ireland
e-mail: melhassan.elsayed@ul.ie

S. Neville
School of Medicine, University of Limerick, Limerick, Ireland

Department of Paediatrics, University Hospital Limerick, Limerick, Ireland

M. E. Abdalla et al. (eds.), *Social Accountability of Medical Schools*,
https://doi.org/10.1007/978-3-031-94435-2_10

being designed to address learning outcomes that are set internally by faculty or implicitly by the institution, the whole curriculum is planned in conjunction with stakeholders to address the top health and social needs that are described by the concerned partners, including the local community [2].

Having a curriculum with social accountability at its core would mean focusing on the social accountability values of relevance, equity, quality, and cost-effectiveness [2]. The ultimate goal of implementing those values includes reducing inequity in society, exposing students to how this impacts health, and equipping them with ways to address such inequities. The implementation of a curriculum with social accountability orientation brings benefits for society and population, benefits for the institutions, and benefits for students. The population will receive more patient-centred care with associated positive outcomes on the health of communities, along with greater accountability of the institution to communities through improved communication and collaboration [3] (see Fig. 10.1). Previous studies have found that students who attend medical schools that employ health equity curricula are more likely to practice in underserved communities [4–6]. By incorporating social accountability principles, institutions will build strong reputations as population health advocates which may result in higher or more competitive student intake. Another benefit to institutions is through enhanced compliance with accreditation standards, which call for institutions to engage with communities and contribute to a more equitable and effective health service [7]. Students of institutions that adopt a social accountability approach will be embedded in their local communities. Through this integration they will acquire other competencies such as leadership, cultural competencies, and a greater understanding of both the social determinants of health and how to mitigate them [8–10].

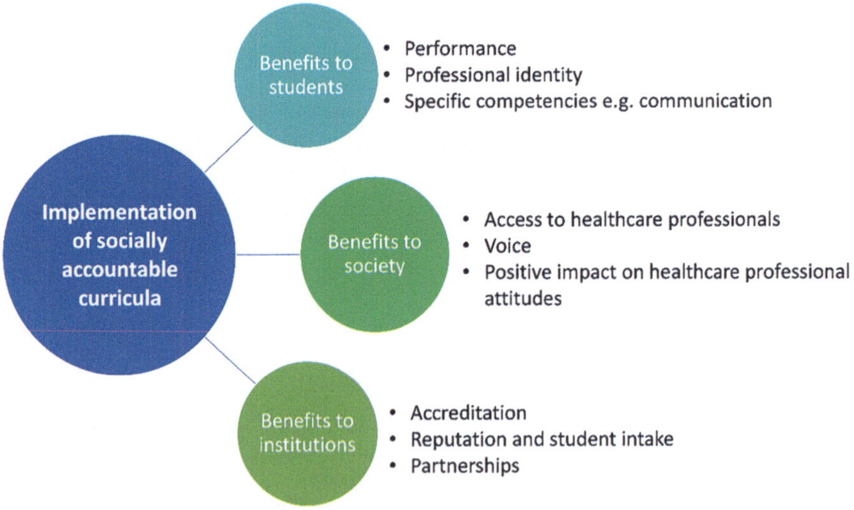

Fig. 10.1 Benefits of socially accountable curricula to students, society, and healthcare profession education institutions

Social accountability principles should be integral to all the activities of a medical education institution, including education, research and service delivery. Despite the pervasiveness of social accountability rhetoric in health professions education (HPE) school strategy documents, the literature detailing the day-to-day actions of schools that translate these principles into reality is often at a theoretical level [11]. Deciding which components of social accountability are included in a curriculum has been identified as an area requiring work [12].

To facilitate the reading of this chapter, the content will be addressed under the headings of one of the common frameworks for curriculum development in health professions education, Kern's Six–Step Approach [13]. The six steps are (i) problem identification and general needs assessment, (ii) targeted needs assessment, (iii) goals and objectives, (iv) educational strategies, (v) implementation, and (vi) and evaluation Fig. 10.2 summarises the application Kern's Six Step approach to designing a socially accountable curriculum. Case studies and examples have been integrated throughout the chapter to show readers examples and practical steps to achieve a socially accountable curriculum.

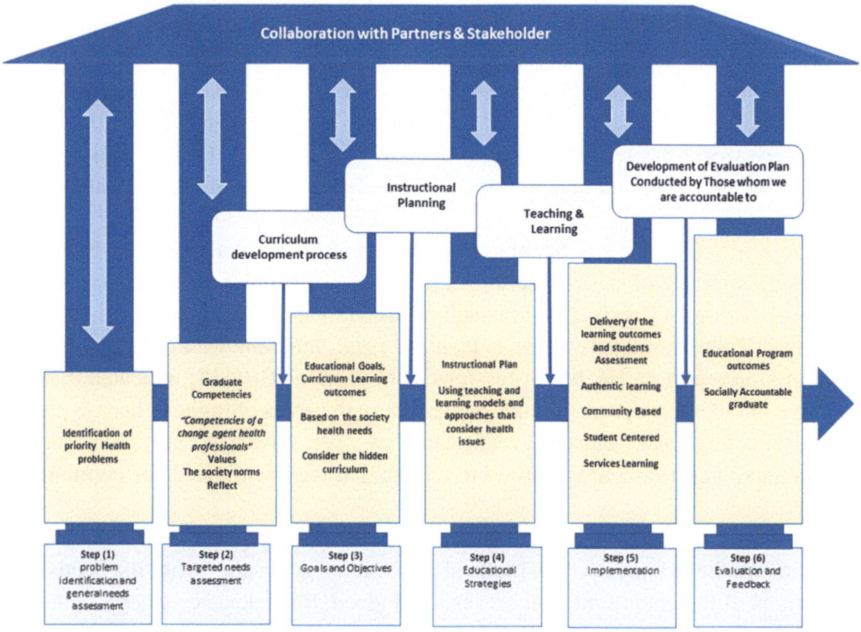

Fig. 10.2 Application of Kern's Six Step approach to designing a socially accountable curriculum

Step 1: Problem Identification and General Needs Assessment

Problem Identification

Social accountability is a broad concept and is interpreted differently in different geographic and cultural settings. For example, HPE literature from North America focuses on pressing social factors such as racial bias, access to care and housing, and food insecurity that can significantly impact people's health [14]. These social factors are known as the social determinants of health (SDH). Literature on SDH from across the globe also includes factors such as economic and political stability, education quality and access, neighbourhood socioeconomic disadvantage, income and working conditions, early childhood development, and health care quality, varying greatly by context [15]. Throughout this chapter we will use examples of curricula that make a concerted effort to contextualise teaching to local public health issues and social determinants of health.

Most health professionals will encounter patients or serve communities of varied socioeconomic and cultural backgrounds yet are not always equipped with the necessary education and tools to assess and address the SDH that influence health outcomes. For this reason, many educators and stakeholders have recognised the integration of SDH into health professions education as essential in preparing health professionals to appreciate and address health inequities and disparities [16]. Healthcare workforces who are aware of SDH and consider it when dealing with health problems are better able to respond to the health needs of the population they are serving [17].

In addition to the above, healthcare systems are facing challenges such as high costs and a shortage of skilled healthcare providers. Curricular exploration of value-based care or cost-effectiveness is usually limited to specialised post-graduate programmes. This shortage is more evident in rural and remote areas. The Lancet Commission report on Health Professions Education in 2010 [18] indicated that the shortage of healthcare professionals is greatest in the areas of highest disease prevalence, reflecting Tudor-Hart's inverse care law [19]. Given workforce shortages, innovations in curricula are required to ensure that the health needs of populations are met.

The World Health Organization's social accountability grid (1995) encourages reflection on the extent to which medical education's goals align with the needs and aspirations of the communities it serves [2]. Indeed, this relevance can be seen as a fundamental essential constituent of a curriculum that aligns with health system needs and the health needs of the societies it serves [20]. We argue that it is essential that HPE schools frame their education and training within the needs of the community and/or region where they are based. Educators must take the global concept of social accountability and adapt it to the local context [21] in order to inculcate the concept in the curriculum and to translate it into learning opportunities for students.

General Needs Assessment

A general needs assessment of social accountability within the curriculum requires thoughtful reflection on the local environment and community, together with the expected evolving roles of health professionals [13]. Many pre-existing national and regional level indicators are helpful for this activity. A "health needs assessment" is a process of determining the health and healthcare needs of any defined population in an area. Recently, a classification system was introduced to standardise the 'measurement' of health, called The International Classification of Functioning, Disability and Health, endorsed in 2001 by all Member States (WHO, 2018c). Other methods have been used by organisations to try to meld multiple SDH and local needs into a core set of health indicators, such as expert panels [22], and co-produced health indices [23, 24]. The reality is that different organisations collect many different population-level health indicators for many different reasons. The Organisation for Economic Co-operation and Development produces useful summaries of the health of countries and regions that are useful for general needs assessments [25]. Some examples of health indicator data that are collected at regular intervals include the European 'Eurostat' [26], and census data e.g. the Office for National Statistics (ONS) in the United Kindgom [27]. Sub-national health indicators vary in availability and the reason for this is complex.

Partnerships are an important aspect of the curriculum development process. Partners and stakeholders should be involved in the planning and implementation of the general needs assessment and indeed in each step of curriculum development. We will explore the role of partnerships in curriculum development further in Step 5. The concept of partnership for social accountability is discussed in more detail in another part of this book.

General Needs Assessment Case Study: College of Medicine-Jazan University [28]

The College of Medicine-Jazan University in Saudi Arabia led a needs assessment with the goal of identifying common health issues to inform the curriculum of the college. The stakeholders consulted included municipality members, military officers, healthcare workers, physicians, civil servants, school teachers, and community leaders. Data was collected through open and closed-ended questions. Faculty members and students worked together to collect the data.

Results of this process identified relevant health and social issues and provided insights about the strategies for control and prevention of such issues within the local community.

Step 2: Targeted Needs Assessment

The literature describes socially accountable educational programmes as having graduates who are change agents, and who produce an impact and change on healthcare by prioritising the health concerns of the community they serve [2].

There is some uncertainty in how a socially accountable health professional comes to be, and it can appear aspirational. The educational perspective is that it can be taught, and the underlying theories on learning from the last 20 years have taken on a helpful socialisation approach [29]. This literature has defined how, as trainees move through their programmes, their social awareness grows alongside their professional identity [30]. This shifts teaching staff from teaching social accountability to looking for ways to support identity development. It is also possible that the desire to address the inequalities in society may be strongly instilled by family and upbringing or innate personality characteristics. As this may be the case, we must look at student selection and recruitment processes, which is outside the scope of this chapter and explored in more detail in other chapters in this book. In this section, we address the assessment of the needs of students to achieve a socially accountable curriculum.

Learner Needs Assessment

The assessment of learner needs often relies on perceived needs—those of the trainees involved, of educators in the field, and/or of national experts. For social accountability curricula, the opinions of other stakeholders must be considered also. It is cautioned that ideally such needs assessments should also involve objective measures that can be performed regularly to be maximally effective for improving learning [31, 32].

The literature demonstrates that undergraduate health professions students are frequently unfamiliar with the construct of social accountability, as are their teachers [33, 34]. Learners typically can identify community-based learning, patient-centeredness, and impact on society as sub-aspects of social accountability [35]. Further aspects sometimes identified by the participants are sustainability, moral issues, and interprofessional collaboration [34]. Students themselves have expressed that programmes are implemented with little appreciation of social accountability and addressing of the local health needs in teaching [12]. Students need to learn about these health problems to be prepared for their future roles. Notably, learners' perceptions of their learning needs is heavily dependent on their previous experiences, including their own socioeconomic/cultural background [36, 37].

Baseline knowledge, skills and attitudes and learner-identified gaps therein may be assessed in many ways, including student surveys, focus groups, and performance in assessments [38–41]. A student-centred approach to education that incorporates participatory collaboration is another way of supporting and promoting critical thinking across the curriculum [42]. The community should be directly

Table 10.1 Examples of types of learner needs assessment

Type of needs assessment	Example
Gap or discrepancy analysis	Comparing the current competencies in the curriculum with the competencies required by the health system.
Reflection on action and reflection in action	Thinking back of the performance of students/graduates and thinking on the actual current performance of students/graduates.
Peer review	Reports from peer institutes or peer professionals regarding the performance of students/graduates. Reports from accreditation visits (if any).
Self-assessment	Voluntary self-assessment or in preparation for accreditation.
Critical incident review and significant event auditing	Review of incidents in hospitals or community settings, e.g. relating to professionalism.
Observation	Making use of the of the educators' and stakeholders' observation of the graduates' performance.
Practice review	Review of reports about practice in hospitals and community health settings.

involved in this step, through engagement around their priority topics for healthcare practitioner training. For example, the Northern Ontario School of Medicine engages in reciprocal dialogue with a local steering committee to inform educational as well as service and research activities [43]. The downstream impacts of such broad approaches to needs assessment on healthcare provision and patient and population health outcomes are vital but challenging to measure, particularly as there are so many confounding factors at play.

Table 10.1 below illustrates a range of needs assessment approaches and examples of their application in socially accountable curricula.

Step 3: Goals and Objectives

Regarding teaching and learning of social accountability, the approach lately is that it should be taught explicitly, by outlining specific competencies or defining core content. This is an important step for encouraging action in educators and learners.

Setting Curriculum Goals and Objectives

Goals and objectives are related to the end towards which the curriculum is developed. According to the Global Consensus for Social Accountability of Medical Schools (GCSA), that end is to graduate health professionals who have the necessary competencies to deal with the changing health needs of the communities they serve, the health system in which they work, and to anticipate the populations' expectations [44]. Setting the right goals and objectives will help in developing curriculum content that reflects social accountability, selecting the appropriate teaching, learning and assessment methods, facilitating the evaluation of the curriculum and, most importantly, facilitating the communication of the curriculum with stakeholders. There is some debate amongst educators about whether social accountability needs to be defined as a competency, and whether it is beneficial to measure it. For example, in Canada, measurement of the competencies of the socially accountable practitioner is being explored [45]. EmiratesMEDs is an example of a competency framework for medical education that has integrated social accountability as a competence [46]. On the other hand, some educators are wary of creating prescriptive measurable standards relating to social accountability, given the importance of context and concerns that they could diminish professional discretion, innovation, and set unrealistic expectations [47, 48].

The process of developing goals and objectives for a socially accountable curriculum needs to consider the four values related to social accountability and the involvement of all stakeholders, including the society themselves; this is crucial to fit within the definition of the concept of social accountability, and to differentiate it from those of social responsibility and social responsiveness, as outlined in the social obligations scale [49]. The involvement of stakeholders, including society, in health professions education is discussed in other chapters of this book.

To help realise the ultimate aim of a socially accountable curriculum, the GCSA asked for future health professionals who are capable of integrating population and individual health, concentrating on health promotion and acting as change agents in the health system to advocate for prevention and rehabilitation [44]. This aim should be reflected in curriculum goals and individual learning outcomes within the curriculum document. Preston et al. (2016) identified the socially accountable curriculum as one that integrates basic and clinical sciences together with population health and social sciences. They recommend that early clinical exposure will add to the relevance of and support theoretical learning. They also argue that graduates are expected to work in underserved areas and contribute to positive impacts on the health and social outcomes of communities [50]. A recent call for introducing Health System Science (HSS) in curriculum may add to the preparation of the needed future health workforce. The HSS is defined as 'the study of how health care is delivered, including how health professionals collaborate and how the health care system can improve patient care and health care delivery' [51].

The CPU model (Conceptualisation-Production-Usability) produced by Boelen and Wollard can act as another framework to inform the development of curricular goals and objectives [52]. The model suggests (among other points) that reference should be to the needs of the population and the health system, aiming at retention of graduates who will have impact on the health needs of the population through a well-designed educational programme [53].

These ideas of the GCSA have blended with the curriculum design literature in medicine, and have in turn drawn on the spiral model developed by Bruner [54]. For example, Harden and Stamper (1999) illustrated how revisiting topics at increasing levels of complexity allows learners to grasp core concepts in the early stages of the University of Dundee medical course before building on these ideas later to achieve more advanced learning [55]. Year 1 focuses on structure, function and behaviour.

In Years 2 and 3, students revisit these concepts when studying abnormal structure, function and behaviour. This knowledge is then related to clinical practice in Years 4 and 5, and finally the theory is put into practice in students' pre-registration year. Besides vertical integration of topics, there are 'network' approaches to the curriculum that promote horizontal connections between different activities in a course, and give the learners some decision-making over their learning activities [56]. The obstacles to implementing a spiral curriculum/horizontal integration are siloed working between disciplines or between pre-clinical and clinical faculty, time constraints, and defining regular assessments that require learners to contextualise new topics with core knowledge.

The Curriculum

There are different versions of the curriculum. The formal curriculum is what is intended to be delivered by the school. However, the classes taken by students may vary within any given course of study. Assessment has a large role in driving learning in the formal curriculum. Aspects of social accountability may be best explained within the formal curriculum, e.g. patient consent and communication skills.

The informal curriculum refers to opportunistic encounters between teachers and learners. This may be placement-based or in simulated scenarios. The nature of the learning is spontaneous and context specific.

The hidden curriculum is neither formal nor informal. It is often the result of working within communities of practice, observing everyday clinical scenarios and social norms in the workplace. While the very nature of the hidden curriculum means it cannot be mandated to deliver the goal and objectives of the taught curriculum, its influence on learner attitudes to social accountability cannot be underestimated [57].

Curriculum goals case study: Ateneo de Zamboanga University School of Medicine [58]

The Philippines is a low-middle income country with reported significant health inequities, with rural areas having poorer health indicators and shortages of health workers compared to urban areas. The goal of the combined degree of medicine and public health (MD-MPH) curriculum is to train physicians with skills and attitudes oriented toward social accountability, intersectoral collaboration, and community participation. The 12 impact programs of the Philippine Department of Health were integrated into the core content of this curriculum. There are mandatory monthly community placements every semester in years one to three and the final year consists of a 10-month community placement. There is evidence that these efforts to immerse students in the rural community have strengthened the health system by increasing motivation to work in the community and involving community stakeholders in education.

Step 4: Educational Strategies

There is a substantial body of literature at an educational strategy level [59–63]. Some scholars in the area emphasise the moral imperative and development of community services, self-awareness, and experiential learning. Other strategies include lecture-style didactic sessions, small group teaching, simulations and reflection. This section will explore more closely a handful of strategies, namely clinical vignettes and case presentations, the use of art and literature, and experiential learning as educational methods for consideration when planning a socially accountable curriculum. A non-exhaustive list of strategies is presented in Table 10.2.

Table 10.2 Examples of socially accountable educational strategies

Example	Educational strategies
Grigore T. Popa University of Medicine and Pharmacy, Isai, was the first medical university in Romania to introduce bioethics as a mandatory subject in its curriculum in the early 2000s. Teaching staff who were educated in a masters program in bioethics at Case Western Reserve University in Cleveland, Ohio, USA, contributed greatly to its development. In the Faculty of Medicine, bioethics is currently taught as a mandatory subject during one semester, with 14 h teaching and 14 h of seminar. The seminar classes have an interactive format, with interactive discussions, debates, scenarios and ethical analyses of simulated cases. The general objective of the bioethics course is to carry out an integrative analysis of bioethical concepts and professional behaviour norms regarding the professional and social responsibility of the medical profession, as well as to build the ability to identify the moral aspects specific to medical practice in medical students. [prof Beatrice Ioan, Grigore T. Popa University of Medicine and Pharmacy, Romanis]	Scaffolding learning via course content and assessment tasks; Interactive discussions and debates; Scenarios and simulated cases; Multiple choice questions
The School of Pharmacy and Biomolecular Sciences, Royal College of Surgeons in Ireland, have designed an innovative elective module aimed to develop the 'eco-literate' student and to allow them to evolve as individuals and as future graduates to become advocates/champions for the adoption of sustainable strategies in their daily lives, and in healthcare delivery. A multimodal delivery method is used to optimise knowledge uptake, to cultivate critical thinking regarding climate change mitigation and adaptation strategies, and to allow exploration and discussion of the role of the healthcare professional therein. Class-based activities include quizzes relating to the United Nations sustainable development goals (UN SDGs), video clips, and interactive data tools to stimulate debate. Clinical cases provide the opportunity to understand how patients, healthcare systems, and national decision-makers must be prepared to adapt to climate impacts, and the inequities in the global distribution of these impacts. Medicines-use case studies focus on the carbon footprint of inhalers, anaesthetics, and how social, green, and blue prescribing can be harnessed to optimise health co-benefits. An off-site immersion in nature activity combines exposure to the biodiversity of plants and the need for their ecological protection. Students are required to submit an evidence portfolio documenting module learnings with opportunities for reflection on how they, as future pharmacists, will answer the urgent call to address climate change. [prof Aisling O'Leary, Royal College of Surgeons in Ireland]	Quizzes, video clips, interactive data tools to stimulate debate; Case studies; Nature immersion—Site visit; Evidence portfolio

(continued)

Table 10.2 (continued)

Example	Educational strategies
Young@heart clinics: Pharmacy students at the University of Newcastle rotate through a community clinic where they conduct blood pressure checks and provide basic healthy lifestyle advice to community members, and signpost to further healthcare supports as necessary. Students are supported in their clinic sessions by an on-site clinical supervisor (a qualified pharmacist) who provides briefing and debriefing for each session. Medical students also join some clinics and students report learning from each others' approaches to the service user interactions. The University collaborated with the local authority to establish the clinic, which started as a voluntary activity and is now embedded as a mandatory part of the curriculum. [University of Newcastle [64]]	Service learning; Interprofessional education (IPE)
The course on primary health care practice and family medicine at the Faculty of Medicine, University of Gezira (FMUG), Sudan, is a longitudinal course extending for four semesters. Students work in primary health care centres and each student is attached to a family in wad Medani town (where the FMUG is located). Students visit these families regularly throughout the course to study their health status and aid them with any medical and psychosocial problems [65].	Community-based education (CBE)
The BMBS programme at the School of Medicine at the University of Limerick (UL), Ireland, has an 18-week longitudinal integrated clerkship (LIC) in general practice through clinical attachment to a university-affiliated primary care teaching practice. This attachment accounts for 25% of students' clinical training and is consistently rated highly by students in feedback. The aim of this longer placement is to facilitate active participation of medical students in patient care in the community setting [66].	Longitudinal integrated clerkship (LIC)

Clinical Vignettes and Case Presentations

Since the 1980s there has been a shift away from didactic methods, favouring small group teaching such as problem-based learning, team-based learning, or flipped classroom type activities, which often rely on clinical vignettes or case presentations. Such scenarios typically begin with the presentation of a medical problem in the form of a patient visiting a medical professional [67], which offers an opportunity to teach social accountability values [44]. The story format of the case prompts students to consider the body's structure and function, and also a patient's social and cultural history [68]. Case details such as the patient's name, ethnicity, and patient's voice can serve the function of providing medical history and social and economic context. They can also, inadvertently or otherwise, contribute to the hidden curriculum, either by being contrived, assigning blame to the patient, or presenting a bias in attitude [69, 70]. These social and cultural narratives provide an opportunity to explore the messy complexities of human experiences that impact healthcare such as moral, environmental, cultural, political, and economic values.

One well researched area with good case writing resources for educators is Problem-Based Learning (PBL) [71–74]. The challenge of accurately presenting

Table 10.3 Selected extracts from case presentations to demonstrate the contrast in approach for a case vignette with a basic science perspective and a case with a social accountability perspective

	Basic sciences perspective	Social accountability perspective
Case outline	Presentation of a young woman to a family planning clinic requesting contraception while breastfeeding a 6-month old child	Presentation of a young woman to a family planning clinic requesting contraception while breastfeeding a 6-month old child
Learning outcomes	Describe the mechanism of action, efficacy and side effects of the different hormonal and non-hormonal methods of contraception	Describe the mechanism of action, efficacy and side effects of the different hormonal and non-hormonal methods of contraception Understand attitudes towards contraception and identify factors that affect contraceptive behaviour use Describe sexual health policies in [country]
Questions to facilitate discussion	What are the risks and benefits of the different contraceptive options? What is the relevant sexually transmitted infection (STI) prevention advice?	What is the minimum age at which it is appropriate to give contraceptive advice? What are the risks and benefits of the different contraceptive options? Are there any cost barriers to women's use of contraception and how might these be overcome? What is the relevant STI prevention advice? What are the sexual and reproductive health services in your area?

the patient perspective on health in case writing is explored in detail in the literature [69, 75, 76]. Four previous studies carried out demographic-based needs assessment of the health issues presented in PBL cases [77–80]. These studies emphasise evolving health care needs such as the increasing burden of chronic diseases like diabetes, the emerging long-term impacts of immune therapies for cancer, the increasingly elderly population with complex multimorbidity and cognitive impairments, and expansion of primary and community health services [77–79]. Another study looked at gender stereotypes reinforced in PBL cases from a feminist perspective [81]. All these studies argue that the needs of society change quickly and keeping the curriculum up to date is an ongoing task. Table 10.3 presents an excerpt from a socially accountable case presentation.

The Use of Art and Literature

Edutainment in this context can be defined as the use of media clips from television programmes, films or other sources as part of health education delivery [82]. Several studies have demonstrated the acceptability of this approach on a variety of topics

[83–86]. Typically, this activity involves some delivery of didactic information, the watching of a video, one or more facilitated discussions on the video, and one or more activities that require further reflection and reaction to opinions on the topic. The technique has been reported to successfully engage students to think about social risks and results in students being able to identify more risks [86].

Film to teach about social determinants of health case study. Cincinnati Children's Hospital Medical Center [86]
This curriculum was developed following a needs assessment and piloting of videotaped social history vignettes. Videos of roleplays of resident physicians with patients screening for SDH were developed, showing appropriate and inappropriate behaviours. A series of "day in the life" videos were also filmed to allow patients and families from the clinic tell their story of how screening, detection, and intervention impacted their family's lives. The educational activities involved a didactic PowerPoint presentation, viewing the appropriate/inappropriate vignettes, engaging in group discussion, viewing the "day in the life" videos, and participating in a final discussion.

Typical learning outcomes:

1. Recognise the barriers to health facing patients and families from diverse socio-economic backgrounds
2. Discuss empathetic engagement of patients and families in an attempt to maximise residents' effectiveness in screening for social determinants of health (SDH)
3. Formulate a plan to mitigate the effects of SDH through referrals to government agencies and/or community resources

Experiential Learning

Not every component of the skills, knowledge and attitudes that a healthcare professional-in-training requires to meet the needs of the community they serve can be delivered in a didactic setting. Experiential learning through hospital or community-based attachments provides an invaluable opportunity to develop these social accountability proficiencies. Once embedded in the clinical setting, healthcare learners must juggle a range of competing priorities with respect to their educational goals and must learn to integrate their prior learning in a holistic manner, tailored to individual patients.

Consider a learner in the clinical setting who has been taught the most appropriate management of a particular condition. They confidently offer this suggestion while on clinical placement but are surprised to find that the patient is prescribed an alternate management plan. Perhaps this management plan is more culturally acceptable to the patient. Possibly the patient cannot afford the suggested medication and an appropriate alternative is available free of charge or subsidised by government/insurance scheme. The learner may discover that the patient accepts the medication, but exploring the potential risks and benefits proves a challenge due to a language or literacy barrier.

Clinical placements allow students to apply their knowledge in the context of the patient before them. Students are invited to reflect upon the social determinants of health when meeting a patient. Suddenly the learner is confronting unforeseen roadblocks, overcoming barriers, and viewing the problem from the patient's perspective [87]. The role of the preceptor here is twofold—one, to guide the student through the clinical encounter using a socially accountable framework to inform decision-making, and two, to facilitate reflection on the part of the trainee about the context and challenges of the case. Critical reflection can support learning of such complex concepts and contribute to the establishment of professional values [88].

Clinical placements in rural, indigenous, or other underserved community settings have been shown to be instrumental in embedding social accountability in the curriculum, through Community-Oriented Medical Education (COME), Community-Based Medical Education (CBME), Community-Engaged Medical Education (CEME), or Longitudinal Integrated Clerkship (LIC) models. In a review of social accountability curricular activities in undergraduate medical education, Mihan et al. found that 80% of socially accountable programmes described community-specific placements [89]. Service learning allows students to know their community and work effectively in society [21]. Other reported competencies include communication, teamwork, leadership, and project management skills, in addition to supporting the position of the institution within the community [90]. Such placements not only allow students to develop specific competencies, but may contribute to their desire to work in underserved communities in their future careers [58, 91].

Experiential learning is not limited to clinical settings. In a spiral "Geomedicine Curriculum" for paediatric residents described by Real et al. (2017), paediatricians-in-training completed a two-week advocacy rotation, which included time spent at a food bank and a public benefit agency, as well as a self-guided tour of an area of extreme socioeconomic disadvantage, where participants had the opportunity to meet with community members [92].

Community Placements Case Study: Nelson R. Mandela School of Medicine [93, 94]

Nelson R. Mandela School of Medicine (NRMSM) in Durban, KwaZulu-Natal Province, South Africa, has designed the module, "making a difference," where students are required to undertake 16 h of community service in disadvantaged communities. The aim of this module is for students to understand the disease profile and determinants of health in the local area, and includes working with non-governmental organisations (NGOs), addressing HIV and tuberculosis and referring on to further services. Community-based primary care clinics mean students diagnose, research, and treat community health issues together with local residents.

Step 5: Implementation

A socially accountable curriculum may be created through design of an entirely new curriculum or by introducing social accountability themes to the existing curriculum structure and content. As such, implementation will differ according to the situation. It is well-known that there are many barriers to curricular change, such as comfort with the status quo, perceived increased workload for both students and educators, lack of resources, and learner perceptions regarding the value of new or additional content [95, 96]. Implementation methods may vary depending on the scale and timeframe of the proposed change. The appreciative inquiry model is an ideal choice to guide change towards social accountability. The model and its application are discussed in another chapter of this book.

Partnerships

Successful implementation of socially accountable curricula must consider the strengthening of institutions' partnerships with stakeholders. The Partnership Pentagram Plus can provide a strong conceptual framework for building, supporting, and maximising such relationships [97]. Collaboration between stakeholders is required to identify the appropriate resources for curriculum implementation, such as the community sites where training will take place. Collaboration is also important to generate the support needed for curriculum implementation and change.

These partnerships can be academic-service working groups, links with the community, or cross-border in nature. Patients, who are seen as "experts by lived experience," value opportunities to "give back" by taking an active role in the education of health professionals. The community development sector has developed numerous participatory methodologies, which have been adapted for the curriculum design process in the education setting [98]. Support from governmental and community organisations can ensure that curricular implementation is aligned with local and national health project goals [99].

There is effort involved in making partnerships successful for everyone. Tensions can be expected when trying to achieve consensus on priority topics, power balances, conflicting agendas and an over-emphasis on job readiness over academic training. Likewise, it is not appropriate to use outside agencies to substitute an in-house curriculum, or for contributions to be experienced as a tick-box activity or out-of-context addition to a curriculum. There is a need to clearly define the roles, responsibilities, and expectations of all involved. The evolving role of health workforce is further discussed in Part I.

Partnerships Case Study: The Northern Ontario School of Medicine, Canada [100, 101]
The northern Ontario School of Medicine (NOSM) has become a landmark for innovative and community-focused medical education. Their curriculum has been shaped through a community consultative process and community partnerships. The program emphasises distributed community engaged learning, with activities spanning over 70 communities, primarily indigenous, francophone, and rural communities.

Reflection for Readers

1. How do you create space for participatory collaboration in curriculum design and planning within your discipline?
2. Who are the interested stakeholders in the educational design process in your discipline/field of practice?
3. How might they be leveraged to support engagement in this process?
4. Can you think of one example of how to engage in participatory collaboration in designing a course or assignment in your field of study?

Procuring Resources

A key aspect of implementation is the development of an effective administrative mechanism for the curriculum; clarifying who will have responsibility to follow the process. For example, will there be a social accountability committee, or will implementation be the responsibility of a specific department? Will implementation require the procurement of additional resources and, if so, through what funding streams? Although the context and organisational culture will vary, the key principle should be that social accountability is embedded within the organisational thinking of all members.

Identifying and Addressing Barriers to Learning

One potential barrier to incorporating social accountability into the health professions' curriculum is the learner's perception of the value of such content. Students may be focused on the acquisition of knowledge and skills and, given the pressure of exams, may not value opportunities to engage with the local community or indeed recognise that such a learning opportunity exists [12]. While on clinical placement, some students may think in terms of 'ticking off' an anthology of medical conditions rather than thinking about the patient before them.

Other barriers to learning in postgraduate training are well documented, including work commitments, financial costs of education, family commitments, lack of classes offered at convenient times, poor perception of the strengths and/or reputations of programmes of interest, length of time since prerequisite courses had been taken, the perception that going back to school means becoming a full-time student, and course work done in a foreign institution not being considered transferable [102]. While not specific to social accountability, their effects will affect student learning regardless of context.

Step 6: Concepts for Evaluating the Effectiveness of the Curriculum

Curriculum evaluation is a collection of activities to judge the effectiveness of a curriculum based on its early set goals and objectives [89]. This section considers the measurement of effectiveness through learner assessment as well as programme/curriculum evaluation. Social accountability within the curriculum can be measured by examining the extent to which it applies the four principles of social accountability during planning, implementation, and impact phases [2, 103]. Evaluation of the concept of social accountability is discussed in detail in the last part of this book; this section will highlight some of the concepts related to curriculum evaluation specifically.

Assessment of Learners

With respect to teaching and learning methods, it is crucial to plan an assessment system that complies with the principles of social accountability, cognisant that assessment drives learning [104]. The validity of a socially accountable curriculum is evidenced as the institution graduates a health workforce who respond to the health needs of the community; appropriate assessment methods will follow this principle [105]. Assessment systems and instruments should consider diversity alongside the four values of social accountability, both in making final judgement about students' progression and during the development of assessment content. For example, the same community representation and avoidance of bias should apply to the development of vignettes for written or clinical examination questions as is outlined in the section on clinical vignettes and case presentations in Step 4 above.

Curriculum Evaluation Frameworks

Many tools have been developed as curriculum evaluation frameworks and serve to benchmark how a curriculum is doing in terms of covering an issue or topic such as social accountability [106]. For example, Wood et al. (2022) and Larkin at al (2013) describe socially accountable frameworks that can be applied to health professions curricula [107, 108]. Another tool is tailored to evaluate a problem-based learning curriculum [109]. The InspirE5 curriculum and evaluation framework provides a foundation for a standardised approach to describe or compare health humanities education in different contexts and across a range of health professions courses; this framework may be adapted around the world to progress health humanities education [110].

Other techniques to develop socially accountable educational practices include Boelen and Heck's (1995) 'planning, doing, impacting' framework [2], also known as the WHO Social Accountability Grid, the CARE model (clinical activity, advocacy, research, education and training) [111], the AIDER model (assess, inquire, deliver, educate, respond) [112], Preston et al's (2016) 'building blocks' framework, which centres on situational elements encompassing the local health system, workforce, and community partners, and the DISCuSS model, which emphasises community engagement as a core step in curriculum development [113]. Accordingly, mapping community needs is an established technique to determine a curriculum. Kelly et al. 2022, presented and example of community health needs with the curriculum content, namely the PBL scenario to make them more socially accountable. Community needs assessments for curriculum development have been previously carried out [114] but the work by Kelly and colleagues is the first application of the combination of techniques of a PBL-specific social accountability inventory together with mapping of local context [115].

Curriculum developers can select the most appropriate tool/model to use, according to their curriculum context. As with every step in the curriculum development process, it is crucial to involve stakeholders in curriculum evaluation as partners in the selection, planning, and implementation of the evaluation. One of the important steps in curriculum evaluation is the development of the evaluation questions. Yazdani et al. (2019) have identified some points to be considered in curriculum evaluation in social accountability, such as the presence of needs assessment in setting the curriculum goal, the presence of field training for students, and the relation of student assessment to the expected role of future doctors [116]. Of course, ethical considerations related to confidentiality are required and appropriate procedures to collect and manage data, such as consent, should be in place. Those ethical deliberations need to be part of the evaluation planning discussions.

Take-Home Messages

The challenge for educators is to continuously evolve the curriculum to meet the changing needs of society and, as such, to be socially accountable.

Integrating social accountability into the curriculum for health professions education requires deliberate reflection by faculty, and we have outlined strategies that can facilitate this reflection, including general needs assessment, learner needs assessment, goal setting, and curriculum evaluation techniques. It is important that curriculum content is based on up-to-date information.

We have outlined teaching and assessment activities that may be useful for educators, whether they are overhauling a curriculum or altering or adding components to their existing curriculum.

Any curriculum change also involves investing in relationships with community partners, procuring resources, and leveraging leadership to overcome barriers to change. There is a need to fund and develop health professions educators who can be leaders and role models in the area of social accountability.

Although each institution's approach to addressing health inequalities and social accountability will be defined and designed locally depending on the circumstances, hopefully the case studies in this chapter offer some key learning points for educators to consider.

References

1. Tanner D, Tanner LN. Curriculum development: theory into practice. Macmillan; Collier-Macmillan; 1975.
2. Boelen C, Heck JE, Organization WH. Defining and measuring the social accountability of medical schools. World Health Organization; 1995.
3. Green-Thompson LP, McInerney P, Woollard B. The social accountability of doctors: a relationship based framework for understanding emergent community concepts of caring. BMC Health Serv Res. 2017;17:1–7.
4. Phelan SM, Dovidio JF, Puhl RM, Burgess DJ, Nelson DB, Yeazel MW, et al. Implicit and explicit weight bias in a national sample of 4,732 medical students: the medical student CHANGES study. Obesity. 2014;22(4):1201–8.
5. Ko M, Heslin KC, Edelstein RA, Grumbach K. The role of medical education in reducing health care disparities: the first ten years of the UCLA/drew medical education program. J Gen Intern Med. 2007;22:625–31.
6. Rabinowitz HK, Diamond JJ, Markham FW, Wortman JR. Medical school programs to increase the rural physician supply: a systematic review and projected impact of widespread replication. Acad Med. 2008;83(3):235–43.
7. Boelen C, Pearson D, Kaufman A, Rourke J, Woollard R, Marsh DC, et al. Producing a socially accountable medical school: AMEE guide no. 109. Med Teach. 2016;38(11):1078–91.
8. Abdalla M, Taha M, Mukhtar WNO, Elsanousi M. Impact of community-based medical education on graduate performance: a qualitative study using a critical incident technique. Health Prof Edu. 2022;8(1):38–44.

9. Strasser RP, Lanphear JH, McCready WG, Topps MH, Hunt DD, Matte MC. Canada's new medical school: the northern Ontario school of medicine: social accountability through distributed community engaged learning. Acad Med. 2009;84(10):1459–64.
10. Woolley T, Ross S, Larkins S, Sen Gupta T, Whaleboat D. "We learnt it, then we lived it": influencing medical students' intentions toward rural practice and generalist careers via a socially-accountable curriculum. Med Teach. 2021;43(1):93–100.
11. Abdalla ME, Boelen C, Osman WN. Development and evaluation of an online course about the social accountability of medical schools. J Taibah Univ Med Sci. 2019;14(3):241–5.
12. McCrea ML, Murdoch-Eaton D. How do undergraduate medical students perceive social accountability? Med Teach. 2014;36(10):867–75.
13. Kern DE, Thomas P, Hughes M. Curriculum development for medical education: a six-step approach. Baltimore, MD: The John's Hopkins University Press; 2016. p. 5–9.
14. Sciences NAo, Health BoG, Health CoEHPtAtSDo. A framework for educating health professionals to address the social determinants of health. 2016.
15. Marmot M, Wilkinson R. Social determinants of health: the solid facts. 2nd ed. Denmark: World Health Orgnization Regional Office for Europe; 2003.
16. Lewis JH, Lage OG, Grant BK, Rajasekaran SK, Gemeda M, Like RC, et al. Addressing the social determinants of health in undergraduate medical education curricula: a survey report. Adv Med Educ Pract. 2020;Volume 11:369–77.
17. Abdalla ME, Taha MH, Onchonga D, Magzoub ME, Au H, O'Donnell P, et al. Integrating the social determinants of health into curriculum: AMEE guide no. 162. Med Teach. 2024;46(3):304–16.
18. Frenk J, Chen L, Bhutta ZA, Cohen J, Crisp N, Evans T, et al. Health professionals for a new century: transforming education to strengthen health systems in an interdependent world. Lancet. 2010;376(9756):1923–58.
19. Tudor HJ. The inverse care law. Lancet. 1971;297(7696):405–12.
20. Prihatiningsih T, Kamal Y, Woollard R, Fisher JD, Abdalla Elhassan M, Boelen C. Social accountability and accreditation: impacting health system performance and population health. Soc Innov J. 2020:3.
21. Oriokot L, Rujumba J, Munabi IG, Mubuuke AG, Kiguli S. Implementation of social accountability in undergraduate medical training at a sub-Saharan African medical school: stakeholders' perspectives. Edu Health. 2024;37(1):30–8.
22. Freitas Â, Santana P, Oliveira MD, Almendra R, Bana e Costa JC, Bana e Costa CA. Indicators for evaluating European population health: a Delphi selection process. BMC Public Health. 2018;18:1–20.
23. Costa C, Santana P, Dimitroulopoulou S, Burstrom B, Borrell C, Schweikart J, et al. Population health inequalities across and within European metropolitan areas through the lens of the EURO-HEALTHY population health index. Int J Environ Res Public Health. 2019;16(5):836.
24. Shandera WX. The bottom quartile for health indices in America vs Europe. J Infect Public Health. 2014;7(5):420–6.
25. Murray ET, Shelton N, Norman P, Head J. Measuring the health of people in places: a scoping review of OECD member countries. Health Place. 2022;73:102731.
26. Eurostat. Weekly death statistics 2024. Available from: https://ec.europa.eu/eurostat/statistics-explained/index.php?title=Weekly_death_statistics&stable.
27. Fitch B. The changing picture of long-term international migration, England and Wales: Census 2021. Office for National Statistics. 2023.
28. El-Naggar MM, Ageely H, Salih MA, Dawoud H, Milaat WA. Developing an integrated organ/system curriculum with community-orientation for a new medical college in Jazan, Saudi Arabia. J Fam Community Med. 2007;14(3):127–36.
29. Monrouxe LV. Identity, identification and medical education: why should we care? Med Educ. 2010;44(1):40–9.

30. Cruess RL, Cruess SR, Boudreau JD, Snell L, Steinert Y. Reframing medical education to support professional identity formation. Acad Med. 2014;89(11):1446–51.
31. Norman GR, Shannon SI, Marrin ML. The need for needs assessment in continuing medical education. BMJ. 2004;328(7446):999–1001.
32. Gonsalves CL, Ajjawi R, Rodger M, Varpio L. A novel approach to needs assessment in curriculum development: going beyond consensus methods. Med Teach. 2014;36(5):422–9.
33. Galukande M, Nakasujja N, Sewankambo NK. Social accountability: a survey of perceptions and evidence of its expression at a sub Saharan African university. BMC Med Educ. 2012;12(1):96.
34. Oudbier J, Boerboom T, Peerdeman S, Suurmond J. How do educational staff and students in a medical school perceive social accountability? A multi-perspective qualitative interview study. Edu Health. 2024;37(1):20–9.
35. Reddy AT, Lazreg SA, Phillips RL Jr, Bazemore AW, Lucan SC. Toward defining and measuring social accountability in graduate medical education: a stakeholder study. J Grad Med Educ. 2013;5(3):439–45.
36. Green AR, Chun MB, Cervantes MC, Nudel JD, Duong JV, Krupat E, et al. Measuring medical students' preparedness and skills to provide cross-cultural care. Health Equity. 2017;1(1):15–22.
37. O'Brien L, Wassall N, Cadoret D, Petrović A, O'Donnell P, Neville S. Perceptions of and preparedness for cross-cultural care: a survey of final-year medical students in Ireland. BMC Med Educ. 2024;24(1):472.
38. Hundey B, Gonzalez A. Conducting focus groups for curriculum review and improvement. 2019. Available from: https://teaching.uwo.ca/pdf/curriculum/Focus-Group-Guide-for-Curriculum-Review-Guide-1.pdf.
39. Satran L, Harris IB, Allen S, Anderson DC, Poland GA, Miller WL. Hospital-based versus community-based clinical education: comparing performances and course evaluations by students in their second-year pediatrics rotation. Acad Med. 1993;68(5):380–2.
40. Grant J. Learning needs assessment: assessing the need. BMJ (Clinical research ed). 2002;324(7330):156–9.
41. DeSilets LD. Needs assessments: an array of possibilities. J Cont Edu Nursing. 2007;38(3):107–12.
42. Boyle FA, Buchanan FM, Ritchie D, Gamage KA. A collaborative curriculum: navigating the risks and rewards of staff-student partnership in curriculum design. Edu Sci. 2023;14
43. Strasser R. Community engagement: a key to successful rural clinical education. Int Elec J Rural Remote Health Res, Edu, Pract Policy. 2010;10:1543.
44. Global Consensus for Social Accountability of Medical Schools. Global consensus for social accountability of medical schools. Canada: Global Consensus for Social Accountability of Medical Schools; 2010.
45. Naidu C, Reid S, Burch V. Development of a CanMEDS-based instrument for evaluating medical students' perceptions of the key competencies of a socially accountable healthcare practitioner. Perspect Med Edu. 2020;9(2):98–106.
46. United Arab Emirates Ministry of Education. Competency framework for medical education EmiratesMEDs. Dubai: United Arab Emirates Ministry of Education; 2022.
47. Strasser R, Kam SM, Regalado SM. Rural health care access and policy in developing countries. Annu Rev Public Health. 2016;37:395–412.
48. Clithero-Eridon A, Albright D, Ross A. Conceptualising social accountability as an attribute of medical education. Afr J Prim Health Care Fam Med. 2020;12(1):e1–8.
49. Boelen C. Why should social accountability be a benchmark for excellence in medical education? Educación Médica. 2016;17(3):101–5.
50. Preston R, Larkins S, Taylor J, Judd J. From personal to global: understandings of social accountability from stakeholders at four medical schools. Med Teach. 2016;38(10):987–94.
51. Bartoletta KM, Starr SR. Health systems science. Adv Pediatr. 2021;68:1–19.

52. Boelen C, Dharamsi S, Gibbs T. The social accountability of medical schools and its indicators. Edu Health. 2012;25(3):180–94.
53. Boelen C, Woollard B. Social accountability and accreditation: a new frontier for educational institutions. Med Educ. 2009;43(9):887–94.
54. Bruner JS. The process of education. Harvard University Press; 2009.
55. Harden RM. What is a spiral curriculum? Med Teach. 1999;21(2):141–3.
56. Efland AD. The spiral and the lattice: changes in cognitive learning theory with implications for art education. Stud Art Educ. 1995;36(3):134–53.
57. Lawrence C, Mhlaba T, Stewart KA, Moletsane R, Gaede B, Moshabela M. The hidden curricula of medical education: a scoping review. Acad Med. 2018;93(4):648–56.
58. Guignona M, Halili S, Cristobal F, Woolley T, Reeve C, Ross SJ, et al. A curriculum for achieving universal health care: a case study of Ateneo de Zamboanga university School of Medicine. Front Public Health. 2021;9:612035.
59. Preston R, Larkins S, Taylor J, Judd J. Building blocks for social accountability: a conceptual framework to guide medical schools. BMC Med Educ. 2016;16(1):227.
60. Barber C, van der Vleuten C, Leppink J, Chahine S. Social accountability frameworks and their implications for medical education and program evaluation: a narrative review. Acad Med. 2020;Sep;95:1945–54.
61. Prideaux D. The global–local tension in medical education: turning 'think global, act local'on its head? Med Educ. 2019;53(1):25–31.
62. Puschel K, Riquelme A, Sapag J, Moore P, Díaz LA, Fuentes-López E, et al. Academic excellence in Latin America: social accountability of medical schools. Med Teach. 2020;42(8):929–36.
63. Bhutta ZA, Chen L, Cohen J, Crisp N, Evans T, Fineberg H, et al. Education of health professionals for the 21st century: a global independent commission. Lancet. 2010;375(9721):1137–8.
64. Abdul-Salam P, Richardson C, Nazar H. Undergraduate pharmacy students' perceptions and experiences of a student-led clinic providing preventative services. Int J Pharm Pract. 2024;32:riae023–321.
65. Mirghani O, El Amin E, Ali M, Osman H, Hamad B. A combined course of primary health care practice and family medicine at the university of Gezira. Med Educ. 1988;22(4):314–6.
66. O'Regan A, O'Doherty J, Green J, Hyde S. Symbiotic relationships through longitudinal integrated clerkships in general practice. BMC Med Educ. 2022;22(1):64.
67. Savin Baden M, Wilkie K. Challenging research in problem-based learning. McGraw-Hill Education (UK); 2004.
68. Schmidt HG. Problem-based learning: rationale and description. Med Educ. 1983;17(1):11–6.
69. MacLeod A. Six ways problem-based learning cases can sabotage patient-centered medical education. Acad Med. 2011;86(7):818–25.
70. Hough L. Hegazi I, vol. 7. Challenging the hidden curriculum through problem based learning: a reflection on curricular design: MedEdPublish; 2018. p. 7.
71. Woodward CA, Ferrier BM. The content of the medical curriculum at McMaster University: graduates' evaluation of their preparation for postgraduate training. Med Educ. 1983;17(1):54–60.
72. Azer SA, Peterson R, Guerrero AP, Edgren G. Twelve tips for constructing problem-based learning cases. Med Teach. 2012;34(5):361–7.
73. Sockalingam N, Rotgans J, Schmidt HG. Student and tutor perceptions on attributes of effective problems in problem-based learning. High Educ. 2011;62(1):1–16.
74. Marchais JED. A Delphi technique to identify and evaluate criteria for construction of PBL problems. Med Educ. 1999;33(7):504–8.
75. Kenny NP, Beagan BL. The patient as text: a challenge for problem-based learning. Med Educ. 2004;38(10):1071–9.
76. Little P, Everitt H, Williamson I, Warner G, Moore M, Gould C, et al. Observational study of effect of patient centredness and positive approach on outcomes of general practice consultations. BMJ. 2001;323(7318):908–11.

77. Majumder AA. Review of PBL'PROBLEMS' and examination questions. Med Teach. 2005;27(5):474.
78. Metsemaker JF, Bouhuisj PA, Snellen-Balendong HA. Do we teach what we preach? Comparing the content of a problem-based medical curriculum with primary health care data. Fam Pract. 1991;8(3):195–201.
79. Finucane P, Nair B. Is there a problem with the problems in problem-based learning? Med Educ. 2002;36(3):279–81.
80. VanLeit B, Cubra J. Student-developed problem-based learning cases: preparing for rural healthcare practice. Educ Health (Abingdon). 2005;18(3):416–26.
81. Phillips SP. Problem-based learning in medicine: new curriculum, old stereotypes. Soc Sci Med. 1997;45(3):497–9.
82. Hoffman BL, Hoffman R, Wessel CB, Shensa A, Woods MS, Primack BA. Use of fictional medical television in health sciences education: a systematic review. Adv Health Sci Educ. 2018;23:201–16.
83. Hoffman BL, Sidani JE, Jonassaint CR, Wolynn R, Donovan AK. Utilizing television clips for graduate medical education anti-racist curricula: an acceptability study. Cureus. 2023;15(7):e41526.
84. Bartlett R, Jøranson N, Breievne G. Using documentary films to teach nurses about gender and the vulnerabilities facing older men with advanced dementia. J Clin Nurs. 2022;31(13–14):1817–25.
85. Baminiwatta A, Fernando R, Williams S. Improving medical students' understanding of dementia using a movie (the father). Education for Primary Care. 2023;34(2):109.
86. Klein M, Beck A, Kahn R, Henize A, O'Toole J, Alcamo A, et al. Video curriculum on screening for the social determinants of health. MedEdPORTAL. 2013;9:9575.
87. Meili R, Fuller D, Lydiate J. Teaching social accountability by making the links: qualitative evaluation of student experiences in a service-learning project. Med Teach. 2011;33(8):659–66.
88. Winkel AF, Yingling S, Jones A-A, Nicholson J. Reflection as a learning tool in graduate medical education: a systematic review. J Grad Med Educ. 2017;9(4):430–9.
89. Mihan A, Muldoon L, Leider H, Tehfe H, Fitzgerald M, Fournier K, et al. Social accountability in undergraduate medical education: a narrative review. Education for Health. 2022;35(1):3–8.
90. Demirören M, Atılgan B. Impacts of service learning-based social responsibility training on medical students. Adv Physiol Educ. 2023;47(2):166–74.
91. Mitra G, Gowans M, Wright B, Brenneis F, Scott I. Predictors of rural family medicine practice in Canada. Can Fam Physician. 2018;64(8):588–96.
92. Real FJ, Michelson CD, Beck AF, Klein MD. Location, location, location: teaching about neighborhoods in pediatrics. Acad Pediatr. 2017;17(3):228–32.
93. Clithero-Eridon A, Albright D, Ross A, Crandall C, Contribution of the Nelson R. Mandela School of Medicine to a socially accountable health workforce. African Journal of Primary Health Care and Family Medicine. 2019;11(1):1–7.
94. Clithero-Eridon A, Crandall C, Ross A. Future medical student practice intentions: the South Africa experience. BMC Med Educ. 2020;20:1–8.
95. Yengo-Kahn AMMB, Courtney E, Lomis, Kimberly D. Medical students' perspectives on implementing curriculum change at one institution. Acad Med. 2017;92(4):455–61.
96. Sklar DP. Implementing curriculum change: choosing strategies, overcoming resistance, and embracing values. Acad Med. 2018;93(10):1417–9.
97. Markham R, Hunt M, Woollard R, Oelke N, Snadden D, Strasser R, et al. Addressing rural and indigenous health inequities in Canada through socially accountable health partnerships. BMJ Open. 2021;11(11):e048053.
98. Sidebotham M, Walters C, Chipperfield J, Gamble J. Midwifery participatory curriculum development: transformation through active partnership. Nurse Educ Pract. 2017;25:5–13.

99. Elsanousi SEM, Khalafallah O, Habour A. Assessment of the social accountability of the faculty of medicine at University of Gezira. Sudan Eastern Mediterranean Health Journal. 2016;22(4):258–66.
100. Strasser R, Hogenbirk JC, Minore B, Marsh DC, Berry S, McCready WG, et al. Transforming health professional education through social accountability: Canada's northern Ontario school of medicine. Med Teach. 2013;35(6):490–6.
101. Ross BM, Cervin C. Northern Ontario school of medicine. Acad Med. 2020;95(9S):S588–S91.
102. Landry LG, Orsolini-Hain L, Renwanz-Boyle A, Alameida M, Holpit L. The nursing educational highway in action: results of a needs assessment and the formation of a collaborative workgroup. Nurs Educ Perspect. 2012;33(4):274–7.
103. Leinster S. Evaluation and assessment of social accountability in medical schools. Med Teach. 2011;33(8):673–6.
104. Fischer J, Bearman M, Boud D, Tai J. How does assessment drive learning? A focus on students' development of evaluative judgement. Assess Eval High Educ. 2024;49(2):233–45.
105. Abdalla ME. Assessment: social accountability and the society. In: Written assessment in medical education. Springer; 2023. p. 169–74.
106. Bates J, Schrewe B, Ellaway RH, Teunissen PW, Watling C. Embracing standardisation and contextualisation in medical education. Med Educ. 2019;53(1):15–24.
107. Wood B, Attema G, Ross B, Cameron E. A conceptual framework to describe and evaluate a socially accountable learning health system: development and application in a northern, rural, and remote setting. Int J Health Plann Manag. 2022;37(Suppl 1):59–78.
108. Larkins SL, Preston R, Matte MC, Lindemann IC, Samson R, Tandinco FD, et al. Measuring social accountability in health professional education: development and international pilot testing of an evaluation framework. Med Teach. 2013;35(1):32–45.
109. Abdalla ME, Dash N, Shorbagi S, Taha MH. Development and validation of inventory tool to evaluate social accountability principles in case scenarios used in problem-based curriculum (social accountability inventory for PBL). Med Educ Online. 2020;26(1):1847243.
110. Carr SE, Harris A, Scott K, Ani-Amponsah M, Hooker C, Phillips B, et al. InspirE5: a participatory, internationally informed framework for health humanities curricula in health professions education. BMC Med Educ. 2022;22(1):490.
111. Meili R, Ganem-Cuenca A, Leung JW-S, Zaleschuk D. The CARE model of social accountability: promoting cultural change. Acad Med. 2011;86(9):1114–9.
112. Sandhu G, Garcha I, Sleeth J, Yeates K, Walker GR. AIDER: a model for social accountability in medical education and practice. Med Teach. 2013;35(8):e1403–e8.
113. Goez H, Lai H, Rodger J, Brett-MacLean P, Hillier T. The DISCuSS model: creating connections between community and curriculum—a new lens for curricular development in support of social accountability. Med Teach. 2020;42(9):1058–64.
114. Karimi S, Zohoorparvandeh V. Need assessment of the general Practitioner's curriculum based on clinical activities, advocacy, research, and education (CARE) model. Future of Medical Education Journal. 2019;9(1):18–24.
115. Kelly D, Hyde S, Abdalla ME. Mapping health, social and health system issues and applying a social accountability inventory to a problem based learning medical curriculum. Med Educ Online. 2022;27(1):2016243.
116. Yazdani S, Akbarilakeh M, Abdalla ME, Charles B, Arbabisarjou A, Moonaghi HK. Measuring social accountability of medical universities' education function-design, development, and validation of instrument. J Evol Med Dent Sci. 2019;8(26):2110–4.

Chapter 11
Longitudinal Clerkships to Promote Social Accountability

Sarah Strasser and Andrew O'Regan

Learning Outcomes

1. Describe the history of LICs and their natural fit for SA.
2. Outline the transformation in medical education with LICs.
3. Describe how to develop, implement and maintain LICs with SA.
4. Outline the potential benefits, opportunities and challenges.
5. Identify areas for further related research and development.

Introduction to Socially Accountable LICs

LICs are "characterized by being the central element of clinical education whereby medical students:

1. participate in the comprehensive care of patients over time,
2. participate in continuing learning relationships with these patients' clinicians,
3. meet most of the year's core clinical competencies, across multiple disciplines simultaneously through these experiences" [1].

LICs have evolved over 50 years, since the original Rural Physician Associates Program. Initially introduced as a workforce initiative in rural and general practice settings, LICs have demonstrated educational and professional benefits for learners [2, 3]. Now LICs can be found in a variety of clinical settings, both rural and urban,

S. Strasser (✉)
University of Waikato, Hamilton, New Zealand
e-mail: sarah.strasser@waikato.ac.nz

A. O'Regan
University of Limerick, Limerick, Ireland

M. E. Abdalla et al. (eds.), *Social Accountability of Medical Schools*,
https://doi.org/10.1007/978-3-031-94435-2_11

where context and continuity are underpinning principles to the LIC experience for all involved [4]. LICs could transform medical education from the traditional clinical clerkships in teaching hospital block rotations [5, 6].

Clinical aspects of medicine have evolved beyond the individual doctor-patient relationship to include the influence of families, carers and populations, with medical curricula adapting to reflect population health and well-being. Medical schools have moved from being purely academic-clinical institutions to being more SA-oriented. This is reflected in their programmes of education, research and their collaboration with clinical services. Accreditation criteria, funding conditions, requirements for research grant proposals are adapted to reflect SA which contributes to the institution's national and international standing. When SA is a high priority for medical schools and universities it is usually referred to in the vision, mission and values statements [7].

These changes have occurred against the backdrop of community connectedness and societal expectations to be more inclusive. LICs where learners live, work and study with their teachers and local community, provide the opportunities for all these interests to be comprehensively included and to provide opportunities for development, through the daily activities, within a guided, relationship-based experience.

What Does Success Look like? LIC Outcomes

Research reports the potential of LICs to mould socially accountable doctors for the future—doctors that deliver high quality care based on a lived understanding of the communities they serve and who advocate for cost effective and equitable health care for all [8]. To be successful, LICs require well-supported teachers, well-supported learners and a well-supported community. In addition, a well-resourced curriculum, aligned selection and assessment criteria and evaluation processes that are co-created, co-designed, co-delivered and co-evaluated by the local community makes for a more readily sustainable program.

In a LIC, these principles come together naturally as it becomes more established; the LIC becomes a devolved, interdependent true partnership with members of the local community providing the leadership for the program. This involves maximising the use of local resources; having the various roles clearly defined; and, with excellent communication keeping everybody well-informed, while the LIC is supported by external agencies and the academic institution. The principle of "nothing about us, without us" means the external players have roles as facilitators rather than leaders, and the community takes on distributed local leadership roles aligned with their strengths and expertise. Research in the LICs has identified an additional socio-economic benefit for the communities with an LIC, where the community is found to be better engaged and has a sense of community empowerment [9, 10]. Text Box 11.1 outlines the expected outcomes at the end of the LIC year for all stakeholders (from a partnership pentagram perspective).

Text Box 11.1 The Expected Outcomes at the End of the LIC Year for All Stakeholders (from a Partnership Pentagram Perspective)
The expected outcomes for the learners at the end of the LIC year:

- They have mastered the key learning objectives set for that clinical year (this is the basis of comparison with their peers in block rotations).
- LIC learners in general practice settings are inspired to be generalists or generalist specialists in community settings (the LIC helps to develop their professional identity formation).
- They can identify the key benefits of long-term relationships for patients and their families with a clinician over time. By seeing patients who are at different stages of an illness and understand the longer-term impact these may have on an individual and the community.
- They think beyond the diagnosis and consider the longer-term consequences of poor health. They may be able to bring their first-hand knowledge and these understandings into their clinical management with patients and within the health care team.
- They have the knowledge and skills, confidence and competence, more than the specified minimum core learning outcomes, having developed a SA-orientation.
- They have a better understanding of the whole health system and how it works together.
- They develop clinical acumen and appreciate the value of supporting patients to master their own control over their illness, health and Well-being in their context.
- They understand the population includes not only the patients they see in the clinical setting but also those living in the community who they do not see in the clinical setting.
- They have a broad experience and first-hand knowledge of the social determinants of health and how the health system works and does not work, to meet the health needs of the community.
- They may have ability to identify the community determined priorities of health needs and the experience of working with community members to address these needs from their research project and portfolio activities.
- They have experienced being in a health care team and value team-based care.
- They have a better understanding of themselves, their leadership and collaboration skills and their own limitations.
- They learn to be resourceful in under resourced settings and increase their confidence and competence in their own ability to live and work in such settings.
- They are well prepared for their next level of learning.

The expected outcomes for the community at the end of the LIC year:

- Individual community members value having learners as "their student doctor" to advocate for them as well as improving their health literacy.
- Collectively, community members gain esteem from contributing to educating future potential health care providers and see the program as a source for recruitment and retention, and so, see the program as a future supply of health professionals.
- Communities contribute to promoting and supporting youth to learn about health and the range of health careers in high school.
- Communities are recognised for helping learners see the social determinants of health at the local level; they benefit from the outcomes of the learner's community engaged research projects/ academic activities (this increases as these projects become more community determined and continued by successive learners).
- Communities contribute to the identity formation by learners.
- Communities may have a role in responding to particular social and personal needs of LIC learners, teachers and their families.
- The LIC opens opportunities that wouldn't be there otherwise, e.g., higher education, capital grants, employment and being part of the research enterprise.
- Financial and social development with funding and empowerment leading to collective self-importance of the community.

The expected research outcomes at the end of the LIC year:

- The research dimension builds capacity and capabilities for all of the above -learners, clinical teachers and community.
- Research in, by and for the community focussed on improving the health outcomes at the community level.
- Learners, clinical teachers and community members learning research skills and being part of the research enterprise.

The expected outcomes of the health service i.e. a Centre or practice in the community and hospital (including administrative staff) providing inpatient care with involvement of the community, at the end of the LIC year:

- Affirmation of the importance of the health care service to the community, the rewards and satisfaction of addressing the health care needs of the community leads to a more stable workforce connected to the community providing learning, teaching and research for the community, enhances quality and effectiveness of service.**The expected outcomes of the academic institution at the end of the LIC year:**

- Learners and clinical teachers are top performing and are undertaking community level research, clinical teachers are proud to be associated with the academic institution and contribute to curriculum development, management etc.

- Higher level of standing amongst their peers as being community connected and engaged.
- They are regarded as more relevant by funders, policy makers and potential applicants who see the LIC as being more personalised and relevant.
- Other programs may take the lead from the example of the LIC to become more community engaged.**The expected outcomes for policy makers at the end of the LIC year:**

- The LIC provides a local connection, this grass roots basis contributes to policy that is more socially accountable, responding to people in community settings, is more effective and efficient.**The expected outcomes for profit/ not-for-profit organisations (NGOs) in the community at the end of the LIC year**

- Economic benefits and rewards of economic development.
- Contributions to the LIC, learners learning and being seen to be part of the community.
- More sustainable with access to a health service

Implementation: Starting or Transitioning to an LIC with SA

Success and sustainability of the LIC as a whole programme hinges on providing an optimal learning environment (formal and informal) and the following are required factors for implementation:

- Selection
- Well supported clinical teachers, learners and community
- Well-resourced curriculum in place
- Assessment
- Evaluation

Selection

Selection of learner, clinical teachers and community are all interrelated and it is essential that selection processes are focussed on SA accountability and the expected outcomes. The more involved community members are in establishing the LIC, the more likely the LIC will become sustainable over the years. Communities are often able to take on challenges that might be overwhelming for clinicians such as finding housing and transport for learners. This type of community engagement and empowerment is variably taken up by medical schools and may be more likely to occur at the local LIC level because of established long-term relationships.

Starting a LIC requires a local champion who is enthusiastic about the concept of LICs and medical education generally. Ideally, they will be well established in a generalist clinical practice. The patient population the practice serves needs to be of sufficient numbers and case mix to ensure learners will have a large enough throughput of patients over the period of the LIC to meet the clinical learning objectives. LIC sites should have clinical space and facilities that accommodate using the parallel consulting model where the learner and clinical teacher both have their own consultation rooms and access to procedural facilities plus internet.

The clinical lead (clerkship co-ordinator) should be respected by their peers and bring other clinical teachers (interprofessional) as a team of local teachers willing to teach and support learners in their practices. They will need an in-depth knowledge of their practice and support from their practice and community with protected time for teaching and administrative duties, including time away from the practice to visit the medical school, and a willingness to be available for LIC business both in and out of clinic hours; it is not a 9–5 job, 5 days a week! Teaching and administration of the LIC needs to be recognised as equivalent to clinical service time.

The local community must be engaged early in the process and be willing to support learners in the community. Civic leaders should be prepared to support and advocate for the program. They might have roles within the community as leaders in local organisations themselves. A hospital in the community is not essential but at least having one nearby which provides a service for this community, so that learners will get a full range of clinical environments from their patient interactions with the local and distant health care delivery services. Learners following patients on their allocated panel of patients may include referrals involving visits to tertiary teaching facilities. Administration in both practice and hospital settings should have a willingness to support learners on site in the first place and also to teach about health services administration and take on responsibilities for learner wellness. This will help the learners appreciate how the health system works and the relationships between each health care service delivery organisation, the patients, the community and their funders that make it a viable, supportive and sustainable network of interdependent practitioners at the local, community level.

It is a whole community commitment to train health professionals, "it takes a village to train a doctor", and full orientation, onboarding, induction and training about the LIC for the team will take time. An absolute criterion for the champion is that they are able communicators and adept at keeping everyone well informed about the LIC and what is happening when. The longitudinal nature of the LIC provides sufficient length of time to develop trustful interdependent relationships and partnerships as described in the symbiosis model of the LIC, as illustrated by Worley's Symbiotic Model [4] or Boelen's Partnership Pentagram [11]. The LIC ethos is about continuity of relationships with whole person care for the patient and family, and about the whole learner, rather than episodic patient centred (or visit centred, transactional) care with the corollary focus on the whole wellbeing of the learner. This can be considered the foundation for SA of clinicians in health professional education.

A local administrator is essential for LIC implementation, someone who not only works well with the clinician lead but also cares about the learners and the program. The person must be committed to keeping everyone well informed and feeling valued. Such a person, ideally also well known within the community, is savvy to the needs of the teachers, learners and community, who knows who to go to for help when required without feeling over or under whelmed by the task. A key characteristic is that learners feel that this person is approachable and available to them, providing an invaluable resource and insightful practical help.

Selection of Learners. Many LICs, rural or urban, are established for the entire class to undertake a LIC where they are immersed in a community to live, work and study during the first core year of clinical training. Some schools have provided LICs for additional years and some the whole full length of education and training as a health professional (undergraduate and postgraduate). Mechanisms that provide learners opportunities to hear from previous students as to what the experience is like, covering both the clinical and social aspects are invaluable. Preparation during the earlier years with opportunities to meet clinical teachers, establishing core clinical skills and experiences with patients in clinical settings is beneficial. The selection process should involve community groups. Forward planning, where a continuum of education and training exists for medical specialties that are needed in a particular region, will ensure better transitions for learners as they progress from medical student to postgraduate training roles, while remaining in the region. Desired healthcare workforce outcomes, e.g., need for rural family medicine physicians, rural generalists, and generalist specialists, should be explicitly included into the design of a LIC [12]. Opportunities for higher training and academic qualifications should be available so that they become highly skilled clinicians and/or clinical academics, as well as clinical teachers and members of faculty, and that in time they contribute to the selection process.

Text Box 11.2 Summary of Key Selection Considerations
Clinical teachers and clinical site attributes for selection:

- Community-orientation—clinical teachers should have a history of close collaboration with community groups and be respected by their own peers.
- Learning environment—Clinical sites should create an atmosphere conducive to questioning, reflection and shared understanding.
- Exposure—Essential for all learning on LICs is that the clinical teacher and clinical site facilitate learner experience a diverse patient population.
- Openness to evaluation—Sustainability on LICs hinges on regular and frequent interaction between clinical teachers and faculty, including site visits and responding to feedback from learners.
- Commitment to education—Clinical teachers should be willing to attend orientation, curriculum and assessment days and to upskill.
- All personnel at the clinical site, including clinical staff, other clinical teacher(s) and non-clinical, administrative staff must work to ensure stu-

dents are integrated into a community of practice and co-operate with the clinical tutor to facilitate handing increased responsibility to the learner.**Learners' attributes for selection**

- Social determinants of health—learners should have interest in and appreciation of social determinants of health.
- Independent learners- learners should be willing and capable of learning independently and to be able to reach educational outcomes without direct faculty input.
- Community-orientated—learners should demonstrate prior interest and experience in working with communities relevant to the LIC.
- Responsive to feedback—Learners should be open to feedback from clinical teachers and community groups with which they will engage.
- Alignment with career plan—future career interests of learners should align with generalist or generalist-specialist occupations.
- Team players—learners should be able to work with teams, both interdisciplinary healthcare teams and as part of peer learning groups.

Well Supported Learners, Teachers and Community

Being well-supported involves targeting personal preferences to make it more meaningful and will result in an improved learning environment to live, work and learn. This will promote recruitment, retention and potential return in the longer term. Ideally the LIC sites should have supports that would normally be found on the university main campus, such as academic support, financial support and health care services i.e. not left to the local clinical team, except for in emergent, urgent and important issues, in particular access to mental health and wellness support. Table 11.1: What Well Supported Looks Like outlines the key areas to consider for support.

Mechanisms must be in place prior to the flagging of problems. The relationship between learners and teachers is more intense in an LIC, and behaviours and attitudes come to light over time. Many LICs have found it beneficial to send learners into LICs in pairs; this not only reduces isolation of learners but also reduces workload on the clinical teachers, as working in pairs allows them to bounce ideas between themselves before escalating the issue to their clinical teacher. Learners are often the first to be aware of any problems being experienced by their peers and they need to know who and how to get help on an urgent, immediate basis when needed. As part of the hand over from 1 year to the next, the individual learners experience in the early years needs to be made available to the LIC director so that the best support can be made available in advance, whether it is academic, health, mental, social or professionally related. Most schools will have well-recognised services available for learners or another identified person who is not involved in assessment of learners, accessible if needed.

Table 11.1 What well supported looks like

What you will see as an outcome of being well-supported: a well connected, continuing LIC community		
Learner—Willingness to undertake an LIC, to live, work and study in the community. A pro-active learner.	**Clinical teacher**- Support for the LIC within the community & academic institution. A fully engaged educator who actively seeks academic progression.	**Community**—Defined and supporting the LIC learners, teachers and health care delivery services & staff. Sustained delivery of LIC.
What support is required:		
• Housing accommodation in the community suitable for learners and adaptable for individuals or families. (house rules clearly stated), • Suitable accommodation for study (clinical & home). • Access to full student services as available on main university campus, on-line or within the community, independent of learner progression. • Connectivity to other students—Main campus or distributed. • Family connections supported. • "Who are you going to call if…worse case scenarios" • Welcomed into the community and clinicians' lives.	• Flexible position description to meet individual needs; allocation of dedicated time sufficient to be able to do the job. • Support roles provided: Admin, research, faculty development and HR services. • Access to university resources: Library and academic mentoring. • Pre- negotiated recognition of work, time & timings of meetings as equivalent to providing clinical services by colleagues, staff and practice; (vice versa with LIC and academic institution.	• Recognised as being the experts in their own local context of themselves and their community. • Development of respectful, trustworthy relationships; listened to, heard and followed up. • Support for active community involvement in the LIC, including equal payments for work done/ time out of regular work (known process reviewed on a regular basis), in particular selection and evaluation. • Included in the decision making of the LIC. • Being well informed about the LIC: Who's who, what they do and when. • Presentations back to the community are developed according to how the community would like to receive them. "Nothing about us, without us". • Debunking the notion of academic institutions as being "an ivory tower"; instead seen as providing answers to questions that make a difference for the better; providing access to resources they would not otherwise have.

(continued)

Table 11.1 (continued)

What you will see as an outcome of being well-supported: a well connected, continuing LIC community		
As a result, when asked, they will be able to report that they are well-supported with evidence from their experience of LIC initiatives:		
• Informed beforehand about community (demographics, communication, transport, food access, social & religious/ belief systems, access to finances), clinical setting, accommodation. • Well prepared from learning activities/ events in preceding years of education & training to be useful in clinical practice. • Opportunity to meet supervisor beforehand & visit the community; information about the practice itself & other health care services in the community, referral patterns, particular interests of supervisor & other teachers. • Clinical—understand and know what to expect: Curriculum in place including information on portfolio requirements, research projects & assessment/ progress. Information about additional learning opportunities. • Knows who to go to, to ask for assistance • Well prepared for their next stage in learning. • Engage in community life/ develop an interest and willingness to investigate public health, patient / community interests in health & wellness. • Notice things that matter ("outside eyes") or from a long-standing connection or personal interest to help the community consider issues that could lead to a preferred future. • Identify the research project of interest through individual or group activity i.e. dialogue with supervisors, patients & community contacts • Willingness to get involved in extra- curricular activities in the community- e.g. engage with school children/ youth in teaching/ sporting activities or support them; engage in other health & wellness initiatives for specific groups of people eg elderly, men's health groups, walking groups etc. • Discuss clinical management and compare/contrast how SDH may impact outcomes, share experiences with colleagues. • Pick up/ follow on from ideas already developed within the community leading to local community driven issues for research project.	• Well informed about the whole LIC program and know how their contribution fits into the whole. • Understand the benefits of teaching/learning to improve clinical practice, teaching & job satisfaction-communicate this to colleagues –bring them along to establish a network or community of practice. • Role model professional and clinical identity & life in this community. • Introduce learner to practice & health care services in the community & the practitioners (& v.v.) • Include learners in your normal daily life/ home; if not yourself identify a 'go-to' person who will holistically care for the students • Include learner in active learning (develop learning plans together) & follow up areas of interest/challenges. • Identify a patient panel of people who intersect with the health sector often or who meet learners' particular interest/needs. • Raise issues from clinical practice & community with learner that might be of interest to them in developing their project while on the LIC. • Share & celebrate LIC with senior/other clinical & academic colleagues to raise level of awareness to (work service learning in place) learning in community settings benefits & challenges, write up experience & attend conferences, engage in decision-making structure/ processes of the institution; establish a presence; develop awards for learners & teachers; develop a network/ community of practice. • Meet with colleagues on a regular basis to share & discuss experiences. • Confident to facilitate dialogue in the community and a strengths-based approach (SBA) to the community's preferred future.	• Informed about the LIC & having HP learners in the community, benefits & challenges. Advocacy for the LIC within different levels of government. • Willingness to actively participate in learners' education & training. • Willingness to introduce & engage with learners in the community eg way of life in the community & be a guide to particular areas of interest: Location, sports, art, volunteer activities, health. & education. Just being friendly. • Willingness to help provide housing accommodation for learners & support their social interests/ aspirations. • Willing to be involved in local research oriented to improving health & wellness in the community • Willing to be involved in dreaming, designing & delivering a preferred future for the community (a fully inclusive strengths-based approach) • Whole community engaged in prioritising goals towards SBA preferred future of an improved health of the community leading to a positive change in the way of life in the community i.e. daily/ monthly activity & review/ refresh towards ultimate goal. • Support a graduated scale of SA activities—From individual patient focus to involving community groups e.g. food availability/food security, health literacy/education, specific group offerings/ project promoting health e.g. walking trails. • Willing to contribute to SBA & make aligned commitments over time that have a positive impact on the LIC. • Involvement in the research enterprise including learning research skills and employment.

LIC Curriculum

SA should permeate every aspect of a medical school curriculum and not confine itself to a particular module. As outlined in chap. 12, integration of SA into medical school curricula is not just beneficial, it is essential. To this end, a curriculum must reflect and promote the link between health care and societal needs and values, thereby ensuring socially conscious future doctors. While clinical teachers in LICs may feel under equipped to teach it, this should be addressed by demystifying the concepts and by demonstrating to clinical teachers that they as health professionals in the community are the most experienced and expert professionals to teach about their needs. They are usually part of the community themselves. Furthermore, while the LIC is often the core clinical year of a medical school curriculum, social accountability activities and formal teaching should be incorporated from the first week of medical school. This might involve in-house modules in combination health systems, ethics and global health as well as early patient contact program described in Table 11.2: Case Studies of Social Accountability on the LIC. SA should not be confined to a single domain of learning; it involves knowledge, skills and attitudes.

Different medical schools have taken the principles of SA and applied them to their LICs to varying degrees, depending on the context of the communities in which they are situated as well as the limitations of the curriculum. Text Box 11.3 describes an example from Scotland of how a community engagement project encouraged students to think about SA during their LIC. The purpose is to ensure that students grow in understanding of both how social determinants in communities affect health and health outcomes and how disease effects communities. This chapter has been informed by interviews with key LIC team members across five medical schools. No one model exists for the LIC; it is a flexible structure containing the core features of continuity and relationship-based education. The organising principal is the person and not the disease. Research has described how over the course of the LIC students are allowed to develop their independence and their level of responsibility, thereby taking more responsibility for their patients [13].

Continuity of Relationships with Patients Learners in many LICs are assigned patients from the outset. In some instances, the learner 'shadows' the patient as they attend hospital and other healthcare appointments. In this way, learners learn about patients across the different healthcare settings they encounter; they learn with the patient about their medical conditions, and they experience the challenges and day-to-day, real-world difficulties their patients encounter. Learners come to understand how their patient may need to navigate public transport where some routes render access and timely attendance at appointments very difficult, while negotiating access to private transport cost, rigid work hours and family relationships may be barriers for others. This level of understanding and way of thinking about health and illness, the difference between cure and care, referred to as person-focused care, can develop over the course of the LIC [14]. As learners progress through the LIC, they are assigned more patients and carry out home visits.

Table 11.2 Case studies of social accountability on the LIC

LIC location	LIC structure	Example of social accountability strategy	Social accountability outcome
ScotGEM, university of Dundee	10-month LIC completed by all students in year 3 (of four). Students are in the same GP practice for the year, accessing further learning in the same local hospitals over the course of the year. They have a weekly small group tutorial with their local mentor. Objectives of the LIC include: • Understanding population health • Community engagement and quality improvement activities • Understanding of generalist medicine; • Understanding of healthcare systems Student in a range of LIC settings with many in rural settings but a number in more urban settings as well.	Community engagement project – Learners partner with a community group to identify a health need – Having identified this need, they then undertake a service learning project with the group. This looks different for each student, but should involve some sort of regular voluntary commitment over the year. – This is a compulsory part of the LIC. – Students must give an assessed presentation at the end of the academic year to their peers and local faculty. This is marked and contributes towards their final grade for the year. – Students who particularly excel may be nominated for academic prizes related to social accountability which also carry a monetary value. – The University of Dundee runs a global citizenship award and ScotGEM LIC students have won this previously in open competition with other entrants.	Students develop awareness of social accountability and social determinants of health. This provides an opportunity for learners to understand the lived experience of patients and communities. Several examples of social accountability based community engagement projects are available.

(continued)

LIC location	LIC structure	Example of social accountability strategy	Social accountability outcome
Stellenbosch University Faculty of medicine and health sciences	Current structure: Students can choose to participate in a rural LIC in final year, where they are placed in a district or small regional hospital serving a rural community. They see the full range of patients attending the healthcare facility, so the curriculum is determined by the patients they see, and have to meet all the final year outcomes of the medical programme through this exposure. The LIC currently accommodates 21 students. Renewed curriculum Two-part structure to the updated LIC: 1. Students attend, as part of a small group, the same urban primary care clinics in years 1–3. (already implemented) 2. In final year, students can choose to undertake a 36-week rural LIC, as part of the final year which is entirely distributed outside of the central tertiary care hospital. (to be implemented in 2027)	Quality improvement project – Students identify a QIP in conjunction with their supervisor while on placement – QIPs included training (usually of personnel), health education posters or pamphlets, or processes to improve care (e.g. waiting time, triage). Hosting family – Families from each community agreed to support their medical students – While students did not stay with the family, meetings with them were organised over the course of the LIC and students were invited to their homes for meals occasionally. Student award – A prize is awarded every year to the student who displays the values of the graduate attributes, including social accountability, while on placement. Adopt a clinic – Students in the LIC are required to adopt a clinic for the time that they there which means visiting clinic on a weekly basis, providing support to nursing staff there, engaging in healthcare, following up patients and getting to know the community. Home visits – Students are encouraged to do home visits when it is relevant, particularly for patients with multiple problems, with disability or with obvious social circumstances that are impacting on their health. – They are required to include a reference to a home visit in some of the patient studies presented for assessment, and also to discuss how they have engaged the broader healthcare team with these patients. Where relevant they are required to do an assessment of the patient using the international classification of function.	Benefits were realised by staff and patients. Students became agents of change. Students reported gaining important insights that deepened their understanding of the host family's health needs. Students also are encouraged to present the QIP at an annual community partnership function which evolves students, healthcare staff and community members across the different professional programmes in the rural clinical school. Attributes, such as volunteerism, engagement with community organisations were recognised and rewarded.

(continued)

Table 11.2 (continued)

LIC location	LIC structure	Example of social accountability strategy	Social accountability outcome
University of Colorado School of medicine	The LIC is set across 16 learning communities in different healthcare systems. The LIC takes place in year 2. (mixed locations)	In service learning – The school partners with over 70 voluntary organisations; students choose one based on their personal interests. Students have already had exposure to a 'health and society curriculum' in years 1 which continues throughout the 4 year medical school curriculum. Accompanying patients on their journey – Students must develop a patient panel of at least 15 patients which they follow longitudinally throughout the LIC year. Students select their own patients to follow. – The student accompanies their patients to all health care appointments across multiple healthcare settings. – The student develops a portfolio of patients and is asked to pick one and do an in-depth mapping of their health experiences. – The student conducts home visits to patients over the course of the LIC developing a sense of community and social determinants not appreciated in the clinical setting. End of year presentations and shared learning. – Over the course of the LIC, students complete a portfolio of the patients they have accompanied. Students present capstone projects at the end of the LIC year – Students collaborate and cross pollinate ideas about their patients and their patients' community.	Students apply their health and society knowledge longitudinally. In service learning helps them to better understand the social determinants of health. It gives them an opportunity to contribute to improving the community's health. Students begin to understand their individual patients' barriers and facilitators to health. Over time, as they gain exposure to more patients, they gain perspective on the entire community: How transport, access, housing all act as social determinants of health. The content of the assessment process demonstrates to students that SA is valued. Through this process, a community resources map is developed, whereby patients' clinical conditions are linked to various social determinants of health identified for that community.

(continued)

Table 11.2 (continued)

LIC location	LIC structure	Example of social accountability strategy	Social accountability outcome
Harvard Medical School (HMS)	The LIC takes place over the entirety of 1 year (Jan to Jan): From mid-year 2 through mid-year 3. This is HMS'S full principal clinical experience (its core clinical year). The LIC is set across the clinics and hospitals of Cambridge health Alliance, HMS'S public health system. LIC students are assigned a panel of up to 100 patients whom they follow across the health system (and sometimes beyond) regardless of the discipline they are attending. Students are also assigned a panel of preceptors with whom they co-manage both the students' longitudinal cohort patients and many hundreds of others who are seen for more acute, episodic, surgical, emergency, or inpatient encounters.	Patient care—"Walking in their shoes" – Students are assigned patients during the year and follow their patients through primary, secondary, and sometimes tertiary care, attending outpatient clinics, hospital admissions with their patient, and providing care in community facilities, shelters, and in their homes. Presenting to faculty, peers, and healthcare team—The sum of all the noticing – Caring for patients, students accumulate a portfolio of practical challenges faced by their patients, information gleaned through 'walking in their shoes.' Students meet in small groups of up to 14, compile their notes on their patients' challenges, and consider solutions to serve their patients, their faculty, their clinical care sites, and the institution as a whole. At the end of the yearlong program, 1–2 students from each group present their recommendations to the student body, faculty, program leadership, departmental leadership, and to the health system's institutional executives.	Students develop understanding of their patients' backgrounds and experiences of illness, of health, and of healthcare. Students grow in empathy and develop realistic perspectives on their patients, their caregivers, and on the health system and community resources. As students accumulate experiences with diverse patients and their breadth of needs, assets, challenges, they powerfully advance their understanding of their community—Its history, culture, demography, barriers, and supports. This educational structure provides broad opportunities for students to engage the lived experience of patients and communities and to serve as advocates for improved health and healthcare with decision makers. Several examples of actions are available.

(continued)

Table 11.2 (continued)

LIC location	LIC structure	Example of social accountability strategy	Social accountability outcome
University of Missouri School of medicine	Students participating in the rural scholars program can opt into the LIC. The rural LIC encompasses the entire third year and is offered at designated rural training sites across three rural health systems. Students develop a continuity patient panel and learning is integrated across disciplines and settings.	Community integration project – students are paired with a community organisation and together they identify, implement and evaluate a project that addresses a community health need. – student responsibilities include required reflection assignments and presentation of projects at an annual poster session. Continuity patient reflection – students complete a reflection assignment describing what they have learned from one of their continuity patients throughout the year-long LIC.	Upon completion of their time in the community, students are able to: • Identify risk factors and health care disparity issues within the community through first-hand experience • Develop and fulfill a commitment to community needs • Identify strategies for improving health care standards/delivery systems • Develop effective communication, cultural competency, and research and evaluation skills • Write reflectively about the service and learning aspects of their experience

Text Box 11.3 The ScotGEM Community Engagement Project: An Example of a SA Orientated LIC

The ScotGEM longitudinal integrated clerkship started initially with a small pilot in 2016 which was offered as an option to students entering year 4 of the 5-year undergraduate medicine course at the University of Dundee. During the LIC, students undertake a community engagement project (CEP)

This service-learning project is compulsory for all students on LIC, whereby they undertake regular volunteering having identified a local community group or need. The CEP is a core component of their portfolio and is a presentation of the CEP forms part of their summative assessment towards the end of the academic year, contributes 25% of their overall portfolio grade (which itself constitutes 20% of their overall grade for the year). Furthermore, the students who do particularly well in their end of year assessment and/or are nominated by their tutor are considered for ScotGEM community engagement prize which attracts formal recognition on their degree transcript and a monetary reward. Students may subsequently be nominated for the ScotGEM social accountability award in their final year which again attracts formal recognition on their degree and is awarded during the school prize giving ceremony at graduation, attracting a substantial cash prize, ensuring that the social accountability of the ScotGEM curriculum receives maximal visibility with the school and university.

The CEP has not been without its challenges. During 2020/21 and the implementation of COVID social restrictions in the UK, limiting the students' ability to undertake their CEP in their local community. Students often ended up undertaking CEPs remotely serving patients and clients from outside their local community. One common example was that of telephone befriending. This was clearly a very important service to deliver during the lonely months of COVID lockdown, however it proved really challenging to students as they were not able to use their experiences to gain a greater understanding of their local community. Some students subsequently struggled to "see the point" of their volunteering as they were often able to see outcomes from their efforts, and struggled to relate their experiences in the CEP to those they were having during clinical experiences in their LIC practice.

After the disruption of COVID, the CEP has become more established within the curriculum and enjoys much better engagement from both students and teaching staff. Responding to the significant commitment made by students, the assessment weighting of the CEP has increased from 10% initially to its current weighting of 25%. A database of student CEPs has been developed to help inspire incoming LIC students to undertake a CEP in which they can really use their skills and talents to the benefit of their local community.

Continuity of Relationships with Clinical Teachers One of the salient features of LICs is the development of strong relationships between learners and their clinical teacher(s). The latter tend to be highly skilled clinicians and medical educators who have a lived experience of the health needs and priorities of the communities they serve and in which they often live themselves. Often clinical teachers show interest in the learners' overall development and in their career progression. Learners get invited to medical meetings, social gatherings and often to meals at the clinical teacher's family home. It is a truly immersive experience, where mentorship and role modelling are strong tools for learning. The so-called hidden curriculum, which has (with good cause) been elsewhere criticised in the past, in this setting can be a huge positive influence on the development of future physicians, as learners observe attributes of patience, understanding and empathy as well as clinical excellence from carefully selected clinician-educators over a prolonged period.

Continuity of Relationships with Community Having a single clinical setting as a base for an academic year or more allows learners to develop links with the community. Often people from the communities are assigned a student to host for up to a year (and, in some cases, more). This may take the format of the learner occasionally visiting a family home for a meal and the family checking in with the learner during the clerkship, to the learner living with a family for the entire duration of the LIC. Some institutions, observe how learners engage with their hosts' community and incorporate this into the grading or create an award for students whose community report an outstanding level of involvement.

Continuity of Clinical Setting Being in the same clinical setting for an extended period, allows learners to identify patterns in patient presentation and how various community-level barriers impact on presentation and/or management. Many medical schools employ quality improvement projects to encourage students to reflect on barriers and solutions to improve quality and equity. Traditional block placements, where time spent in any one location is limited by the fragmented structure, are less amenable to this type of learning. The structure of LICs allows learners not only to experience challenges in the community but to become agents of change while they are on placement. Furthermore, strong evidence supports the strategy of involving learners in communities of practice in which they become co-providers of health. Support is needed, through clear guidance on which responsibilities and tasks take priority. One such example is the University of San Fransisco California PISCES (Parnassus Integrated Student Clinical Experience) guidelines for scheduling longitudinal patient care [15].

Assessment at the LIC

The challenge for the LIC in assessment is "educational programs emphasize recent scientific and technical developments in health sciences, but proportional representation is given to education concerning priority health needs" [11]. Given the wide geographical distribution of LIC learning hubs, the concern is whether these sites can maintain the integrity of the assessment process and that assessors are objective. The best way to manage this is to have several approaches:

1. Provide faculty development training on assessment within the LIC community of practice including consensus statements of expectations for pass, borderline and fail.
2. Engage the LIC team of clinical teachers in developing a suite of assessments specific to SA. LICs are suited to workplace assessment modalities such as direct observation of consultations and clinical skills, mini-CEX and 360-degree (involving multiple assessors on the LIC) evaluations.
3. Encourage assessment that promotes learners to reflect on the health needs of the community and social determinants of health, including portfolios, quality improvement initiatives, reflective essays and case presentations involving group work or community groups.
4. Include LIC clinical teachers on curriculum and assessment committees so they can advocate for these types of assessment.
5. Train a group of LIC clinical teachers to be assessors.
6. Invite outside observers from the main school.
7. Ask questions directly as to what is in the exams with regards to SA: "What is the evidence they are assessed on the inverse care law?"(Catherine Todd, ScotGEM 2024.)

Evaluation

The Social Accountability Grid from the WHO describes the values of social accountability: relevant, high quality, equity and cost-effectives across the domains of education, research and clinical services and provides for progression of being socially accountable from planning, to doing and providing an account of impact [11]. Several frameworks have been developed from this baseline with regards to SA in the medical school, which can be adapted for a LIC, including:

1. IFSMA toolkit, which has a useful rubric; as well as ones for health care service delivery organisations [16].
2. The SAFHWT, illustrated with examples; and, as part of accreditation of the academic institution or health service delivery organisation with an overlap on management of partnerships and community engagement [17].

The benefit of having active community engagement and empowerment to drive LICs is that they provide the local long term knowledge of the community, including promises made and not kept, what works, what does not and why, ensuring a more effective and sustainable LIC. Therefore, selection of outcomes under evaluation and metrics employed should involve community representatives. Core LIC outcomes include improved clinical education, increased recruitment and retention of physicians in underserved communities and social accountability advocacy fostering a community-engaged education [18]. Research has reported that LICs have improved recruitment of physicians in both underserved urban [19] and rural areas [20]. However, the processes that bring about these outcomes are much more complex to evaluate. Therefore, evaluating what the literature refers to as the 'black box' of the process of education in LICs is a priority for future study.

Conclusion

The experiential mode of learning, with the support of experienced clinical teachers and faculty, fosters understanding of the SA pillars of relevance, equity, quality and cost-effectiveness. As they progress through the LICs, learners hold simultaneous roles as students and student-doctors, they develop into more active participants and contribute to the healthcare setting, they come to appreciate social accountability both in terms of education and health service delivery. Sustainability of socially accountable LICs requires an appreciation of its value and then buy-in at all levels. Government bodies, including departments of health and higher education, regional funding bodies, hospital, public health and primary care networks, local area services must recognise the importance of the long-term capacity of LICs to mould socially accountable doctors for the future—doctors that deliver and advocate for high quality care based on a lived understanding of the communities they serve.

Acknowledgements The authors wish to thank sincerely our esteemed colleagues who provided key information over online conversations as well as valuable feedback from reviewing relevant aspects of the chapter.

Llyod Thompson, Fiona Graham, Catherine Todd of ScotGEM, University of Dundee and St Andrew's Scotland.

Jennifer Adams, Professor and Dean, University of Colorado School of Medicine.

Ian Couper, Director: Ukwanda Centre for Rural Health, Professor of Rural Health, Department of Global Health, Faculty of Medicine and Health Sciences.

Dave Hirsch, Professor and Associate Dean, Undergraduate Medical Education, Harvard Medical School/ Cambridge Health Alliance.

Jana Lee, Programme Director, University of Missouri.

Roger Strasser, Professor of Rural Health, Founding Dean Emeritus, NOSM University, Canada.

References

1. Hirsh D, Walters L, Poncelet AN. Better learning, better doctors, better delivery system: possibilities from a case study of longitudinal integrated clerkships. Med Teach. 2012;34(7):548–54.
2. Poncelet AN, Mazotti LA, Blumberg B, Wamsley MA, Grennan T, Shore WB. Creating a longitudinal integrated clerkship with mutual benefits for an academic medical center and a community health system. Perm J. 2014;18(2):50–6.
3. Mazotti LA, Adams JE, DeWitt DE. A value analysis of longitudinal integrated clerkships: consideration of costs and benefits. Education for. Prim Care. 2024;35:1–7.

4. Worley P, Couper I, Strasser R, Graves L, Cummings BA, Woodman R, et al. A typology of longitudinal integrated clerkships. Med Educ. 2016;50(9):922–32.
5. Teherani A, Irby DM, Loeser H. Outcomes of different clerkship models: longitudinal integrated, hybrid, and block. Acad Med. 2013;88(1):35–43.
6. Myhre DL, Woloschuk W, Jackson W, McLaughlin K. Academic performance of longitudinal integrated clerkship versus rotation-based clerkship students: a matched-cohort study. Acad Med. 2014;89(2):292–5.
7. Boelen C, Dharamsi S, Gibbs T. The social accountability of medical schools and its indicators. Edu Health. 2012;25(3):180–94.
8. Brown ME, Ard C, Adams J, O'Regan A, Finn GM. Medical student identity construction within longitudinal integrated clerkships: an international, longitudinal qualitative study. Acad Med. 2022;97(9):1385–92.
9. Hogenbirk JC, Robinson DR, Strasser RP. Distributed education enables distributed economic impact: the economic contribution of the northern Ontario School of Medicine to communities in Canada. Heal Econ Rev. 2021 Jun 9;11(1):20.
10. Strasser RP, Joe Lipinski CPA. The economic contribution of the northern Ontario School of Medicine to communities participating in distributed medical education. Can J Rural Med. 2015;20(1):25.
11. Boelen, Charles, Heck, Jeffery E & World Health Organization. Division of Development of Human Resources for Health. (1995). Defining and measuring the social accountability of medical schools / Charles Boelen and Jeffery E. Heck. WHO. https://iris.who.int/handle/10665/5944
12. Bartlett M, Couper I, Poncelet A, Worley P. The do's, don'ts and don't knows of establishing a sustainable longitudinal integrated clerkship. Perspect Med Edu. 2020 Feb;9:5–19.
13. Dubé T, Schinke R, Strasser R. It takes a community to train a future physician: social support experienced by medical students during a community-engaged longitudinal integrated clerkship. Can Med Edu J. 2019 Jul;10(3):e5.
14. Starfield B. Is patient-centred care the same as person-focused care? Perm J. 2011;15(2):63–9.
15. UCSF PISCES program. University of California san Fransisco. Guidelines for scheuduling Longitudinal Patient Care https://meded.ucsf.edu/md-program/current-students/curriculum/foundations-2/clerkships-continuity. Last accessed 9 September 2024.
16. IFSMA Toolkit. International Federation of Medical School Associations https://ifmsa.org/pre-departure-training/. Last accessed 8 August 2024.
17. Anawati A, Ramsoondar N, Cameron E. The SAFE (social accountability as the framework for engagement) for health institutions project: rapid evidence narratives. Can Fam Physician. 2023 Sep 1;69(9):630–4.
18. Strasser R, Hirsh D. Longitudinal integrated clerkships: transforming medical education worldwide? Med Educ. 2011 May;45(5):436–7.
19. Adams JE, Ard C, Cunningham JM, Jiménez S, Lockspeiser T, Hirsh DA, Kulasekaran V. Preliminary workforce outcomes of an urban longitudinal integrated clerkship. Acad Med. 2023 Dec 1;98(12):1420–7.
20. Strasser R, Hogenbirk JC, Minore B, Marsh DC, Berry S, McCready WG, Graves L. Transforming health professional education through social accountability: Canada's Northern Ontario School of Medicine. Med Teach. 2013 Jun 1;35(6):490–6.

Part V
Monitoring Outcomes and Measuring Impact

Chapter 12
Socially Accountable Research: An Emerging Framework

Maxwell Kennel, Kerri Delaney, Jessica Jurgutis, Joseph LeBlanc, Sarah Larkins, Karen Johnston, and Erin Cameron

Learning Outcomes

1. Recognise the role of research within the WHO's definition of Social Accountability, beyond education and service.
2. Differentiate between the outcome-focused and process-focused goals of Socially Accountable Research using critical reflexivity.
3. Recognize how Social Accountability principles influence research design, methodology, team composition, and implementation.
4. Identify potential case studies within institutional or regional contexts for applying Socially Accountable Research principles.
5. Describe a conceptual framework for Socially Accountable Research and its relevance in advancing medical education.

M. Kennel · K. Delaney · J. Jurgutis
Dr. Gilles Arcand Centre for Health Equity, NOSM University, Sudbury, ON, Canada

J. LeBlanc
NOSM University, Sudbury, ON, Canada

S. Larkins · K. Johnston
James Cook University, Douglas, QLD, Australia

E. Cameron (✉)
Human Sciences Division, Dr. Gilles Arcand Centre for Health Equity, NOSM University, Sudbury, ON, Canada
e-mail: ercameron@nosm.ca

M. E. Abdalla et al. (eds.), *Social Accountability of Medical Schools*,
https://doi.org/10.1007/978-3-031-94435-2_12

Introduction: Social Accountability (SA) and Research

As others in this volume have explored, SA arose in the 1990s as a value and principle meant to guide medical schools in addressing the priority health needs of the specific communities and societies they are tasked to serve. The original and oft-quoted definition of SA from Charles Boelen and Jeffrey Heck's 1995 document "Defining and measuring the social accountability of medical schools" suggests that Social Accountability pertains to three domains: education, research, and service [1]. The first and last domains of the Social Accountability of medical schools have been studied in great detail since the mid-1990s, with many policy documents and scholarly works [2, 3] focusing on how SA ought to be pursued in the contexts of *education* and *professional service*. However, the precise way the principle of SA conditions *research* has been understudied, at least in the western context.

Boelen and Heck's definition of SA further states that, in terms of health care reform, it seeks to align medical education with the priority needs identified by "governments, health care organizations, health professionals and the public." [1] In 1995, the WHO also published a document called "Developing Protocols for Change in Medical Education," which emphasized the need to educate doctors to serve people's needs, insisting that "Physicians must now address fundamental issues such as equity of access to health care; quality of care; consumer satisfaction; rationing of resources; individual versus community rights; environmental determinants of health; technology assessment; cost containment; and competition with other health care providers [see Chap. 2 for more details on the evolving role of future physicians]. The search has begun for a new model that integrates all these factors." [4]

Although the search for new models has been a perennial part of education reform, these two 1995 documents (and several that preceded and followed them, including the 1992 "Towards the assessment of quality in medical education") [5] represent a beginning point for a conversation that has grown and transformed up to the present. In the year 2000, the Partnership Pentagon (later called the "Partnership Pentagram" and then the "Partnership Pentagram Plus") was developed by Charles Boelen in a working paper called "Towards Unity for Health" [6]. The goal of the series of models that led to the Partnership Pentagram Plus was to conceptualize community engagement in the context of Social Accountability. Its five contact points started with policymakers, health professionals, academic institutions, communities, and health managers (or administrators). This model was later expanded to include linked sectors (which include those with interests in health like non-profits and NGOs) and eventually retitled the "Partnership Pentagram Plus." [7]

But even this revision does not fully account for how the category of "community" cuts across and includes all aspects of the Partnership Pentagram Plus, given that policymakers, health professionals, academic institutions, health administrators, and those in linked sectors are all part of the society and its communities which medical educators and practitioners are tasked to serve [8]. Further discussion about the pentagram can be found in Chap. 3. The discourse on SA has struggled to conceptualize the relationship that the medical profession ought to have with society and its communities. One example of this struggle is the often-vague use of the term "community" to authorize certain forms of knowledge and assertion see Chap. 6 for more elaboration on this. This vague use of "community" contrasts with the difficult work required to treat these individuals as equal partners at the table where medicine's relationship with society is discussed and decided [9].

Amidst this storied history and struggle to become more accountable, responsive, and responsible for society's health needs, research has often taken a back seat to the more urgent demands of medical training and public and professional service. However, research has also been part of the conversation on SA from the start. For example, we can look at the claim in the 2001 document "Universities and the Health of the Disadvantaged" that:

> Priority should be given to research on the special health problems of disadvantaged communities, on understanding the underlying determinants of poverty and inequity, and on approaches to reducing the disparity in health status between disadvantaged and well-off communities. Exploitation of disadvantaged communities and disadvantaged patients for research purposes should specifically be avoided. Attention should be given to obtaining informed consent from both individuals and communities. Members of disadvantaged groups should be included on university committees with research oversight [10].

As early as the 1991 document "Changing Medical Education: An Agenda for Action," the place of research was central to the call that Boelen and his colleagues made for universities to identify the "priority health management problems in and with their community," [11] to develop a "management system to ensure smooth, productive, and mutually beneficial inter-faculty or inter-departmental collaboration," and to build "a strong partnership with the key actors in the community where the initiative is to be centred—local civic authorities, health authorities, professional groups, voluntary organizations, etc.—and serve as the coordinating catalyst among them." [10] Already in 1991, the place of research in the context of community partnership was present in the precursor documents that would inform the 1995 definition of Social Accountability and eventually the Partnership Pentagram Plus.

In the 2010s and 2020s, the conversation continued alongside calls for accountability within and beyond the healthcare systems by Indigenous, Black, and other marginalized communities. The relationship between SA and Social Justice—accompanied by essential movements toward Antiracism, Disability Justice, Decolonization, and EDI—challenged the fundamental bases of SA as a concept and practice and advanced its goals in context-dependent ways. These movements drew on strategies both inside and outside academic and educational institutions and, over the last several decades, have transformed academic knowledge production in better informed and validated ways by those with lived experience of discrimination and inequity.

In many ways, while SA has been identified as a powerful paradigm shift in reorientating medical schools and meeting workforce needs, SA as a *research movement* has still largely been under-studied. To date, SA literature has been primarily focused on and defined by institutional, educational, and graduate outcomes, but there are growing calls to expand this body of literature. To address this gap and acknowledge the rich history of community-based research and relevant methodologies, we now seek to engage in understanding the diversity of approaches to, within, and across socially accountable research and their differing visions of health, well-being and social transformation. Here we provide two case studies of research projects that exemplify this diversity in unique ways by taking SA as a guiding principle as they conceptualize and enact change. The first case study concerns research that was undertaken by a group of institutions that were each founded upon a social accountability mandate. The research was not only in the name of SA but also intended to gather evidence about the impacts of socially accountable medical schools. The second case study is entirely different in that it builds upon a community need, identified in a specific region, and led by a group of people working together to address the need. As you will see in the descriptions below, arguably, both case studies provide important considerations when conceptualizing and enacting socially accountable research.

Socially Accountable Research Across the Local-Global Axis: Two Case Studies

Case Study 1: Research on Social Accountability Across Institutions: THEnet

The Training for Health Equity Network (THEnet; thenetcommunity.org) is a community of practice of 14 medical and health professional schools across six continents that share a mission of socially accountable health professional education (Table 12.1).

Founded in 2008, THEnet brings together these small medical schools, located primarily in rural and underserved areas in a mix of eleven low and high-income

Table 12.1 Training for Health Equity Network (THEnet) partner health professional schools

Training for Health Equity Network (THEnet) partner health professional schools
1. Ateneo de Zamboanga University School of Medicine, The Philippines[a]
2. Ghent University, Belgium[a]
3. Flinders University, Australia[a]
4. Imperial College, United Kingdom
5. James Cook University, Australia[a]
6. Latin American School of Medicine (ELAM), Cuba[a]
7. Northern Ontario School of Medicine University, Canada
8. Patan Academy of Health Sciences, Nepal
9. Walter Sisulu University, South Africa[a]
10. University of Gezira, Sudan
11. University of New Mexico, USA
12. University of the Philippines, Manila, School of Health Sciences, Leyte, The Philippines[a]
13. University of Sherbrooke, Canada
14. University of Texas, El Paso, USA

[a]Founding School

countries, that share a commitment to producing and supporting a health workforce that will meet the needs of the populations they serve [12]. Although the strategies used by these schools vary in response to their context, specific approaches are shared across partner schools to achieve this commitment:

1. Recruiting students (and faculty) from under-served and under-represented populations;
2. Providing primary care-focussed curricula; delivering medical programs mainly in community settings and under-served communities and;
3. Providing postgraduate training pathways according to local health workforce needs.

An articulated mission where understanding the local population and their needs, orienting learning, research and service activities of the population served (particularly under-served and marginalized populations), and strong, charismatic leadership in the pursuit of workforce outcomes are also important [13].

When THEnet was formed as a community of practice, the seven founding schools (Table 12.1) set an initial task of developing an evaluation framework and a program logic (Fig. 12.1), for use by schools and their communities to critically reflect on the degree to which the school had reached its social accountability goals. This framework, developed based on earlier work by the WHO [14], was divided into three (later four) domains: (i) Who do we serve, and what are their needs?; (ii)

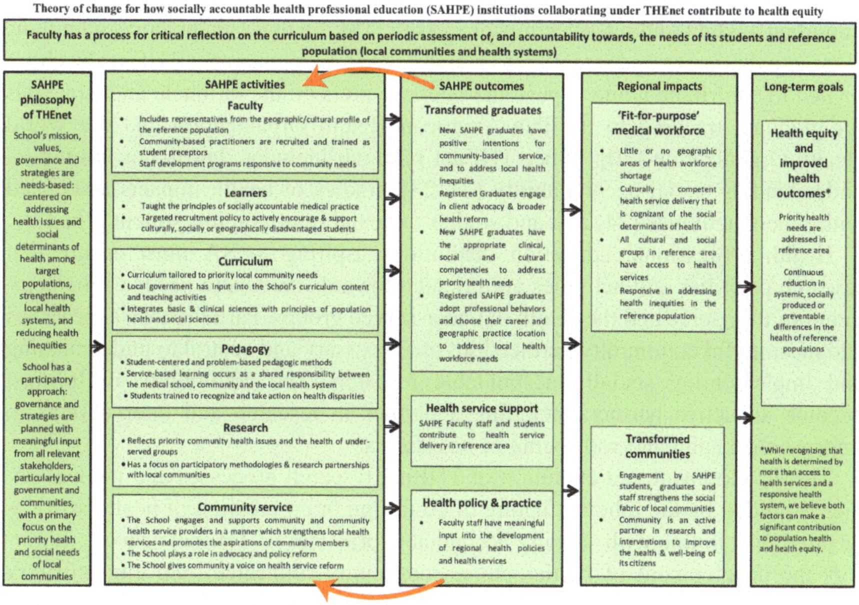

Fig. 12.1 Program logic model for socially accountable health professional education (SAHPE). https://thenetcommunity.org/wp-content/uploads/2017/04/Program-Logic-Model-1.pdf

How does our school work?; (iii) What do we do? and (iv) What difference do we make? [15].

Several agreed-upon principles underpin THEnet's proposed approach to collaborative research and evaluation. Firstly, SA is an aspirational goal rather than an arbitrary level that can be achieved, with a requirement of ongoing critical reflection and improvement by faculty required. Secondly, performance against all the measures in these domains needs to be reviewed by the communities themselves rather than just by faculty or education academics. Thirdly, to deliver SA health professional education, producing competent graduates alone is not enough; institutions need to hold themselves accountable for delivering fit-for-purpose health professionals and working in partnership to strengthen the health system and the quality of care it provides. This principle implies that schools need to measure graduate outcomes, in terms of location and type of practice against need, but also their impact on the health system and, ultimately, health and social impact on under-served populations [15]. These three principles have driven the collaborative program of research of THEnet over the past 15 years (summarised in [15]).

After developing the THEnet evaluation framework for social accountability in health professional education and its successful implementation [16], THEnet led the development of a collaborative graduate outcome study (GOS); a prospective cohort study with more than 6000 learners now enrolled from nine partner schools across seven countries [17]. This was designed to collect demographic details and practice intention data from learners at entry and exit to medical school and then follow them longitudinally with actual practice location and discipline data on four occasions until ten years after graduation from medical school. This has led to important insights about selection processes [18], changes in practice intentions [19], actual practice and intention to emigrate [17]. Consequently, THEnet has been invited to contribute white papers and book chapters on the rationale and strategies for graduate tracking to the Pan American Health Organization and the World Health Organization [20]. Other THEnet research includes, but is not limited to, understanding social accountability [21–23], studies of health impacts associated with school activities [24, 25], and studies of social return on investment [26, 27].

Health professional education institutions aspiring to SA must ensure that research priorities and activities are oriented towards the health needs of the communities they serve and the health of under-served groups. Participatory approaches and meaningful community partnerships are necessary and central to understanding and implementing socially accountable research. The community itself must become an active partner, including a partner in research and interventions to improve the health and well-being of its citizens.

The development and evolution of THEnet research processes and methodologies is guided by the inherent nature of co-design or co-creation of health services or programs, in line with socially accountable practices of THEnet schools. It mirrors the development of participatory, community-connected, and emancipatory research approaches in First Nations health research across countries, and rural and remote health approaches. Some schools work with other under-served groups in their contexts, for example, the Muslim minorities in the islands of southwestern

Mindanao, in the Philippines, as shown in the outcomes of the Philippines social return on investment study [24]. In the context of the THEnet community of practice, our collaborative research involves conscious attention to decolonizing principles, where lower-income schools are supported to develop, own and publish their research rather than to be minor partners in collaborations with those from higher-income settings (usually in the global north).

These principles collectively imply conducting research "from, in, with, and for" under-served communities and should spur—health professional education institutions aspiring to SA returning to the WHO partnership pentagram to truly partner with communities, health services, policymakers and others to conduct research that both improves health and health services for under-served communities and is viewed by the community themselves as something that meets their needs.

In conclusion, THEnet uses research to advance SA by studying the impact of health professional education and school activities on population health and the social and graduate outcomes of the communities they serve. At the same time, THEnet is exemplary in how it partners with communities to address the priority health and health service needs of underserved populations—making it a manifestation of Socially Accountable Research that is both concerned with the topic of Social Accountability and a form of Socially Accountable Research.

Case Study 2: Socially Accountable Research Within a Region: The Nourishing Health Education Coalition

The Nourishing Health Education Coalition is a research network based in Northern Ontario, Canada. It emerged formally in 2022 and although it is connected with the Dr. Gilles Arcand Centre for Health Equity at NOSM University, its organizational structure is distributed beyond a single institution. Its origins date back nearly two decades within the region's Indigenous and local food systems. Members have worked within the region's food security and sovereignty movements and have gradually formed the research coalition as an extension and evolution of their practice.

The combination of *health* and *research* is critical as the health policy upstream impacts of Social Accountability are meant to retain medical graduates, provide a return on social investment, impact career choices, impact practice locations, and strengthen healthcare resources and alignment of education. The Nourishing Health Education Coalition attempts to merge health and research by bridging the enterprise of research, healthcare, and SA within and beyond the context of NOSM University. Through embedded research systems, programs like The Nourishing Health Education Coalition can take a collective impact approach to addressing food insecurity and sovereignty while addressing the challenges presented in defining "community."

Members of this coalition are Northern Ontarians. Some are also the medical university's faculty, while others are alumni, and some are both alumni and faculty. Some members work in public health, some educate in public health, while others work and educate in public health at the medical university. Some members are Indigenous community members who are also alumni, faculty, and leadership. The common thread is regional: all of our community members in northern Ontario eat, live, and breathe the direct impacts of high rates of food insecurity and the associated erosion of food sovereignty [28]. They have committed to the principles of practising—through immersion in collaboration—to (1) work slowly and intentionally, (2) centre their relations on reciprocity, (3) live and centre in a different narrative (*Mino bimaadiziwin*, "the good life"), (4) listen and take direction from community, and (5) use the collective knowledge of the region and its partners for change.

In 2020, five local food actionists facilitated planning to convene regional and community assets and strengths to address the wicked problem of food insecurity within the region. Supported by the national Nourish leadership initiative [29], this cohort developed the following theory of change (Fig. 12.2).

This model was rooted in the need to address the high rates of food insecurity in the North through indigenous knowledge of food systems and sovereignty. Working with the understanding that *Mino bimaadiziwin* [30] is what had sustained life in this place since time immemorial, the features of this model were focused on which resources were shared equitably in the context of right-relation, including with non-human community members. We are aware, through our practice as health professionals, educators and researchers within the region, that this life still exists and that it still provides security and wellness to countless households throughout the region. We also know that—from education to service to research—*local solutions to local problems lead to impactful outcomes and community wellness*. Through practices such as sharing, respect, reciprocity, and the focus on local knowledge, we could,

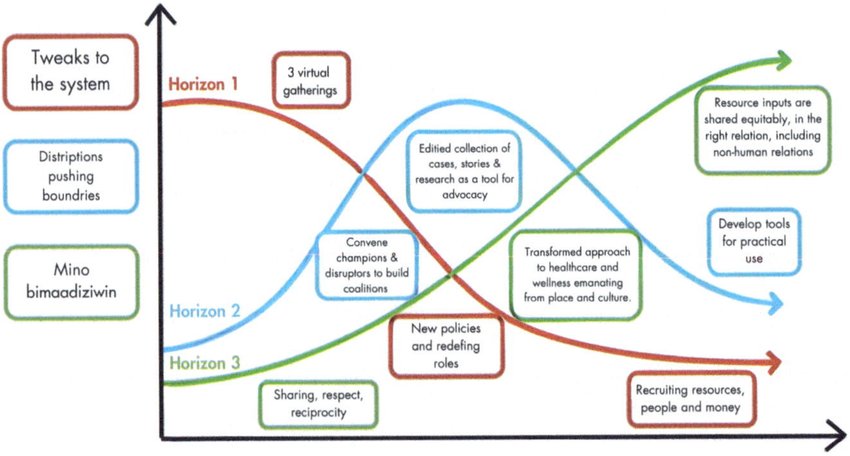

Fig. 12.2 The Nourishing Health Education Coalition's Three Horizons

over time, implement actions across three horizons that would lead to sustained change.

The three horizons presented above should not be read as sequential, nor are they necessarily completely independent. Instead, they represent specific actions' initial and long-term impacts (a change on the *y*-axis over time). These particular actions were grouped into ideas that represented tweaks to the system, ideas and actions that disrupted the system and pushed boundaries, and others representing the existence of *Mino bimaadiziwin*. Across time, having gatherings in 2020 meant that we, by necessity, started virtually, but this evolved to intentional, in-person gatherings we later termed "summits."

Holding a gathering of any kind in the context of a medical institution and in the name of research in and of itself is not a revolutionary act. It is what *happens* at those gatherings, who is invited, and who speaks that allows us to start pushing the boundaries of Socially Accountable Research. Our gatherings intentionally focused on convening champions—both in the audience as well as in speakers—and disruptors that were meant to build this coalition. We saw this process as a calling-in. Through these gatherings, we sought to highlight where *Mino bimaadiziwin* existed and where we could share our knowledge with respect and reciprocity by highlighting local initiatives that met these criteria. The research components related to sharing the stories for use in education and disseminating the impacts of this approach are being collected in an edited collection of cases and stories with expected publication in 2025.

Some of the key elements highlighted are where existing roles, such as programmatic universally funded positions, could be adapted and redefined by local needs, leading to positive health outcomes and impacts in relation to access to food and food sovereignty. We see this transformed approach to healthcare and wellness emanating from place and culture through the collection and the stories that are shared of individuals working within their roles, making small tweaks to the systems, pushing boundaries to develop new policies and supporting tools for practical use as well as recruiting people and resources to support this movement. Putting our attention toward the wicked problems we confront requires having a way of convening the health professionals and educators who are embedded in the community. The coalitional approach outlined above, where our members move beyond their professional roles and become more than the sum of our parts, means that we bring people together on the theme of food sovereignty in ways that extend beyond restrictive categories that stand in the way of Socially Accountable Research.

Socially Accountable Research: An Emerging Framework for Consideration

With growing calls for research to respond to complex societal problems, characterizing Socially Accountable Research is timely and relevant. The two case studies above show that approaches to socially accountable research can be distinctly different, acting uniquely to serve the target communities. In attempts to further study ways of conducting socially accountable research and research on SA,, a scoping review has been undertaken by a group of researchers, educators, administrators, policymakers, institutions, and organizations. This section will detail some preliminary findings from the scoping review's title/abstract search and from the discourse that has surrounded the review process, resulting in an emerging framework.

Approximately 2800 English articles were included in the scoping review. By sorting through the titles and abstracts of these articles, three common themes were identified.

1. There are numerous studies of SA apart from the discourse on SA in medical education, including largely autonomous discourses on Corporate Social Responsibility (CSR), Teacher Education and Pedagogy, civil and civic forms of Social Accountability focused on voting and anti-corruption (often led by the World Bank), and more.
2. It is difficult to discern whether research has authentically been conducted in a socially accountable manner—both because measures of SA are diverse and sometimes performative or tokenistic, and because it is difficult to verify claims to SA in the presentation of research results.
3. There is a widespread use of the term "Social Responsibility" in abstracts and lists of keywords in research generally, but this does not necessarily reflect a deep and sustained strategy of community responsiveness and engagement on the part of researchers or institutions.

At this point in the history of the concept of SA, several key linkages are clear. Research is a vital part of both education and service, for what would education be without the research that backs it? And what good is research if it is not a form of public service? Based on the assumption that research must inform education and that good research performs a public service (with significant debate about what counts as a public service, and which communities benefit from such service across the species-barrier and into ecology), the main question of this chapter is: *What makes research socially accountable?*

This question is not—however—unique to the discourse on SA. Just as there is a parallel conversation on SA in the context of governance, civic engagement, and anticorruption (exemplified by the publications of the World Bank and others, see Chap. 1), there are many parallel conversations on what makes research socially accountable in areas like Community based participatory research (CBPR), and in Indigenous Methodologies wherein the social bonds and forms of accountability that define them are often less stratified than they are in western colonial institutions (as we see in Case Study 1). We note this here because it is often the temptation of some social scientific discourses to proceed without acknowledgment of parallel conversations in adjacent fields that are concerned with similar questions.

Socially accountable research is dynamic and can go by many names, which makes it challenging to characterize. Moreover, there is a need to characterize socially accountable research and extend those insights into research network formation and maintenance domains in a global context. Again, in the early stages of the above scoping review, an emerging framework has been conceptualized based on the discourse surrounding the inclusion/exclusion criteria for the review. This framework can be seen in Fig. 12.3 below.

Like any heuristic set of distinctions, the three terms in the outer circle above will often overlap and combine and should, therefore, not be understood as ideal types that perfectly capture what they refer to. With this in mind, the three categories above allow us to begin distinguishing between research that focuses *on* the practice of SA, research that talks *about* social accountability, and research that itself *is* socially accountable—all conditioned by critical questions about what specific communities and constituencies researchers are accountable to.

One could imagine a research project that would be described by all three categories, and it is also easy to think of examples of research projects that only pertain to one or two of the three categories. It is essential to distinguish between Socially Accountable Research, Research *on* Social Accountability, and Research *about* Social Accountability because there is no guarantee that because research is focused on the topic or advancement of SA, its methodology, method, approach, and execution proceed in socially accountable ways. Socially Accountable Research or *"the how"* refers to research based on methodologies that encourage SA *as a condition that must influence the research process*, whether at a particular stage or as a whole. For example, research that takes its primary questions and directions from

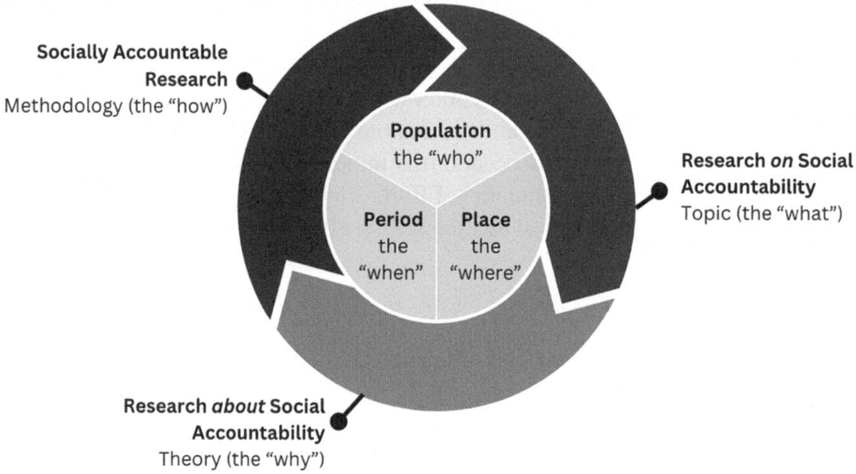

Fig. 12.3 Conceptual framework for studying socially accountable research

self-identified community needs. Research *on* Social Accountability or *"the what"* refers to research that studies the practice of Social Accountability *but may or may not conduct itself in a socially accountable manner*. For example, by measuring the SA of a medical school or its graduates. Lastly, research *about* social accountability, or *"the why,"* refers to research and writing that explores theories of SA and the *rationale behind the concept and practice*. For example, op-eds or commentaries that discuss whether SA is a virtue, professional competency, or a social contract.

The inner circle of Fig. 12.3, *the who, when and where* of socially accountable research, should be considered when talking about socially accountable research, research *on* social accountability or research *about* social accountability. The "*who*" of Socially Accountable Research is essential because it requires partnerships—for example, those detailed in the Partnership Pentagram Plus—to define and decide whether Socially Accountable Research has been done or done well. As mentioned earlier, even what we consider a "community" partner is decisive in how Socially Accountable Research is designed and executed. For example, communities beyond the category of the "human" in animal, natural, and more-than-human worlds are often better understood through Indigenous methodologies and forms of life. The bonds formed between and across the distinctions above are worthy considerations for all researchers seeking to become more socially accountable, for example, in the goals of the OneHealth Approach [31] or in new movements toward planetary health [32]. Rather than separating the activity of doing Socially Accountable Research from ecological accountability, new approaches push past artificial and constructed distinctions between researchers and communities.

The "*when*" of socially accountable research is an important reflection of cultural context. How you approach a community, timing, method, and place should all depend on when the cultural context is most appropriate. The "when" also allows tracking socially accountable research efforts over time. Since the terming of SA [1], tracking publications in white and grey literature can elude any progress in socially accountable research. Lastly, *where* socially accountable research, or research on/about social accountability, happens should be considered. *The where* should be tightly tied to *the who* but is often driven by capacity. Ideally, socially accountable research occurs in the location where *the who* reside. However, prominent research groups from outside these regions often conduct the research when communities cannot. When this occurs, it is important for researchers not to take advantage of or tokenize communities. Efforts should always be made to educate and build community capacity so that the lasting effect of research is beneficial for all who are involved.

Conclusion

In their paper "Social Accountability in Medical Education: A Bibliometric Analysis" Mohamed Elhassan Abdalla and his colleagues identify five clusters of themes in Social Accountability, globally: "SA indicators and medical school accreditation, medical students' attitudes towards underserved populations, the role of physicians in translating SA into medical education, the impact of socially accountable medical education, and preparing medical students for achieving SA in medical education." [33] Through bibliometric analysis—a form of research that holds its conclusions to account to a stable numerical standard—these findings show how research in this area can be undertaken for the sake of furthering Social Accountability while also being accountable to empirical research findings.

Research is essential to advance the aims of SA because no institution or professional can call themselves socially accountable without research-based evidence to back up such a claim. However, the design and practice of research itself also must become more socially accountable if it is to have integrity as part of a professional's responsibility to educate students and serve society. This means embedding community consultation and representation all the way from the selection of a research question, to the design of methodology and selection of a method, to the execution of the project, to the communication of its results, all in the context of the community-academy nexus.

Examples of how to design Socially Accountable Research, as explored above, include Forming partnerships and networks across communities, institutions, regions, and nations, focusing those partnerships on guiding questions like "Who do we serve, and what are their needs? How does our school work? What do we do? and What difference do we make?"; understanding the difference and overlap between Socially Accountable Research, Research on Social Accountability, and Research about Social Accountability; forming coalitional connections with other adjacent discourses and researchers (from those who work on civic engagement to community-engaged researchers); combining horizons of gathering, policy-formation, coalition-building, tool-development, resourcing and recruitment, and publication; and exploring how local solutions to local problems lead to impactful outcomes and community wellness.

Understanding the relationship between SA and research in reciprocal, self-reflexive terms is essential for advancing the conversation on the relationship between Social Accountability and research. In conclusion, we call on the medical education community to invest in researching various topics *for the sake of* SA and transforming methodologies *toward* the ideal of socially accountable research. It emphasizes that while embracing SA is vital, understanding it through the lens of rigorous research—so that research informs claims of SA and that SA conditions research—is what truly propels it from a conceptual ideal to a tangible, impactful reality in medical education.

Take-Home Message

Research on Social Accountability, Research about Social Accountability, and Socially accountable Research are three distinct but overlapping categories that can help researchers and medical educators clarify how research informs their claims about Social Accountability and how the values of Social Accountability can positively influence their research, from design to completion.

References

1. Boelen C, Heck JE, World Health Organization. Defining and measuring the social accountability of medical schools [Internet]. Division of Development of Human Resources for Health. https://iris.who.int/handle/10665/59441
2. Schrewe BM. Medical citizenship and the social right to health care in Canada: a genealogy of medical education discourses. 2023 [cited 2024 Jul 24]. https://doi.library.ubc.ca/10.14288/1.0434651
3. Barber C. Aligning education to societal needs: evaluating social accountability in health professions education [Internet]. Maastricht University; 2023 [cited 2024 Jul 24]. https://cris.maastrichtuniversity.nl/en/publications/6a09b5b5-e2d1-4297-b939-37cbfc26616b
4. Boelen C, Marchais D, Jacques E, Dohner CW, Kantrowitz MP, World Health Organization. Developing protocols for change in medical education: report of an informal consultation [Internet]. Division of Development of Human Resources for Health; 1995. https://iris.who.int/handle/10665/62083
5. Boelen C, Bandaranayake R, Bouhuijs PAJ, Page, GG, Rothman AI. Towards the assessment of quality in medical education [Internet]. 1992. https://iris.who.int/bitstream/handle/10665/61680/WHO_HRH_92.7.pdf?sequence=1
6. Boelen C, Glasser J, Gofin J, Lippeveld T, Orobaton N. Towards unity for health: the quest for evidence [Internet]. 2007. https://pubmed.ncbi.nlm.nih.gov/18058698/
7. Markham R, Hunt M, Woollard R, Oelke N, Snadden D, Strasser R, et al. Addressing rural and indigenous health inequities in Canada through socially accountable health partnerships. BMJ Open. 2021;11(11):e048053.
8. Dempsey SE. Critiquing community engagement. Manag Commun Q. 2010;24(3):359–90.
9. Joseph M. Against the romance of community [Internet]. University of Minnesota Press; 2002. https://www.jstor.org/stable/10.5749/j.ctttt4ng
10. World Health Organization. Universities and the health of the disadvantaged [Internet]. 2000. https://iris.who.int/handle/10665/66711
11. World Health Organization. Changing medical education: an agenda for action [Internet]. 1991. https://iris.who.int/bitstream/handle/10665/60494/WHO_EDUC_91.200.pdf?sequence=1
12. Pálsdóttir B, Neusy A-J, Reed G. Building the evidence base: networking innovative socially accountable medical education programs. Educ Health [Internet]. 2008 Sep 12;21(2) http://www.educationforhealth.net/
13. Pálsdóttir B, Neusy AJ. Global health: networking innovative academic institutions. Infect Dis Clin N Am. 2011;25(2):337–46.
14. Boelen C, Woollard B. Social accountability and accreditation: a new frontier for educational institutions. Med Educ. 2009;43(9):887–94.
15. Larkins SL, Preston R, Matte MC, Lindemann IC, Samson R, Tandinco FD, et al. Measuring social accountability in health professional education: development and international pilot testing of an evaluation framework. Med Teach. 2013;35(1):32–45.
16. Ross S, Preston R, Lindemann I, Matte M, Samson R, Tandinco F, et al. The training for health equity network evaluation framework: a pilot study at five health professional schools. Educ Health. 2014;27(2):116.
17. Johnston K, Guingona M, Elsanousi S, Mbokazi J, Labarda C, Cristobal FL, et al. Training a fit-for-purpose rural health workforce for low- and middle-income countries (LMICs): how do

drivers and enablers of rural practice intention differ between learners from LMICs and high income countries? Front Public Health. 2020;8:582464.
18. Larkins S, Michielsen K, Iputo J, Elsanousi S, Mammen M, Graves L, et al. Impact of selection strategies on representation of underserved populations and intention to practise: international findings. Med Educ. 2015;49(1):60–72.
19. Larkins S, Johnston K, Hogenbirk JC, Willems S, Elsanousi S, Mammen M, et al. Practice intentions at entry to and exit from medical schools aspiring to social accountability: findings from the training for health equity network graduate outcome study. BMC Med Educ. 2018;18(1):261.
20. Hogenbirk J, Ross S, Larkins S, Woolley T. Chapter 4. Where do graduates go? Developing a graduate tracking system: the experience of THEnet. In: World Health Organization, editor. Strengthening the collection, analysis and use of health workforce data and information: a handbook. Geneva: World Health Organization; 2002. p. 325.
21. Ellaway RH, Van Roy K, Preston R, Greenhill J, Clithero A, Elsanousi S, et al. Translating medical school social missions to student experiences. Med Educ. 2018;52(2):171–81.
22. Preston R, Larkins S, Taylor J, Judd J. Building blocks for social accountability: a conceptual framework to guide medical schools. BMC Med Educ. 2016;16(1):227.
23. Preston R, Larkins S, Taylor J, Judd J. From personal to global: understandings of social accountability from stakeholders at four medical schools. Med Teach. 2016;38(10):987–94.
24. Halili S, Cristobal F, Woolley T, Ross SJ, Reeve C, Neusy AJ. Addressing health workforce inequities in the Mindanao regions of the Philippines: tracer study of graduates from a socially-accountable, community-engaged medical school and graduates from a conventional medical school. Med Teach. 2017;39(8):859–65.
25. Reeve C, Woolley T, Ross SJ, Mohammadi L, Halili S, Cristobal F, et al. The impact of socially-accountable health professional education: a systematic review of the literature. Med Teach. 2017;39(1):67–73.
26. Woolley T, Cristobal F, Siega-Sur J, Ross S, Neusy AJ, Halili S, et al. Positive implications from socially accountable, community-engaged medical education across two Philippines regions. RRH [Internet]. 2018 Feb 11 [cited 2024 Jul 26]. https://www.rrh.org.au/journal/article/4264
27. Woolley T, Halili SD, Siega-Sur JL, Cristobal FL, Reeve C, Ross SJ, et al. Socially accountable medical education strengthens community health services. Med Educ. 2018;52(4):391–403.
28. Burnett K, Hay T. Plundering the North: a history of settler colonialism, corporate welfare, and food insecurity [Internet]. 2023. https://uofmpress.ca/books/plundering-the-north
29. Nourish [Internet]. 2024. https://www.nourishleadership.ca/
30. Gross LW. Anishinaabe ways of knowing and being [Internet]. Taylor & Francis. https://www.google.ca/books/edition/Anishinaabe_Ways_of_Knowing_and_Being/9BwGDAAAQBAJ?hl=en&gbpv=0
31. Atlas RM, Atlas RM, Maloy S, Maloy S, editors. One health: people, animals, and the environment [Internet]. ASM Press; 2014. https://www.wiley.com/en-us/One+Health%3A+People%2C+Animals%2C+and+the+Environment-p-9781683673460
32. Planetary Health Aliance. Planetary Health [Internet]. 2024. https://www.planetaryhealthalliance.org/planetary-health
33. Abdalla ME, Onchonga D, Taha MH. Social accountability in medical education: a bibliometric analysis. 2024;16(3):5–19. https://doi.org/10.21315/eimj2024.16.3.2, https://eduimed.usm.my/EIMJ20241603/EIMJ20241603_02.pdf

Further Reading

Boelen C, Dharamsi S, Gibbs T. The social accountability of medical schools and its indicators. Educ Health. 2012;25(3):180–94. https://doi.org/10.4103/1357-6283.109785.

Kennel M. "Institutional social accountability from medical education to accreditation and public policy," Introduction to a special issue on "Institutional journeys toward social accountability in medical and allied health institutions: from policy influence to accreditation transformation". Soc Innov J. 2024;26. https://socialinnovationsjournal.com/index.php/sij/article/view/8556

Pasquino G, Pelizzo R. The culture of accountability: a democratic virtue. London: Routledge; 2023.

Ritz S, Beatty K, Ellaway R. Accounting for social accountability developing critiques of social accountability within medical education. Educ Health. 2014;27(2):152–7. https://doi.org/10.4103/1357-6283.143747.

Ross BM, Cameron E. Socially accountable medical education: our story might not be yours. High Educ Stud. 2021;11(1) https://doi.org/10.5539/hes.v11n1p114.

Schrewe B. Medical citizenship and the social right to health care in Canada: a genealogy of medical education discourses. Vancouver: University of British Columbia; 2023. https://open.library.ubc.ca/soa/cIRcle/collections/ubctheses/24/items/1.0434651

Chapter 13
Social Accountability in Medical Schools: The Role of Participatory Health Research

Anne MacFarlane

Learning Outcomes

1. Explain the significance of WHO policies in promoting community involvement in health research to address health inequities.
2. Define the Participatory Health Research (PHR) paradigm and identify criteria for meaningful partnerships between researchers and communities.
3. Analyze the alignment between participatory health research and social accountability principles.
4. Explore strategies to optimize participatory health research in medical schools through participatory structures, methods, tools, and capacity-building initiatives.

Involving Communities in Health Research

The WHO's Alma Ata [1] advocates that people have the right and responsibility to be involved in decisions about their health. This includes individual involvement in decision-making during healthcare consultations and ***community involvement i***n the development of services, policies and research.

One main rationale for this WHO policy and its recent reiteration [2] is that we need to understand the *lived experience* of people's health to fully understand what is needed to optimize health for all. The social determinants of health—the conditions in which people are born, grow, live, work and age—shape health status,

A. MacFarlane (✉)
Participatory Health Research Unit and WHO Collaborating Centre for Participatory Health Research with Refugee and Migrants, School of Medicine & Health Research Institute, University of Limerick, Limerick, Ireland
e-mail: anne.macfarlane@ul.ie

M. E. Abdalla et al. (eds.), *Social Accountability of Medical Schools*,
https://doi.org/10.1007/978-3-031-94435-2_13

access to healthcare and health outcomes [3]. We know that the social determinants of health are variable across and within populations. This leads to unfair and avoidable differences in health between certain groups. These health inequities need to be addressed. Acknowledging the expertise that people have from their lived experiences of health inequities is a fundamental way to do just that. It transforms our focus from people as being passive victims or groups who have inherent vulnerability to a focus on people as being resourceful, agents of change who can guide or lead the changes that are needed to eliminate health inequities [4, 5]. They can use their lived experience to elucidate to researchers, clinicians and policy makers who do not have that experience, the complexity and nuances of any problems and potential solutions [6].

However, despite decades of attention to this vision of the WHO, communities are not routinely involved in a meaningful way in decisions about their health [7]. Focusing on the specifics of community involvement in research, it is true that more and more health funders advocate for such involvement [8, 9]. There is growth in activity and a keen interest in measuring the impact of research partnerships [10, 11]. Yet, it is still not the norm in health research. There are too many examples of certain groups and populations being excluded or considered' hard to reach' by researchers. There are still too many accounts of tokenistic practices [12]. Tokenism is when the invitation to be involved is not genuine or is not followed through in an authentic way. This may be because decision making remains in the hands of academics or academics carry on with "business as usual" without thinking critically about what structures and methodologies may be needed to authentically share power about decision making. Arnstein's *Ladder of Participation* [13] is a classic in the field because of its visual representation of how activities or initiatives rate from non-participation to meaningful participation. Arnstein's Ladder of Participation is a model that illustrates different levels of citizen involvement in decision-making. It consists of eight rungs, ranging from non-participation (manipulation and therapy) to tokenism (informing, consultation, and placation) and ultimately to true citizen power (partnership, delegated power, and citizen control). This framework helps assess the extent to which communities have a meaningful role in shaping policies and initiatives that affect them. See Chap. 6 for more details about Arnstein's Ladder of Participation.

Participatory Health Research

The ***Participatory Health Research*** paradigm has emerged to provoke radical transformation from tokenism to meaningful involvement of people in health research. Participatory research is defined *centralizing the involvement of those whose lives or work is affected by the issue being investigated in research from start to finish* [4, 14]. It reflects the higher rungs of Arnstein's ladder. In simple terms, participatory health research paradigm is about *research with*, not on/to/for people. It is an umbrella term for a broad family of approaches such as community based participatory research [5], participatory rural appraisal and participatory learning and action research [15], among others. While these approaches have different names, they share a heritage that has a fundamental interest in addressing health inequities by dismantling power structures that mean community members do not have a voice or in relation to their health or research about their health [16]. They share important values that can guide researchers' practices because the values are explicitly about reversing power dynamics that exist between the academy and broader society. These values include a commitment to mutual respect, trust, transparency in decision making and promoting community ownership [4, 5, 14, 17].

It is important to know how to put these values into action. What concrete steps can researchers take to *enact* these values? The minimum criteria are that community members share decisions with academics about the research question, research governance by being part of the steering group, data interpretation and research dissemination [14]. Further, there is evidence that researchers can commit to the use of methods, tools and techniques enact these values because they create 'spaces for participation' that are more equitable than "business as usual" [18]. The concept of ***participatory space*** as applied to research shines a light on the physical, temporal and social aspects of research projects [7, 18]: where is the research being planned and carried out? What time frame is involved—is there ample time to create meaningful partnerships at the start and to pay attention to the quality of the partnership as the project unfolds? What actions are taken to pay explicit attention to power dynamics between partners who come from different backgrounds and how have different social status? Are community members reimbursed for their time using financial payment or other appropriate resources? Do the community members in the research partnership have the confidence and 'permission' to question the views of a senior Professor leading the research? Is the fieldwork planned in a way that gives the research team time to introduce the study to potential participants and to understand any concerns they may have about it? Taken together, asking these kinds of questions gives academic researchers an insight into the way that they need to change the way they work so that the research space (time, venue, attitudinal disposition) is congruent with the values of participatory health research [19].

A final word on the participatory health research paradigm: There are some misconceptions that participatory health research is the same as qualitative research or that it can only be used for qualitative research. This is not the case. Participatory health research as a paradigm, in terms of the family of approaches that are available, is about how research is done *irrespective of what the study design is* [4]. In fact, in line with quality and excellence in all research, the research design should develop based on the research question: what design is needed to answer the research question. This does not change just because a project is a participatory project. There are important examples of participatory projects across different types of preclinical and clinical research [20, 21].

Participatory Health Research Promotes Social Accountability in Medical Schools

The values of social accountability (SA) are relevance, cost effectiveness, quality and equity. As we have seen in Chap. 1, it is common to think about the need for Medical School's to align their curriculum goals with these values in order to create social responsive doctors. In this Chapter, our attention is on how these values align to the *research goals* of Medical Schools. Let's explore how participatory health research actually promotes each of the four values of SA.

First, if decisions about what topics should be researched are co-designed with local community members, then they are likely to respond to their immediate and anticipated health needs. This is essential for the ***relevance*** of research in medical schools. Second, the involvement of communities in medical school research decision-making is ***cost effective*** because it means that resources are directed to research about health needs that the community think are important rather than being wasted on issues that are not. Third, the value of ***quality*** asserts the commitment to upholding impeccable standards in every facet of health research. As mentioned above, like any research paradigm, participatory health research is committed to excellence in terms of standards to ethics and methodological quality and rigour. Participatory studies can incorporate guidance for study design e.g., for systematic reviews and the design of trials and complex interventions [22]. Furthermore, participatory researchers have developed guidance to build capacity for researchers to do high quality participatory research [23, 24]. Such guidance encourages researchers to develop reflective skills to plan and evaluate research partnerships and their impacts. Finally, the most defining feature of participatory health research is its desire for ***equity.*** As we have seen earlier, this paradigm arose precisely because of evidence of unfair health outcomes and a desire to bridge health disparities [4, 5]. This is why participatory health research calls for a radical transformation in health research so that people with lived experience of disparities are regarded as experts who are 'at the table' on an equal footing with other, usually more powerful actors i.e. medical doctors and academics working in health research. What does this radical transformation actually mean or what does it look like? In the next section, we will look at examples of participatory structures, methods and tools that can be used to optimize the participatory health research—and SA—in Medical Schools.

Optimising Participatory Health Research in Medical Schools

A radical transformation in health research in Medical Schools means that we need to consider changes to the structures and processes that support our research. There is a rich literature in the field of participatory health research about structures, methods and tools that are particularly good at creating spaces for participation that are accessible for, and welcoming to, communities (e.g., [25–28]). This is because they are designed to pay explicit attention to power asymmetries and to support dialogues that address the hierarchies between, for example Medical School Faculty and patient or community groups who have been socialized to think that 'doctor knows best'. This kind of hierarchy can be compounded between Medical School Faculty and the wider community if the Faculty does not represent a diversity of groups in terms of socio-economic position, ethnicity or migration status.

Each structure, method and tool is unique in its own way and offers different potential for the voices of community members to be heard and integrated into meaningful dialogues with these more socially powerful research partners. These dialogues can lead to important learning for action and advocacy. Here are examples from primary care research in Medical Schools in North America and Europe.

Participatory Structures

A ***community advisory board*** is an example of a governance structure that has been used. In the late 1980s, a Canada indigenous community approached a primary care doctor/academic at McGill University, Montreal asking for research to explain why diabetes was so prevalent in their community and to do something about it. This led to the celebrated the award-winning Kahnawake Schools Diabetes Prevention Project (http://www.ksdpp.org). The community advisory board has been in place for over thirty years and the membership—community, academic and health partners—oversee a programme of research primarily about diabetes prevention and health promotion. The partnership has resulted in real world changes in the community in terms of diet, exercises and lifestyle. It has resulted in over 80 scientific publications, delivery of hundreds of community and school-based health promotion interventions, and the training of eight PhDs and 22 Masters and six postdocs from three Canadian university Health/Medical Faculties (McGill, Queen's University, University of Montreal), as well as two Kahnawake community advisory board members receiving honorary doctorates from McGill and Queen's Universities. This reveals the ways in which the mutual needs of community and academic partners can be met. An analysis of the dynamics in this partnership using social network analysis methods showed that the ownership for decision-making moved from academic to community members over time [17]. In this way, Thus, the Kahnawake project encapsulates the ultimate goal in participatory health research: that community members initiate the research, participate equally in its development and dissemination. Further, they hold/develop leadership positions in the research programme. The Kahnawake project has been an inspiration to research and capacity building activities in the North American Primary Care Research Group, the largest academic primary care network in the world (napcrg.org). Thus, it is shaping new generations of researchers across multiple Medical Schools.

How do we know that the community members that come forward/get involved are representative of the broader population? What if they are only thinking about themselves and "skew" the dialogues in that way? An innovative project in a Medical

School in Leeds, England about Patient Participation Groups in English general practices was co-designed by a ***co-research group***, comprising seven members of the public with different experiences of Patient Participation Groups s and two GPs. They co-designed an intervention that was tested in two general practices (one in Leeds, one in Manchester) to see if there were ways for the practice staff and some of their patients to co-design a survey that would yield information from the broader practice population about the development of the practice. Using a combination of qualitative and quantitative methods (discrete choice experiment) in a participatory way led to important insights into the ways that patients can influence decision making, championing patient-centered service improvement priorities that were actionable in their local general practice [29]. This intervention can be used in other practices to diversify the membership of Patient Participation Groups and, thus, improve the opportunity for general practices to respond comprehensively to their broad patient population.

Participatory Methods and Tools

In the USA, an urgent need was identified by researchers for patient-centred outcome research in practice-based research networks with diverse ethnolinguistic communities [30]. The research team designed a study to explore whether researchers, clinicians and patients would achieve consensus on [4] a common set of clinical problems that were applicable across a practice based research network and [14] potential clinical interventions to address those problems to inform a patient-centred outcomes research study in a similar research network. The study was designed using ***participatory learning and action (PLA)*** research methods and techniques were used to do just that. PLA is an adaptive research method that brings diverse actors together so that they can participate in dialogues, to learn from each other and co-design actions to bring about real-world change [15, 26]. PLA methods are interactive and use visual maps and charts to generate and analyse data 'on the spot'. In this US study, patients from diverse ethnolinguistic communities and clinicians from seven practices in a practice based research network discussed preferences for patient centered outcomes research that was responsive to patients and the clinicians who serve them in language-discordant settings. The research leads were focused on identified research about clinical priorities, for example diabetes or heart disease. In fact, when the space for discussing priorities was opened up, local communities revealed that *their priority was for research to improve care processes* i.e., their access to care vis better experiences at the reception desks, more support for language differences, more time with their GP doctors to explore their health concerns. These findings are being used to inform new relevant research about care processes to reduce inequities in uptake of colon rectal cancer screening. They also highlight the feasibility of innovation participatory methodologies in practice based primary care research showing how we can expand the repertoire of methodologies in our field.

The rich literature on ***arts-based methods*** in participatory health research provides further scope for such expansion—let's consider photovoice [31]. This is a method where participants take photographs and produce narratives to accompany them. This means that they become central owners of the data generation process and lead data interpretation as well. As photographs and narratives are shared by participants, they work together and with the researchers to elicit key, recurring themes for qualitative analysis. The opportunities for dissemination move beyond the standard academic conference presentation or paper because it is possible to curate an exhibition in-person or using social media to make the findings available in innovative ways and to wider, more diverse audiences. The Optimising Health Literacy and Access (Ophelia) public health project in Portugal is an example of this [32]. Academic and community partners co-designed a timely and relevant research question about health literacy needs in migrant communities. They combined the use of a survey in seven languages with Photovoice as a culturally attuned method that gave participants from Angola, Bangladesh, Brazil, Cape Verde, China, Guinea-Bissau, India, Nepal, Pakistan, Syria and Ukraine the opportunity to take part and inform a health literacy intervention. This is another important example of innovative methods being used by researchers in Medical Schools and reminds us that it is incumbent on use to be open to learning about new methods, such as PLA and arts-based methods, if we are seriously committed to transforming health research in Medical Schools.

To conclude this chapter, I am going to focus on a case study from Ireland that describes capacity building to enable researchers in a medical school to undertake such transformative health research.

Building Capacity for Participatory Health Research in Medical Schools

The School of Medicine in Limerick is maverick in its approach to primary healthcare. Its curriculum has the longest community clerkships in Ireland. Further, it hosts a Participatory Health Research Unit, which is a WHO Collaborating Centre for Participatory Health Research with Refugees and Migrants. The work of the Unit is about *doing* participatory health research projects to generate evidence to inform service delivery and policy. It also focuses on *generating evidence about this paradigm* to guide best practice and to understand the impacts of this way of researching. The Unit has a broad, interdisciplinary membership spanning general practice, nursing, physiotherapy, speech and language therapy, music therapists drawing on disciplines such as biostatistics, health promotion sociology, anthropology and arts practice. The Unit has

- Expertise in arts based research
- Specific goals to build capacity for participatory health research
- Expertise in participatory health research with refugees and migrants

In line with UL strategic goals and the university research strategy, the Unit has worked with the School of Medicine to incorporate doing research with people into its Strategic Plan. The Unit has worked with the University of Limerick Research Office to consider strategic ways to promote the involvement of communities in research across the Departments and Faculties. As a result, through the Health Research Institute, the Unit has led a theme about this way of working and established an annual national Summer School that enables academics, community members and health sector colleagues to meet and learn together about meaningful involvement.

The Unit represented the University of Limerick in landmark capacity building initiatives that were developed by the HRB and IRC to promote public and patient involvement in health research in Ireland. The Unit co-ordinated the co-design of six workshops that are now embedded in the University Training and Development scheme in Human Resources. These cover an introduction to participatory health research, ethics, funding research partners, collaborative grant development and collaborative dissemination. The Unit now represents the University in a newly established national PPI Ignite Network (2021–2026). With a central office in the University of Galway, UL is one of the lead sites working on activities to advance capacity building in UL itself and around the country. Combined, the activities are focused on training for community partners, developing new undergraduate and postgraduate curriculum, critical analysis of policies to enable partnerships, including the essential issue of clarifying appropriate payment methods for partners.

In line with the Participatory Health Research Unit's specialist research knowledge, a School of Medicine PhD examined trust dynamics in the national network and revealed that trust is multi-dimensional, changes over time and that trust building can be dominated by those who have most resources to 'show up' at events etc. usually academics or larger organizations [33]. This cutting-edge doctoral knowledge has been presented at the aforementioned premier primary healthcare conference—the North American Primary Care Research Group annual scientific meeting.

Finally, through its WHO Collaborating Centre, the Unit provides international and national leadership about the specifics of doing participatory research with refugees and migrants. Combining leadership roles in Ireland and with the WHO, the International Collaboration for Participatory Health Research, the European Public Health Association and the North American Primary Care Research Group, results in rich and dynamic networks of academics, community organisations, migrants and health sector planners and policy makers. These actors are working together to optimize migrants' health using participatory health research. For example, in 2023, the Unit started a new Refugee and Migrant Health Partnership with the Department of Health and the WHO. The goal is to involve migrants in public health policy making in Ireland. This includes work to improve their participation in research about their health in Ireland. In line with national PPI Ignite Network's Equality, Diversity and Inclusion strategy, and the Network's interest in responding to the arrival of Ukraine Beneficiaries of Temporary Protection in Ireland from February 2022 after the war on Ukraine started, there was an opportunity to align the work of the Refugee and Migrant Health Partnership with the national PPI Ignite network.

Discussions focused on how to build capacity for more refugee and migrant involvement in research in Ireland. An arts based project called PPI INCLUDES was co-designed with NGO Doras. Here, the use of the arts centered on the use of music and singing, drawing and creative writing to create a participatory space that was welcoming to refugees, migrants, academics and healthcare workers. Working together they generated a vision and action plan to improve refugee and migrants' involvement in health research in Ireland [34]. The implementation of this action plan will be supported by the Refugee and Migrant Health Partnership.

Clearly, the capacity building work in the University of Limerick and across the national PPI network in Ireland is about attention to current and emerging researcher's knowledge, skills and behaviors. However, it is also about *changing the health research eco-system* so that the processes and procedures that enable the enactment of meaningful partnerships are in place. This is on-going and challenging work that requires collaborative working within and across universities, funding agencies and health services. It is essential work that will, ultimately, support radical transformation of research practice in Medical Schools to promote SA.

Take-Home Message

The WHO Alma emphasizes people's right to be involved in decisions about their health, including research. This will help generate evidence to address health inequities.

The resonance between participatory health research and SA is clear and strong. It is necessary to see the synergy between the research activities of Medical Schools and SA so that future doctors are not only care givers but people who can generate comprehensive evidence in equitable ways.

It is necessary to change the way we do research so that research is also co-created with community members. It is imperative to use the evidence from the Participatory Health Research paradigm and make a transformative commitment to meaningful partnerships from start to finish.

There are exemplars in many Medical Schools of a commitment to participatory health research and the use of important methodologies and tools to enact meaningful partnerships. The goal is to make these exemplars the norm rather than the exception—for this institutional level capacity building is needed with equal attention to changes in the national and international health research eco-system. This is vital for support radical transformation to research practices in Medical Schools, promote SA and, thus, ensure that no population group is left behind.

References

1. World Health Organisation. The Alma Ata Declaration. Geneva: World Health Organisation; 1978.
2. World Health Organisation. Declaration of Astana. Geneva: Global Conference on Primary Care; 2018.
3. Marmot M, Friel S, Bell R, Houwelling TA, Taylor S. Closing the gap in a generation: health equity through action on the social determinants of health. Lancet. 2008;372(9650):1661–9.
4. International Collaboration for Participatory Health Research. Position paper no 1: what is participatory health research? Berlin: ICPHR; 2013.
5. Wallerstein NB, Duran B. Using community-based participatory research to address health disparities. Health Promot Pract. 2006;7(3):312–23.
6. Popay J, Whitehead M, Ponsford R, Egan M, Mead R. Power, control, communities and health inequalities I: theories, concepts and analytical frameworks. Health Promot Int. 2021;36(5):1253–63.
7. MacFarlane AE. Optimising individual and community involvement in health decision-making in general practice consultations and primary care settings: a way forward. Eur J General Pract. 2020;26(1):196–201.
8. Gilfoyle M, MacFarlane A, Hannigan A, Niranjan V, Hughes Z, Salsberg J. The public and patient involvement imperative in Ireland: building on policy drivers. Front Public Health. 2022;10:1038409.
9. Denegri S, Coldham T, Eglin S, Frost R, Kerridge L, Matthews R. Going the extra mile: improving the nation's health and wellbeing through public involvement in research. London: NIHR; 2015.
10. Oetzel JG, Wallerstein N, Duran B, Sanchez-Youngman S, Nguyen T, Woo K, et al. Impact of participatory health research: a test of the community-based participatory research conceptual model. Biomed Res Int. 2018;2018:7281405.
11. Russell J, Fudge N, Greenhalgh T. The impact of public involvement in health research: what are we measuring? Why are we measuring it? Should we stop measuring it? Res Involv Engagem. 2020;6:63.
12. Beresford P. Public participation in health and social care: exploring the co-production of knowledge. Front Sociol. 2019;4:73.
13. Arnstein S. A ladder of citizen participation. J Am Inst Plan. 1969;4:238–50.
14. Jagosh J, Macaulay AC, Pluye P, Salsberg JON, Bush PL, Henderson JIM, et al. Uncovering the benefits of participatory research: implications of a realist review for health research and practice. Milbank Q. 2012;90(2):311–46.
15. Chambers R. PRA, PLA and pluralism: practice and theory. In: Reason P, Bradbury H, editors. The SAGE handbook of action research. Sage; 2008. p. 297–318.
16. Nguyen T, Graham ID, Mrklas KJ, Bowen S, Cargo M, Estabrooks CA, et al. How does integrated knowledge translation (IKT) compare to other collaborative research approaches to generating and translating knowledge? Learning from experts in the field. Health Res Policy Syst. 2020;18(1):35.
17. Salsberg J, Macridis S, Garcia Bengoechea E, Macaulay AC, Moore S, Committee KSTP. The shifting dynamics of social roles and project ownership over the lifecycle of a community-based participatory research project. Fam Pract. 2017;34(3):305–12.
18. Cornwall A. Making spaces, changing places: situating participation in development. Institute of Development Studies; 2002.
19. MacFarlane A, Huschke S, Marques MJ, Gama A, Kinaan W, Hassan A, et al. Normalising participatory health research approaches in the WHO European region for refugee and migrant health: a paradigm shift. Lancet Reg Health Eur. 2024;41:100837.
20. Fox G, Fergusson DA, Daham Z, Youssef M, Foster M, Poole E, et al. Patient engagement in preclinical laboratory research: a scoping review. EBioMedicine. 2021;70:103484.

21. Sacristan JA, Aguaron A, Avendano-Sola C, Garrido P, Carrion J, Gutierrez A, et al. Patient involvement in clinical research: why, when, and how. Patient Prefer Adherence. 2016;10:631–40.
22. Skivington K, Matthews L, Simpson SA, Craig P, Baird J, Blazeby JM, et al. A new framework for developing and evaluating complex interventions: update of Medical Research Council guidance. BMJ. 2021;374:n2061.
23. Collins M, Long R, Page A, Popay J, Lobban F. Using the public involvement impact assessment framework to assess the impact of public involvement in a mental health research context: a reflective case study. Health Expect. 2018;21(6):950–63.
24. Staniszewska S, Brett J, Simera I, Seers K, Mockford C, Goodlad S, et al. GRIPP2 reporting checklists: tools to improve reporting of patient and public involvement in research. BMJ. 2017;358:j3453.
25. Chambers R. Participatory workshops: a sourcebook of 21 sets of ideas and activities. London: Earthscan; 2002.
26. de Brun T, O'Reilly-de Brun M, Van Weel-Baumgarten E, Burns N, Dowrick C, Lionis C, et al. Using Participatory Learning & Action (PLA) research techniques for inter-stakeholder dialogue in primary healthcare: an analysis of stakeholders' experiences. Res Involv Engagem. 2017;3:28.
27. MacFarlane A, Galvin R, O'Sullivan M, McInerney C, Meagher E, Burke D, LeMaster JW. Participatory methods for research prioritization in primary care: an analysis of the World Cafe approach in Ireland and the USA. Fam Pract. 2016:cmw104.
28. Morrison C, Dearden A. Beyond tokenistic participation: using representational artefacts to enable meaningful public participation in health service design. Health Policy. 2013;112(3):179–86.
29. Drinkwater J, MacFarlane A, Twiddy M, Meads D, Chadwick RH, Donnelly A, et al. Patient influence on general practice service improvement decision making: a participatory research mixed-methods intervention study. Br J Gen Pract. 2024;74(745):e552–9.
30. LeMaster JW, Lutgen CB, Matharoo J, MacFarlane AE. Refugee and migrants' involvement in participatory spaces in a US practice-based research network study: responding to unanticipated priorities. Health Expect. 2023;26(4):1596–605.
31. Suprapto N, Sunarti T, Suliyanah S, Wulandari D, Hidayaatullaah HN, Adam AS, et al. A systematic review of photovoice as participatory action research strategies. Int J Eval Res Educ. 2020;9(3)
32. Dias S, Gama A, Maia AC, Marques MJ, Campos Fernandes A, Goes AR, et al. Migrant communities at the center in co-design of health literacy-based innovative solutions for non-communicable diseases prevention and risk reduction: application of the OPtimising HEalth LIteracy and Access (Ophelia) Process. Front Public Health. 2021;9:639405.
33. Gilfoyle M, Salsberg J, McCarthy M, MacFarlane A, MacCarron P. Exploring the multidimensionality of trust in participatory health partnerships - a network approach. Front Public Health. 2022;10:925402.
34. MacFarlane A, Papyan A, Garry F, Hassan A, Phelan H. PPI INCLUDES: Public and Patient Involvement Ignite Network Action Plan to include refugees and other migrants in health research. A joint report of Doras and the Participatory Health Research Unit & WHO Collaborating Centre for Participatory Health Research, School of Medicine and Health Research Institute, University of Limerick; 2024.

Further Reading

International Collaboration for Participatory Health Research. Position paper no 1: what is participatory health research? Berlin: ICPHR; 2013.

International Collaboration for Participatory Health Research. Position paper no 6: participatory health research with migrants: opportunities, challenges and the ways forward. Berlin: ICPHR; 2021.

Chapter 14
Appreciative Inquiry: Catalyzing Progress Towards Social Accountability

Cassandra Barber and Robert Woollard

Learning Outcomes

1. Explain the principles and applications of ApI in medical education.
2. Compare ApI's strengths-based approach with traditional problem-solving methods.
3. Identify how ApI promotes social accountability by addressing community health needs.
4. Apply the 5-D cycle to initiate and sustain institutional improvements.
5. Evaluate ApI's impact through measurable outcomes and sustainable practices.
6. Design strategies to integrate ApI into institutional planning and operations.

Introduction

Appreciative Inquiry (ApI) plays a transformative role in medical education by advancing positive change through practical examples and a strong focus on measurable outcomes and continuous improvement. In the current medical education landscape, community needs are central to social accountability. Medical schools must adapt to the evolving health needs of the communities they serve, ensuring that their educational outcomes are closely aligned with societal needs [1,2].

To facilitate this essential transformation, ApI offers a powerful alternative to traditional, problem-centric methods that often focus on deficits and shortcomings

C. Barber (✉)
School of Health Professions Education (SHE), Maastricht University, Maastricht, The Netherlands
e-mail: cassandra@metrein.com

R. Woollard
Department of Family Practice, University of British Columbia, Vancouver, BC, Canada

M. E. Abdalla et al. (eds.), *Social Accountability of Medical Schools*,
https://doi.org/10.1007/978-3-031-94435-2_14

[3, 4]. Instead, ApI advocates for a strengths-based perspective, strategically utilizing existing positive aspects within an organization as a foundation for transformative change [4].

ApI consistently excels in addressing *complex* challenges by adopting a problem-solving *approach* tailored to the dynamic nature of biological and social contexts [4]. Unlike *complicated* problems, which are inherently difficult but bounded by predictability within such things as the laws of physics, *complex* problems require flexibility, adaptive strategies, relationships, and feedback loops [5]. For example, landing a person on the moon involves significant challenges that follow specific laws of physics. Even when an attempt fails, a detailed analysis can be undertaken to decipher the cause, which can be corrected in the next attempt. In contrast, complex challenges, such as building and conducting a medical school that consistently addresses the evolving health priorities of the communities it serves, are not bound by particular "laws." Instead, they are subject to constant feedback loops and behaviour modifications, making them more akin to raising a child [5, 6]. Successes and failures (or triumphs) experienced with one's first child may not apply to a second child due to innate differences and context [6].

This chapter explores how ApI can enhance social accountability in medical education by shifting the focus from identifying problems to amplifying and building upon existing strengths, fostering a positive framework conducive to substantial change [4]. This approach is both theoretical and practical, offering tangible methods for institutions to achieve social accountability objectives [4]. Applying ApI requires a humility approach in situation analysis and proposals for positive change. This involves searching for evidence or current successes, analyzing why these elements work, and using this analysis to expand the elements of success across an institution's culture [4–6].

Defining Appreciative Inquiry in the Context of Social Accountability in Medical Education

Developed in the 1980s [7], ApI represents a departure from traditional approaches to organizational change. Rather than focusing on problems, deficiencies, and what is lacking within an organization, ApI emphasizes exploring, amplifying, and leveraging the existing strengths and successes [3]. The premise that every organization has strengths or effective practices, and these can serve as the foundation for future growth and improvement-principles particularly relevant in the context of social accountability in medical education.

Social accountability of medical schools refers to the obligation medical schools have to focus their educational programmes, services, and research efforts on meeting the priority health needs of the communities they serve [1]. The concept necessitates that medical schools must produce competent graduates who are prepared to address and respond to societal needs [1].

Key Assumptions of ApI

- **Learning from the Past**: Building the future based on lessons learned from the best of the past [6].
- **Enriching Future Visions**: Seeking new knowledge to enrich future possibilities [4].
- **Collective Action**: Acknowledging that collective effort is vital for enacting the values and vision of a group, an organization, or society [8].
- **Imagining New Realities**: Realizing that human systems can create what they imagine [9].

The 5-D Cycle of ApI

The ApI model is structured around five phases, known as the "5-Ds" [4, 6–9].

1. **Define**: Clarify the goals and outcomes of the change process. This critical phase establishes the foundation by accurately describing what needs to be accomplished.
2. **Discovery**: Identify and celebrate what is working well within current practices.
3. **Dream**: Envision what could be possible by building on existing strengths.
4. **Design**: Develop strategic plans to turn these dreams into practical realities.
5. **Destiny**: Implement and sustain these plans, integrating them into the institutional culture and operations.

It is important to recognize that ApI is not about avoiding looking at problems—quite the contrary. Instead, ApI combines philosophical principles with flexible methodologies. An appreciative stance, rooted in ApI philosophy, can be adopted even during problem-solving. This stance encourages focusing on and giving energy to best practices and successes, despite our natural tendency to focus on threats and deficits. Skilled mindfulness can help reinforce this appreciative stance. While this approach may seem counterintuitive initially, it becomes easier with practice. The following observation is worth keeping in mind:

> *...there is an important distinction between ApI philosophy and ApI methodology. Because they've grown up together, sometimes the philosophical principles of ApI are confused with the methodology of ApI. While the first is foundational, the other is infinitely malleable. An appreciative stance—which flows from the philosophy—can always be present, even if the method of choice is problem-solving. Does this sound counter-intuitive? It shouldn't be, because even when solving problems, it's possible to remember to notice and give energy to the best practices and successes that emerge. Given our competence at seeing deficits, this may be very difficult to do in practice. But there's no reason why skilled mindfulness cannot help us get better at maintaining an appreciative stance* [10].

Applying ApI to Social Accountability of Medical Schools

ApI fosters profound engagement with all stakeholders in medical education, including students, faculty, healthcare partners, community members and, in the best case, policymakers and managers [11]. This inclusive approach ensures that institutional advancements not only reflect institutional goals but also resonate deeply with community needs and expectations. Leveraging the positive core of existing practices that align with social accountability goals, ApI fosters an environment where strategic innovations are not only imagined but actively realized.

To fully achieve these outcomes, it is essential that medical schools actively promote all five realms of scholarship defined by Boyer: *discovery, learning, application, integration,* and *engagement* [12]. Discovery focuses on generating new knowledge through research, while learning ensures the dissemination of that knowledge through education. Application involves using academic insights to address real-world health challenges, and integration encourages interdisciplinary collaboration to solve complex issues. Engagement fosters partnerships between medical schools and communities [12], aligning education with societal needs and contributing to public health improvements. Although institutions often focus on the first two realms, it is important to emphasize the fifth realm, which is central to social accountability [13].

Moreover, ApI's focus on positive dialogue and collaborative visioning aligns seamlessly with the principles of social accountability, which emphasize mutual responsiveness to societal health needs [4]. Through ApI, medical schools can transform their educational frameworks to be more dynamically and effectively aligned with the evolving health landscape, thus fulfilling their social contract with society [14–16].

Overall, ApI offers a robust, positive, and inclusive framework for fostering social accountability in medical education. Focusing on strengths, envisioning new possibilities, designing strategic initiatives, and ensuring sustainable implementation, ApI empowers medical schools to meet their societal obligations more comprehensively and effectively.

Strengths-Based Approach for Advancing Social Accountability

ApI's strengths-based approach differs from traditional problem-solving methods that often focus on identifying and addressing deficits. Instead, ApI emphasizes recognizing and amplifying existing strengths and successes within an organization. Focusing on what works well, ApI cultivates a positive, proactive environment, which is essential for fostering a culture of continuous improvement [3] and social accountability.

Core Phases: Define, Discovery, Dream, Design, and Destiny

ApI's methodology is encapsulated in the '5-D' cycle: Define, Discovery, Dream, Design, and Destiny. Recently, greater emphasis has been placed on the initial ***Define*** phase. This underscores the importance of clearly defining the *intent* of the exercise [3, 4]. For example: How do we *design* a new curriculum? How do we *implement* it? How do we *resource* it? The inclusion of the Define phase invites all stakeholders to actively describe the objectives of the initiative, ensuring alignment and shared understanding, which is critical for successful change management [4]. Each phase plays a critical role in fostering social accountability within medical education (depicted in Fig. 14.1).

1. **Define**: The Define phase is foundational, as it clarifies the objectives and outcomes of the change process [3]. During this phase, all stakeholders—students, faculty, community members, and healthcare partners—collaborate to define what needs to be accomplished. Whether the goal is creating a new curriculum or restructuring community engagement, this phase ensures clarity and alignment of expectations [4]. Involving everyone early in the process during the Define phase lays the groundwork for mutual understanding, reducing resistance, and ensures that the entire institution is working toward a shared vision [6].
2. **Discovery**: The Discovery phase involves identifying and appreciating what currently works well within the institution. This phase encourages stakeholders to share stories of success and positive experiences, highlighting the strengths that can be built upon [6]. In the context of medical education, this could involve identifying successful community engagement initiatives, effective teaching

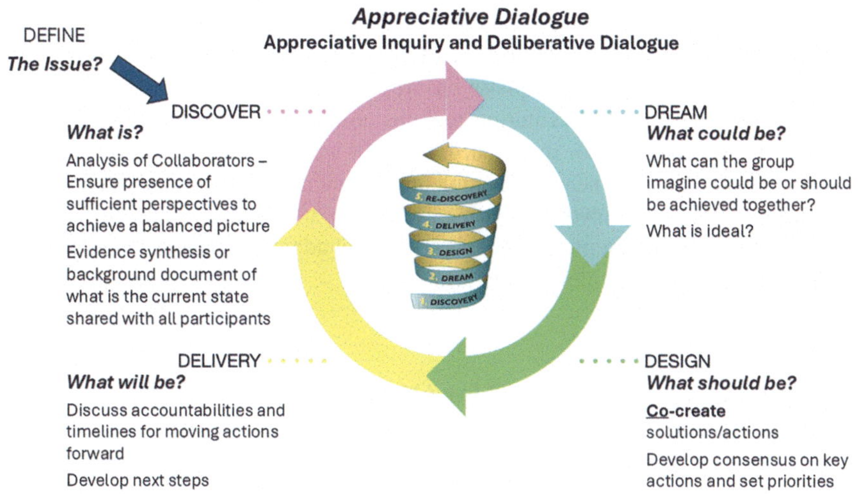

Fig. 14.1 The 5-D Cycle of Appreciative Inquiry for Fostering Social Accountability in Medical Education

methods, and impactful health programs. Carefully exploring what aspects of the undertaking are currently succeeding (because *something* will be) is far more productive than asking the question, "Why are we not succeeding in this area?" The latter often leads to finger-pointing and excuse-making that drains energy rather than sparking excitement at possible joint accomplishment. Acknowledging these positive aspects, institutions can create a foundation for future growth and improvement.

3. **Dream**: In the Dream phase, stakeholders envision what the institution could achieve if its strengths were fully leveraged. This phase is characterized by creativity and aspiration, allowing participants to imagine a future where social accountability is fully realized [4]. This is an expansive phase that invites collective creativity by serially asking the questions, "What if…?" instead of the dampening exploration of "Why we can't…" For health professional schools, this might involve envisioning innovative curricula that address community health needs, enhanced partnerships with local health organizations, or advanced research initiatives that contribute to societal well-being.
4. **Design**: The Design phase translates the aspirations from the Dream phase into actionable plans. Stakeholders collaboratively develop strategic initiatives and concrete steps to achieve the envisioned future [3]. This phase involves creating detailed plans for curriculum development, community engagement, student and faculty selection, promotion, and training. It also involves resource allocation that aligns with social accountability goals. The collaborative nature of this phase ensures that plans are realistic, achievable, and supported by the community. At this phase, the traditional "When the rubber meets the road…" excuses for failure and blame-finding sharpens to questions about, "We know what we want to accomplish, so how ***DO*** we get there?" In complex systems, this process is rarely straightforward with a clear road map. Rather, ApI invites institutions to embark on a self-correcting process: *What? So What? Now What?*
5. **Destiny**: The final phase, Destiny (or Delivery), focuses on implementing and sustaining the changes. This phase ensures that the designed initiatives are put into action and that the institution remains committed to ***continuous improvement*** [6]. It calls forth the question, "How will we know that we are on the right track?" and adjusts as needed to maintain alignment with their goals. In medical education, this could involve ongoing evaluation of educational outcomes, regular feedback from community stakeholders, and adaptive changes to ensure that the initiatives remain relevant and effective.

Strengths of Leveraging ApI for Organizational Culture Transformation Toward Greater Social Accountability

ApI provides a powerful tool for transforming organizational culture in ways that significantly advances social accountability in medical education. Focusing on existing strengths and successes, ApI fosters a positive, proactive environment that enhances engagement and collaboration among all stakeholders. This section explores the numerous benefits of leveraging a strength-based approach for organizational transformation, emphasizing its role in fostering a positive organizational culture, enhancing stakeholder engagement, promoting continuous improvement, and aligning institutional activities with societal needs. Through ApI's strength-based approach and its '5-D' cycle, medical schools can better serve their communities and fulfill their social obligations, ultimately contributing to the overall health and equity of society.

- **Fostering a Positive Organizational Culture**: ApI fosters a positive organizational culture by focusing on strengths and successes, rather than deficiencies. This positive approach can enhance morale, engagement, and collaboration among leadership, faculty, staff, and students. A positive organizational culture is critical for fostering an environment where social accountability can thrive [3].
- **Enhanced Stakeholder Engagement**: ApI's inclusive approach ensures that all stakeholders, including students, faculty, healthcare systems and partners, and community members are involved in the change process. This engagement fosters a sense of ownership and commitment to social accountability initiatives, making the changes more sustainable and impactful [4].
- **Promoting Continuous Improvement**: Emphasizing continuous improvement and adaptive change, ApI ensures that institutions remain responsive to evolving community health needs. This adaptability is critical for maintaining social accountability in a dynamic health landscape [6].
- **Alignment with Core Values**: ApI ensures that institutional activities are aligned with the institution's core values and mission, ensuring that education, research, and service initiatives are consistently geared towards improving community health and well-being [3].

If an individual, a group, or institution wishes to increase its effectiveness in enhancing health and well-being, they should not assume the mantle of "saviour" or be motivated by simple charity with its asymmetrical power relationships in "*doing good*" <u>FOR</u> others. Instead, it is essential to establish a collective stance, working <u>WITH</u> those they wish to serve. This is a core assumption that students often find intuitive when curricula focus on fostering relationships with the communities in which they learning—both within the medical school and in the community [17]. While emphasizing the vulnerability of others can be temptingly satisfying, analyzing and engaging their strengths through the "5-D" approach establishes a more enduring and effective response to factors that compromise their health and well-being. This strengths-based approach also helps institutions adapt more effectively by using the experiences of students and communities to shape the school's evolution [18].

Overcoming Resistance to Change: The Role of ApI

ApI has been used as an effective tool for overcoming resistance to change within the context of medical education. Focusing on strengths, potential, and positive engagement rather than problems and deficits fosters a more collaborative and optimistic atmosphere, reducing the tension often associated with change [19, 20]. Below are specific strategies and examples of how ApI has been utilized to manage resistance to change in education.

1. **Setting a Clear Purpose in the Define Phase**
   The **Define** phase is a critical first step in overcoming resistance to change. This phase focuses on clearly describing what needs to be accomplished and involves stakeholders in clarifying shared objectives. In medical education, this is particularly important during curriculum reforms, where resistance often stems from uncertainty or fear of the unknown. Engaging stakeholders early in defining the goals helps to create alignment, reduce ambiguity, and establish a common understanding of the desired outcomes, thus minimizing resistance [4]. For example, during leadership transitions or curriculum changes, setting a clear purpose can help reframe resistance as constructive feedback. Previous literature suggests that early personal communication and knowledge-sharing during the Define phase fosters a more open and receptive environment for change [19].
2. **Creating a Positive Narrative to Ease Resistance**
   After the Define phase, ApI moves into the Discovery phase, where the focus shifts to identifying what is already working well. This strengths-based narrative is critical in reducing anxiety related to change. In medical schools, where curriculum reforms often provoke uncertainty, ApI highlights successful practices and experiences that enable stakeholder to see the value in proposed changes. Focusing on positive outcomes from similar reforms or success stores from other institutions, ApI helps stakeholders feel more confident in the process [3]. This positive narrative reframes resistance into a willingness to explore new possibilities.
3. **Engaging Stakeholders in Co-Creation to Build Commitment**
   ApI's inclusive nature ensures that stakeholders are engaged throughout the process. From the **Discovery** to **Dream** phases, ApI actively involves faculty, students, administrators, and community partners in joint development of a vision for the future. This co-creation approach fosters a sense of ownership over the change, reducing resistance that often stems from a perception of exclusion from decision-making. Ensuring that all voices are heard, ApI diminishes opposition [19]. In the context of medical education, interviews with faculty and students can reveal underlying beliefs and values that contribute to successful programs [20, 21], allowing institutions to create a future that resonates with community values.
4. **Fostering a Strengths-Based Culture to Build Confidence**
   Resistance to change is often driven by fear—fear of the unknown, fear of failure, or fear of loss. ApI counters this by fostering a strengths-based culture.

During the **Define** and **Discover** phases, ApI encourages institutions to focus on what is already working well. This helps build confidence and reduces the negative emotional responses associated with change. In medical education, this might involve recognizing effective teaching methods or successful community engagement programs that align with the institution's mission [6]. Amplifying these positive aspects, ApI shifts the culture toward one that is proactive and open to change, making the transition smoother for all involved.

5. **Building Trust and Reducing Fear Through Collaboration**
   AI's collaborative approach plays a critical role in building trust, a key factor in managing change. In educational settings, where long-standing traditions and practices may be threatened by change, building trust is essential. Involving all stakeholders from the **Define** phase onward, ApI fosters a culture of transparency and inclusivity, reducing the fear that often accompanies change. In medical education, where curriculum reforms may feel threatening, ApI creates a platform for dialogue that nurtures mutual trust and understanding [7].
6. **Demonstrating Quick Wins to Sustain Momentum**
   Demonstrating early successes or "quick wins" during the **Discovery** phase is an effective way to reduce resistance to change. These quick wins serve as proof that the change process is not only feasible but beneficial. In medical education, ApI might highlight improvements in student engagement or community health outcomes resulting from pilot initiatives. Such early successes encourage further participation and reduce skepticism about the broader change efforts [22].
7. **Aligning Change with Core Values to Enhance Acceptance**
   The Define phase is crucial in ensuring that changes are aligned with the institution's core values. Resistance often arises when stakeholders perceive changes as conflicting with the organization's mission or identity. ApI helps address this by explicitly linking the proposed changes to the institution's mission and values [3]. For example, in medical education, ApI can demonstrate how changes in the curriculum or pedagogy align with the institution's commitment to social accountability.
8. **Sustaining Momentum Through Continuous Feedback and Iterative Improvement**
   ApI emphasizes the importance of continuous feedback and iterative improvement throughout the 5-D cycle. This continuous engagement helps maintain momentum and addresses resistance as it arises. Regularly engaging stakeholders during all phases, from Define to Destiny, allows institutions to adapt their approach based on feedback. This helps ensure that the changes are sustainable, and that resistance is managed constructively [6]. In medical education, ApI has been used to shift from a diagnostic approach that focuses on fixing problems to a nurturing approach that emphasizes growth [19].

ApI offers a practical framework for medical schools to implement social accountability by focusing on strengths and reducing resistance to change. Fostering a mindset shift from "What's wrong and how can we fix it?" to "What's working well and how can we build on it?" encourages faculty and staff to embrace change, rather than resist it. This strengths-based approach empowers individuals and leverages institutional successes, helping medical schools more effectively fulfill their social accountability mandates [23].

Appreciative Inquiry in Action: Practical Applications

While the above sections may sound unhelpfully theoretical, it is important to recognize that ApI has been validated in a wide variety of applications in the organizational spheres—from business through organizational change to academic development. These applications have been successful across a wide range of resource availability, from the most constrained (e.g., Nepal) to the wealthiest (e.g., Canada).

Case Study: Transformative Change Through ApI

In the case of Nepal, the very successful development and engagement of the Patan Academy of Health Sciences (PAHS) [24] over the past two decades is a sterling example. Conceived and deployed on the broad framework of social accountability, it has proven to be a national treasure in deploying health training and services to rural and lower caste health, with particular relevance to responses to the major earthquake in 2015 and the subsequent Indian blockade. The COVID-19 pandemic starting in 2020 provided further affirmation of PAHS as a national resource.

The planning for the Academy began in 2004, when the nation was still in a civil war. In its development it employed the combined approach of engaging the World Health Organization (WHO) “Pentagram Partnership Model” [25] and prepared the students for community deployment by establishing a strength-based perspective. The students (admitted directly from secondary school or careers in community service) were deployed to rural communities within their first year and stayed with members of the national network of female community health volunteers. Their assignment was to engage, get to know and reflect upon the strengths of the community in which they were placed.

Now PAHS is the only school known to the authors that has the word ‘love’ in its mission statement:

> *PAHS is dedicated to sustained improvement of the health of the people in Nepal, especially those who are poor and living in rural areas, through innovation, equity, excellence and love in education, service and research* [26].

In the initial meeting with the class after their return to the home base in Patan/Lalitpur, when asked what they had learned, their first response was, “We had no idea how much love there was in these communities.” Subsequent evaluations and visits confirmed that these sentiments and strength-based (appreciative) approach and perspective made these pioneering classes very effective and impactful in both the development of the curriculum and their predominant career pathways. Notably, prior to PAHS admitting its first batch, 85% of graduates from other schools left the country within two years, with very few entering rural services. Not only are the majority of PAHS graduates over the last decade still in the country, but they are better distributed and capable in the realm of rural health services. It is difficult to tease out the precise role that this ApI approach, coupled with attention to the partnership pentagram has had, but it is reasonable to conclude that, along with a sophisticated selection process, the school has produced cohorts of graduates that approach their careers and practices very differently than those who preceded and those who currently surround them.

A more direct example of the utility and efficacy of ApI can be seen in the development of the *Rural Coordination Centre in British Columbia*, Canada (*RCCbc*) [27]. The *RCCbc* is a tripartite network (government/professional association/university) that came into being early in this century as a response to severe shortages of medical practitioners and rural services in British Columbia. It arose as a rurally focused response and has evolved as a very impactful network devoted to enhancing the health of rural citizens and their communities. An excellent example of the thoughtful use of an appreciative approach coupled with broad system engagement is the calling of a virtual summit in 2020 led by the *RCCbc* in conjunction with the *First Nations Health Authority* (*FNHA*) [11, 28, 29].

This paper provides a detailed outline of a process that not only was grounded in ApI but, through that approach, gained levels of commitment and enduring collaboration that are having palpable impacts on policy. During this engagement of populations and places marginalized by existing services—most notably Indigenous peoples and communities—the *RCCbc* and the *FNHA* have developed an effective collaboration in positively enhancing the health of rural peoples and communities. The process resulted in a reimaging of the WHO's "*Pentagram Partnership*" [25] by adding civil society and local business sectors to make a "*Pentagram Partnership Plus*" (PPP) [11] (presented in Fig. 14.2).

The PPP model has spawned a quarterly standing meeting with the Deputy Minister of Health for the Province (the prime public sector leader). This constructive network has had an impactful influence on the development, deployment, assessment, and modification of policy. It serves as a prime example of active social accountability for all stakeholders involved.

Bringing about positive change in complex systems at various scales is no small task and requires a high level of context specificity. However, it is reassuring that positive change can be found across a wide range of scales and varying levels of resource availability. The *PAHS* and *RCCbc* approaches have demonstrated positive outcomes and can be modified in other contexts. The world is in dire need of such optimism, and the literature contains ideas and evidence to support this optimism.

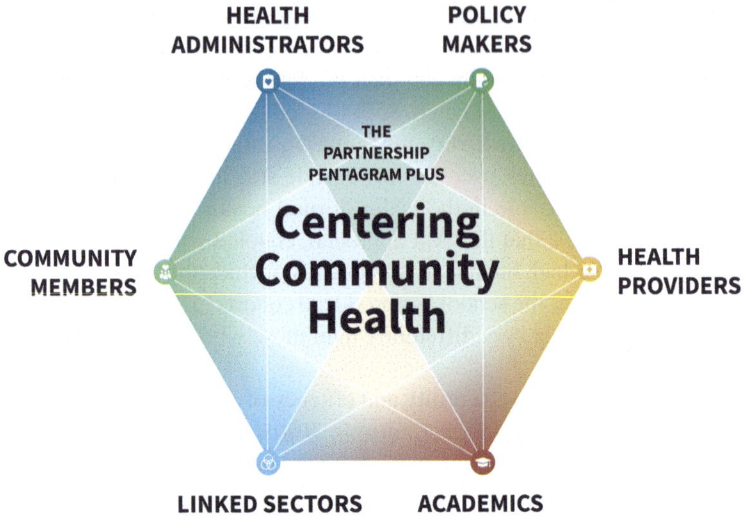

Fig. 14.2 The Pentagram Partnership Plus (PPP)

Impacts of ApI on Social Accountability

ApI has emerged as a transformative approach in medical education, enhancing social accountability by shifting the focus from traditional problem-solving to identifying and amplifying existing strengths. This shift fosters a more inclusive, participatory, and positive educational environment. This section summarizes how ApI can be evaluated using a mixed-methods approach and highlights how sustainability can drive continuous quality improvement and broader social benefits.

ApI has had a measurable impact on promoting social accountability in medical education. Through the evaluation of its influence, the presentation of measurable outcomes, and a reflection on sustainability, it has the potential to foster a culture of continuous improvement and engagement. Medical schools that embrace ApI principles are better equipped to meet their social responsibilities and contribute meaningfully to the health and well-being of the communities they serve.

Evaluation of ApI on Promoting Social Accountability Within the Context of Medical Education

The impact of ApI on promoting social accountability in medical education can be evaluated through various metrics, including the extent to which it has influenced curriculum development, faculty engagement, student outcomes, and community partnerships. Shifting the focus from problem-solving to strength-based approaches encourages a more inclusive and participatory model of education [7, 30].

Evaluations can be conducted through surveys, interviews, and analysis of institutional data to assess changes in these areas.

A key attribute of social accountability is the alignment of educational programs with community health needs [1]. Medical schools can track how well their curricula address the priority health concerns of the communities they serve. Additionally, the engagement levels of faculty and students in community-based projects can also be evaluated to better understand ApI's effectiveness in fostering a sense of social responsibility.

Improvements in Community Engagement and Health Outcomes

The implementation of ApI in medical education has led to improvements in both community engagement and health outcomes. For example, medical schools adopting ApI principles have reported increased student participation in community health projects and higher levels of satisfaction among community partners [11]. These institutions have also seen a greater number of students choosing to work in underserved areas, contributing to improved health outcomes [11].

Quantitative data, such as the number of community health initiatives launched, the participation rates of students and faculty, and the health indicators of the populations served, can also provide evidence of ApI's impact. Qualitative feedback from community members and healthcare providers can further support the positive changes facilitated by ApI-driven programs. Success stories and case studies from institutions like Nepal's *PAHS* and *RCCbc* in British Columbia, Canada, highlight how ApI has fostered transformative change and improved community health.

Sustainability of Changes Implemented Through ApI

Sustainability is a key consideration when evaluating the long-term impact of ApI on social accountability in medical education. Its strengths-based approach fosters a culture of continuous improvement, which is essential for maintaining the momentum of positive changes [6]. The sustainability of initiatives can be assessed by examining the longevity of community partnerships, the retention rates of graduates in underserved areas, and the ongoing adaptation of curricula to meet evolving health needs.

Institutions that have successfully integrated ApI into their operations often report that the positive changes are self-sustaining [19, 31]. This is because ApI encourages an inclusive, participatory approach that involves all stakeholders, creating a sense of ownership and commitment to the initiatives [29]. Regular feedback mechanisms and adaptive strategies ensure that ApI-driven programs remain relevant and effective over time [31].

Moreover, the institutional support for ApI principles, such as continuous professional development for faculty, active student engagement in community projects, and alignment of institutional goals with societal needs, plays a critical role in sustaining these changes. Embedding ApI into the core operations and strategic planning of medical schools ensures that the impact on social accountability remains strong and sustainable.

Leveraging ApI for Continuous Improvement

Continuous improvement is paramount in medical education, and ApI serves as a structured approach to identifying and amplifying institutional strengths. This process ensures that medical education remains responsive to the evolving health needs of society, fostering a culture of excellence and innovation.

Importance of Continuous Improvement in Medical Education

Continuous improvement in medical education requires ongoing efforts to enhance every aspect of educational practice, from curriculum development to faculty training and student outcomes [32]. ApI facilitates this process by promoting a positive, strengths-based approach [19]. Focusing on what works well encourages institutions to build upon existing successes, thereby fostering a proactive and dynamic learning environment. This approach not only enhances the quality of education but also aligns educational practices with societal health needs, ensuring that medical graduates are well-prepared to meet contemporary health challenges [1].

Strategies for Maintaining Momentum and Ensuring Sustainability to ApI Principles

To ensure the sustained impact of ApI initiatives, it is essential to develop strategies that maintain momentum and secure long-term commitment from all involved stakeholders. Continuous professional development for faculty and staff ensures that ApI principles remain at the core of educational practice. Involving students, faculty, and community partners in the process fosters a sense of ownership and commitment to continuous improvement. Institutional leadership must actively support these initiatives by providing adequate resources, recognition, and rewards for successful implementation. Regular feedback from all stakeholders helps to refine ApI processes, ensuring they remain relevant and effective.

Integration of ApI into Operational Reviews and Strategic Planning

For ApI to have a lasting influence, it must be integrated into the regular operational reviews and strategic planning processes within educational institutions [19]. This involves using strength-based evaluation metrics to assess the effectiveness of educational programs and initiatives, ensuring that ApI becomes a core part of the institution's continuous improvement process.

Challenges and Considerations

While ApI offers numerous benefits, its application in the context of social accountability in medical education is not without challenges. Understanding and addressing these challenges is essential to maximize the effectiveness of ApI initiatives. Faculty and staff may resist ApI initiatives due to a preference for traditional problem-solving methods or a lack of understanding of its principles. Implementation requires time, effort, and financial resources, which may be limited in some institutions. Additionally, ApI's principles may not easily translate across different cultural contexts, requiring careful consideration to local norms and values. Ensuring sustainability can be challenging, particularly in environments with high staff turnover or limited long-term planning.

Practical Tips for Overcoming Common Challenges

To overcome resistance and build understanding, institutions can offer thorough training on ApI principles and practices. Starting with small, manageable projects can demonstrate success and build momentum for larger initiatives. Engaging a broad range of stakeholders from the outset can help ensure that initiatives are culturally sensitive and contextually appropriate. Regularly evaluating initiatives and ensuring effective feedback loops helps identify areas for improvement, ensuring that programs remain effective and relevant. This honors the fact that one is dealing with *complex* adaptive systems and not just auditing *complicated* outcomes.

Considerations for Adapting ApI in Different Contexts

For ApI initiatives to be effective across various settings, it is crucial to adapt them to different cultural and institutional contexts. This ensures they are relevant and embraced by all stakeholders involved. ApI processes must reflect local cultural values and norms to be accepted and effective. Additionally, designing ApI initiatives with the institution's mission, vision, and strategic goals helps secure 'buy-in' from leadership [33]. Methodologies should remain flexible to accommodate the unique challenges and opportunities of different institutional contexts.

Conclusion

This chapter highlights the transformative potential of ApI in promoting social accountability in medical education. Focusing on strengths and successes, it offers a powerful framework for driving continuous quality improvement and fostering a positive organizational culture. ApI has the power to catalyze significant, positive changes in medical education, driving institutions towards enhanced social accountability. Embracing ApI principles allows medical schools to better align their educational practices with societal health needs, ultimately contributing to the overall well-being of the communities they serve.

ApI has demonstrated its meaningful potential to foster a culture of continuous improvement and engagement in medical education. Leveraging ApI principles enables medical schools to significantly enhance their social accountability, better addressing the health needs of their communities. Embracing ApI not only drives systemic change and creates a more inclusive, participatory educational environment, but as medical schools strive to be socially accountable, ApI emerges as a powerful tool for achieving lasting, meaningful impact on the health and well-being of the communities they serve. Institutions are encouraged to adopt it as a cornerstone in their efforts to advance social accountability and promote continuous improvement.

Summary of Key Points

- ApI's strengths-based approach contrasts with traditional problem-solving methods, emphasizing the amplification of existing successes.
- ApI facilitates continuous improvement by promoting a positive and proactive environment.
- Strategies for maintaining momentum and ensuring long-term commitment to ApI principles include regular training, stakeholder engagement, institutional support, and robust feedback mechanisms.
- Challenges in applying ApI include resistance to change, resource constraints, cultural differences, and sustainability issues.
- Practical tips for addressing these challenges include comprehensive training, incremental implementation, stakeholder involvement, and continuous evaluation.

- Adapting ApI to different cultural and institutional contexts requires cultural sensitivity, institutional alignment, and methodological flexibility.

Take-Home Message

ApI offers a powerful, strengths-based approach that can significantly enhance social accountability in medical education. Focusing on existing successes and envisioning future possibilities promotes a culture of continuous improvement that aligns educational practices with societal health needs. The key to sustaining these positive changes lies in integrating ApI principles into the core operations of educational institutions, ensuring that medical schools not only respond to current community health challenges but are also well-equipped to adapt to future demands. The chapter encourages institutions to embrace ApI as a fundamental strategy for fostering social accountability and driving meaningful, lasting change in medical education.

References

1. Boelen C, Heck JE. Defining and measuring the social accountability of medical schools. Geneva: World Health Organization; 1995.
2. Boelen C, Pearson D, Kaufman A, Rourke J, Woollard R, Marsh DC, Gibbs T. Producing a socially accountable medical school: AMEE Guide No. 109. Med Teach. 2012;34(11):899–913.
3. Cooperrider DL, Whitney D. Appreciative inquiry: a positive revolution in change. San Francisco, CA: Berrett-Koehler Publishers; 2005.
4. Watkins JM, Mohr BJ, Kelly R. Appreciative inquiry: change at the speed of imagination. 2nd ed. San Francisco, CA: Pfeiffer; 2011.
5. Snowden DJ, Boone ME. A leader's framework for decision making. Harv Bus Rev. 2007;85(11):68–76.
6. Bushe GR. Appreciative inquiry: theory and practice. In: Kessler EH, editor. Encyclopedia of management theory. Thousand Oaks, CA: Sage; 2013. p. 41–5.
7. Cooperrider DL, Srivastva S. Appreciative inquiry in organizational life. In: Pasmore WA, Woodman RW, editors. Research in organizational change and development, vol. 1. Greenwich, CT: JAI Press; 1987. p. 129–69.
8. Ludema JD, Cooperrider DL, Barrett FJ. Appreciative inquiry: the power of the unconditional positive question. In: Reason P, Bradbury H, editors. Handbook of action research. London: Sage; 2001. p. 189–99.
9. Barrett FJ, Fry RE. Appreciative inquiry: a positive approach to building cooperative capacity. Chagrin Falls, OH: Taos Institute Publications; 2005.
10. Rose L. Appreciative inquiry and problem solving: contradiction or complimentary? Coracle Consulting; 2001.
11. Markham R, Hunt M, Woollard R, et al. Addressing rural and Indigenous health inequities in Canada through socially accountable health partnerships. BMJ Open. 2021;11(11)
12. Boyer EL. Scholarship reconsidered: priorities of the professoriate. Princeton, NJ: Carnegie Foundation for the Advancement of Teaching; 1990.

13. Community-Campus Partnerships for Health (CCPH). Linking scholarship and communities: report of the Commission on community-engaged scholarship in the health professions. Seattle, WA: CCPH; 2005.
14. Cruess SR, Cruess RL. An overview of the origins of the social contract between physicians and society, with expectations and demands on both parties. Virtual Mentor. 2004;6:185–8.
15. Cruess RL, Cruess SR. Expectations and obligations: professionalism and medicine's social contract with society. Perspect Biol Med. 2008;51:579–98.
16. Cruess R, Cruess S. Updating the Hippocratic Oath to include medicine's social contract. Med Educ. 2014;48:95–100.
17. Harini S, Prasad R, Dharmarajan S, Arpana R. Integrating community-based education into the medical curriculum: a model for social accountability. Med Educ. 2010;44(11):1105–14.
18. Aiyer H, Walling E, Yeo L, Woollard R. Proposing the community triad model to action social accountability in medical schools. Med Teach. 2024;47(3):534–40. https://doi.org/10.1080/0142159X.2024.2351585
19. Whitney D, Trosten-Bloom A. The power of appreciative inquiry: a practical guide to positive change. Berrett-Koehler Publishers; 2010.
20. Rama JA, Falco C, Balmer DF. Using appreciative inquiry to inform program evaluation in graduate medical education. J Grad Med Educ. 2018;10(5):587–90.
21. Sandars J, Murdoch-Eaton D. Appreciative inquiry in medical education. Med Teach. 2017;39(2):123–7.
22. Bear AJ, Simpson D, Brown D, Bragg D, Marcdante K. Faculty and students perceive common tenets associated with medical student curriculum reform. Int J Med Educ. 2013;4:186–92.
23. Abdalla ME. Application of the appreciative inquiry model for managing change towards social accountability of medical schools. Soc Innov J. 2019. https://socialinnovationsjournal.org/editions/issue-55-1/75-disruptive-innovations/2981-application-of-the-appreciative-inquiry-model-for-managing-change-towards-social-accountability-of-medical-schools
24. Patan Academy of Health Sciences. https://www.pahs.edu.np
25. Boelen C. The partnership pentagon: working together for health. Geneva: World Health Organization; 2000.
26. Foundation of Orthopaedic and Trauma Care. The Academy. https://www.foph.org/academy. Accessed 10 July 2024.
27. Rural Coordination Centre of BC (RCCbc). https://rccbc.ca/
28. Markham R, Graham S, Hunt M, Betkus G, Woollard B, Snadden D, et al. Social Accountability in Practice: Breathing and Weaving Together to Build Relationships and Transform Rural Health Services. Soc Innov J. 2022;14(4). Available from: https://socialinnovationsjournal.com/index.php/sij/article/view/2151
29. First Nations Health Authority. FNHA signs MOU with RCCbc to promote rural health collaboration. https://www.fnha.ca/about/news-and-events/news/fnha-signs-mou-with-rccbc-to-promote-rural-health-collaboration
30. Cooperrider DL. Positive image, positive action: the affirmative basis of organizing. In: Appreciative inquiry: an emerging direction for organization development. Stipes Publishing; 2001.
31. Williamson PR, Baldwin DC, Cottingham AH, Frankel R, Inui TS, Litzelman DK, Mossbarger DL, Suchman AL. Transforming the professional culture of a medical school from the inside out. In: Leading change in healthcare. CRC Press; 2022. p. 265–307.
32. Wong BM, Headrick LA. Application of continuous quality improvement to medical education. Med Educ. 2021;55(1):72–81.
33. Boyatzis RE. An overview of intentional change from a complexity perspective. J Manag Dev. 2006;25(7):607–23.

Further Reading

Foundational Texts on ApI

Bushe GR. Appreciative inquiry: theory and practice. In: Kessler EH, editor. Encyclopedia of management theory. Thousand Oaks, CA: Sage; 2013. p. 41–5. A comprehensive overview of ApI's theoretical underpinnings, this entry offers insights into how ApI has evolved as a management and organizational change tool.

Cooperrider DL, Whitney D. Appreciative inquiry: a positive revolution in change. San Francisco, CA: Berrett-Koehler Publishers; 2005. This foundational text introduces ApI, exploring its principles, philosophy, and potential for driving positive change within organizations.

Whitney D, Trosten-Bloom A. The power of appreciative inquiry: a practical guide to positive change. San Francisco, CA: Berrett-Koehler Publishers; 2010. This guide provides practical strategies for applying ApI in various settings, with real-world examples and tools for fostering sustainable organizational transformation.

Application of ApI in Education and Healthcare

Abdalla ME. Application of the appreciative inquiry model for managing change towards social accountability of medical schools. Soc Innov J. 2019. https://socialinnovationsjournal.org. This paper highlights how medical schools have utilized ApI to enhance social accountability by aligning their educational practices with community health needs.

Rama JA, Falco C, Balmer DF. Using appreciative Inquiry to inform program evaluation in graduate medical education. J Grad Med Educ. 2018;10(5):587–90. This paper explores how ApI can be applied to program evaluation in graduate medical education, demonstrating its effectiveness in identifying strengths, fostering positive change, and improving educational outcomes.

Case Studies on ApI

Ludema JD, Cooperrider DL, Barrett FJ. Appreciative inquiry: the power of the unconditional positive question. In: Reason P, Bradbury H, editors. Handbook of action research. London: Sage; 2001. p. 189–99. This case study examines how ApI has been applied in various organizations, with a focus on its capacity to foster large-scale positive change.

Markham R, Hunt M, Woollard RF, et al. Addressing rural and indigenous health inequities in Canada through socially accountable health partnerships. BMJ Open. 2021;11(11). This paper offers an example of how medical schools and healthcare institutions can apply ApI to address health inequities in rural and Indigenous populations.

Chapter 15
Assessing Medical Schools' Compliance with Social Accountability Principles and Values

Cassandra Barber and Saad Chahine

Learning Outcomes

1. Discuss the concept of social accountability in medical education and its significance in aligning medical schools' activities with community health needs.
2. Identify various frameworks and models that assess and enhance social accountability in medical education.
3. Analyze the strengths and limitations of these frameworks in guiding medical schools toward fulfilling their social obligations.
4. Apply the principles of social accountability in developing strategies for continuous improvement within medical institutions.
5. Evaluate case studies that illustrate the practical application of social accountability frameworks in different global contexts.

Overview of Key Terms

Compliance: In the context of medical education, compliance refers to the extent to which medical schools adhere to established standards and principles, particularly those related to social accountability. Compliance involves aligning the institution's educational, research, and service missions with the health needs of the communities they serve [1, 2]. It ensures that medical schools are not only responsive to

C. Barber (✉)
School of Health Professions Education (SHE), Maastricht University, Maastricht, The Netherlands
e-mail: cassandra@metrein.com

S. Chahine
Queen's University, Kingston, ON, Canada

M. E. Abdalla et al. (eds.), *Social Accountability of Medical Schools*,
https://doi.org/10.1007/978-3-031-94435-2_15

societal needs but also actively engaged in addressing these needs through their education, research, and service activities.

Social Accountability Core Values: These values are the foundational principles that guide the actions and decisions of medical schools in their pursuit of social accountability [1]. The core values include:

- **Relevance:** Ensuring that educational programs and research initiatives address the most pressing health concerns of the community.
- **Equity:** Promoting fair access to healthcare and medical education, with a focus on underserved and marginalized populations.
- **Effectiveness:** Striving for measurable outcomes that positively impact community health.
- **Quality:** Maintaining high standards in medical education, research, and service delivery, ensuring that care provided is evidence-based, comprehensive, and culturally sensitive.

Social Accountability Principles: These principles outline that medical schools have a fundamental responsibility to direct their activities towards addressing the health priorities of the populations they serve [1]. This includes integrating community health needs into the curriculum, engaging in relevant research, and providing services that improve public health outcomes. Social accountability principles emphasize the proactive role of medical schools in not just reacting to, but also anticipating and responding to, societal health challenges [2]. They guide institutions in fulfilling their mission to contribute positively to the health and well-being of the community, ensuring that their education, research, and service activities are aligned with societal needs.

Introduction

Social accountability has emerged as a foundational principle in medical education worldwide. Initially introduced by the World Health Organization (WHO) in 1995, social accountability refers to the obligation of medical schools to direct their education, research, and service activities towards addressing the priority health concerns of the communities they serve [1]. This concept was further expanded by the Global Consensus for Social Accountability (GCSA) in medical schools, emphasizing that social accountability should be a measurable activity, a proactive response to current and future health needs and challenges [2].

This chapter builds on the foundational concepts discussed in previous chapters, providing a detailed overview of various frameworks and models designed to help medical schools demonstrate and enhance social accountability. Here, social accountability is framed as a continuous evaluative process, essential to ensuring that educational outcomes align with community health needs [3]. Assessment plays a critical role in this process, providing essential data that validates how well schools meet their accountability mandates and guides ongoing improvements.

Employing a data-driven approach, schools can systematically evaluate their practices, identify strengths, and address areas for enhancement. This proactive evaluation is critical for developing competent medical graduates committed to community well-being.

Throughout this chapter, various models and frameworks are explored, including the WHO Social Accountability GRID, the Partnership Pentagon Model, the CPU Model, and the GCSA, among others. These frameworks provide different perspectives and methodologies for assessing and improving medical schools' performance across key areas, such as governance, curricular relevance, community engagement, and health outcomes. The chapter also presents case studies from around the world to demonstrate how medical schools have successfully implemented these models to enhance their social accountability. These case studies provide valuable insights into the practical challenges and successes of aligning educational programs with community health needs.

Social Obligation in Medical Education

The medical profession is entrusted with certain responsibilities and privileges by the public, creating an intrinsic social contract between medicine and society [4, 5]. A key aspect of this contract is the obligation of the medical profession to be accountable to society for its actions. Through legislation, regulation, and accreditation, medical schools are tasked with educating competent physicians, prepared to meet societal needs [6]. This relationship represents a social contract between medicine and society, where medical schools are accountable not only to the medical profession but also to the public, including patients, families, communities, and society at large [7]. Additionally, medical schools are not only accountable for the quality of their graduates, service activities, and research, but also for addressing future healthcare needs [2].

Social accountability of medical schools represents a continuous commitment to society, obligating all medical schools, whether they explicitly acknowledge it or not, to align their educational, research, and service activities with the health needs of their communities [7]. This obligation extends to all health professions programs and institutions responsible for preparing the future healthcare workforce [1]. However, social accountability should not be confused with social responsibility.

To clarify these distinctions, the Social Obligation Scale was developed to help evaluate how well medical schools fulfill their social contract [8]. The scale differentiates what it means to be socially responsible, responsive, and accountable, each representing an increasing commitment to addressing community health needs and societal outcomes. Social responsibility refers to the ethical obligation of medical schools to recognize their role in addressing the health needs of the community [8]. It reflects an acknowledgement of the institution's responsibility, but without active measures. Social responsiveness involves proactive actions by medical schools to meet community health needs [8]. At this level, schools engage in specific programs and policies designed to address these needs, moving beyond mere recognition to tangible efforts. Social accountability is the highest level of commitment, requiring medical schools to demonstrate measurable outcomes that reflect their societal impact. Schools at this stage employ systematic evaluation, using data-driven approaches, and engage in continuous improvement to ensure the effectiveness of their programs [8]. They also commit to transparency through public reporting, showcasing their contribution to improving public health (see Chap. 1 for more details on the scale).

Compliance in Social Accountability

In medical education, compliance with social accountability can be understood as a proactive commitment to aligning the educational, research, and service activities of medical schools with priority community health needs [1, 9]. Integrating social accountability into compliance mandates of schools shifts the perspective from being an ideal or aspirational goal to an essential requirement [10]. Such a shift ensures that medical schools are not only responsive to societal needs but also actively engaged in addressing them [1, 2]. This approach highlights the importance of creating a sustainable impact on community health outcomes through targeted educational objectives that promote the four core values of social accountability: relevance, equity, effectiveness, and quality in education, research, and service [1].

Broader Implications of Compliance for Medical Schools

Compliance with social accountability has broader implications for both medical schools and the communities they serve. For medical schools, compliance involves fostering an environment where curriculum development, faculty recruitment, and student admissions are all aligned with the goal of meeting community health needs [4, 11]. This may include widening access through more inclusive admissions processes [12–17], implementing curricular reforms that reflect the social determinants of health [18–21], integrating community-based clinical experiences [22–25], focusing research initiatives on local health issues [1, 8], and collaborating with local health providers and policymakers [1] to ensure that graduates are well-prepared to serve their respective communities effectively.

From the public's perspective, effective compliance leads to greater access to culturally competent healthcare professionals who are attuned to local health challenges [26]. The alignment between medical schools and the communities they serve can lead to improved healthcare delivery and outcomes, particularly in underserved areas [1, 8]. Moreover, when medical schools commit to social accountability, they often become drivers of broader societal change by advocating for policies and practices that address social determinants of health, reduce disparities, and promote greater health equity [27].

Measurement Approaches

As medical schools worldwide strive to align with social accountability principles, effective measurement and evaluation of their compliance have become increasingly essential. This section introduces practical frameworks and models, referred to as 'tools' for simplicity, that medical schools can use to guide their efforts in being socially accountable. These tools offers unique approaches that enable medical schools to integrate social accountability principles into their education, research, and service activities. Additionally, various national frameworks, institution-specific documents and accreditation standards have also emerged to assist schools in embedding social accountability into their mission and practices [28–31]. Accreditation frameworks play a critical role in ensuring that medical schools meet established standards of quality and accountability, including being socially accountable to the communities they serve [8].

WHO Social Accountability GRID

The WHO Social Accountability GRID is one of the earliest formal frameworks for assessing social accountability in medical education. Grounded in the core values of relevance, quality, effectiveness, and equity, the GRID provides a structured approach for evaluating how well medical schools align their educational, research, and service activities with community needs [1]. The GRID aims to improve health outcomes, enhance the relevance of educational programs, promote equity, and foster collaboration across the healthcare system. It operates at three levels: planning, doing, and impacting, which guide schools in setting objectives, implementing strategies, and assessing outcomes to ensure they meet community health priorities [1].

The utility of the GRID has been demonstrated in various contexts, such as the University of Gezira in Sudan [32] and Qassim University in Saudi Arabia [33], where it helped align curricula with local health priorities and identify areas for improvement in community service and research. These studies demonstrate the practical value of the GRID as a tool for medical schools to assess and strengthen their alignment with societal health needs.

Global Consensus for Social Accountability of Medical Schools

The Global Consensus for Social Accountability (GCSA) of Medical Schools is an internationally recognized framework that guides medical schools in aligning their activities with societal needs. It identifies ten key areas essential for achieving social accountability [2]. These areas include anticipating society's health needs, partnering with health systems and stakeholders, and establishing robust governance and leadership structures. They also involve curriculum development, fostering diversity in student recruitment, faculty development, and ensuring adequate resource allocation for social accountability initiatives. Additionally, the areas encompass engaging in community health research, policy advocacy for health equity, and ensuring the adoption of continuous evaluation processes [2]. The GCSA offers a structured and comprehensive approach for medical schools to align their activities with societal needs, promoting health equity, and preparing graduates to address complex health challenges.

ASPIRE-to Excellence Award for Social Accountability

The ASPIRE-to-Excellence Award, established by the Association for Medical Education in Europe (AMEE), recognizes medical schools that excel in key areas, including social accountability [34]. This award serves as a global benchmark, highlighting institutions that successfully integrate social accountability into their core activities.

The ASPIRE Award assesses schools across five key areas: community engagement and partnership, curriculum development, research and scholarship, faculty development, and institutional governance [35, 36]. Medical schools recognized with the ASPIRE Award serve as exemplars of best practices (shown in Table 15.1), providing models for others aiming to enhance their social accountability practices.

Towards Unity for Health (TUFH) International Social Accountability Toolkit (ISAT)

The Towards Unity for Health (TUFH) International Social Accountability Toolkit (ISAT) is a comprehensive framework developed to assess and enhance the social accountability of medical schools [38]. ISAT emphasizes community engagement, curriculum relevance, research and service, and institutional governance. It serves as a self-assessment tool, helping institutions evaluate their progress toward greater social accountability and identify areas for improvement. The toolkit evaluates institutions through four phases, from limited attention to social accountability to full integration and demonstration of impact [38]. The ISAT model provides a

Table 15.1 Social Accountability ASPIRE Award Recipients, 2013–2023

Year	Institution name	Country
2013	Southern Illinois University School of Medicine	United States
2013	Hull York Medical School	United Kingdom
2013	Northern Ontario School of Medicine	Canada
2014	Memorial University of Newfoundland	Canada
2014	University of New Mexico, School of Medicine	United States
2016	East Carolina University, Body School of Medicine	United States
2016	Florida International University, Herbert Wertheim College of Medicine	United States
2016	Leaders in Indigenous Medical Education (LIME) Network	New Zealand
2016	University of Leeds, School of Medicine	United Kingdom
2017	Faculté de Médecine de l'Université Laval	Canada
2018	University of Saskatchewan	Canada
2018	Imperial College London School of Medicine	United Kingdom
2019	Faculté de Médecine, Université de Montréal	Canada
2020	The University of the Wester Indies, Mona	Jamaica
2023	University of Miami Miller School of Medicine	United States

Note: Data retrieved online [37]

comprehensive roadmap for health professions education institutions seeking to enhance their social accountability, ultimately leading to better health outcomes for the communities they serve.

CPU Model

The Conceptualization, Production, Usability (CPU) Model offers a structured approach for medical schools to enhance their social accountability by focusing on three critical domains: Conceptualization, Production, and Usability [8]. This model ensures that a school's activities are aligned with societal health needs, resulting in outputs that are relevant, effective, and impactful.

Conceptualization involves defining the institution's mission and strategic goals, governance and policies, and stakeholder engagement. *Production* focuses on implementing educational, research, and service activities, including curriculum development, faculty and student recruitment, and research and service activities. *Usability* assesses the societal impact and applicability of the institution's outputs, such as graduate outcomes, impact on community health, and continuous monitoring and feedback [8].

The CPU Model has been implemented at the Faculty of Medicine, Suez Canal University, where it was used to better align educational programs with community health priorities and to highlight areas needing improvement [39].

THEnet Evaluation Framework

Building on the CPU Model, the Training for Health Equity Network (THEnet) Evaluation Framework is a comprehensive tool designed to enhance the social accountability of medical schools. The tool focuses on community engagement, educational relevance, and positive health outcomes, particularly for underserved and marginalized populations [40, 41]. It emphasizes recruiting students from underserved backgrounds, developing curricula that address social determinants of health, fostering interprofessional learning, and engaging in community-based education and research to achieve health equity. This framework also places emphasis on understanding the local context, building community partnerships, developing supportive governance structures, and on continuous monitoring and evaluation [40].

The tool offers a structured and practical approach for medical schools to align their educational, research, and service activities with community health needs through a set of measures and standards. This framework has been tested across various contexts, including Ateneo de Zamboanga University, Flinders University School of Health Sciences, James Cook University School of Medicine, Northern Ontario School of Medicine (NOSM), the School of Health Sciences, University of the Philippines, Leyte, and Walter Sisulu University. The practical application of the tool confirmed its utility and applicability in helping institutions align their activities with community health needs [40, 41].

Social Accountability Survey

The Social Accountability Survey is a comprehensive tool designed to evaluate how effectively medical schools align their activities with community health needs [42]. The survey assesses critical aspects of medical education, including program mission statements, admissions processes, curricular content, and educational outcomes [42]. It helps schools identify strengths and areas for improvement in their social accountability practices, guiding strategic planning and policy development. This tool enables medical schools to conduct thorough evaluations of their programs and align their educational strategies with community priorities.

Social Mission Score

The Social Mission Score was designed to evaluate and enhance the social contributions of medical schools, initially focusing on the production of primary care physicians, service to underserved areas, and the graduation of underrepresented students [43]. These three areas collectively produced a quantitative score of how well medical schools meet their social obligations. The framework has since expanded to include a broader health equity model comprising eight measures: institutional mission statements, pipeline programs for underrepresented populations, admissions and selection processes, tuition management, curriculum content, clinical experience locations, mentorship programs, and postgraduate engagement [44, 45]. This expanded framework offers a more comprehensive view of social accountability and its impact on society.

The integration of social mission activities in medical schools is increasingly recognized as vital for promoting diversity, primary care selection, and equitable physician distribution [45, 46]. This framework provides practical methods for schools to evaluate and strengthen their social mission, ultimately contributing to improved health equity outcomes [46].

Partnership Pentagon Model

The Partnership Pentagon Model is a strategic framework designed to enhance collaboration among key stakeholders in healthcare and education [47]. It aims to improve health outcomes and ensure equitable access to healthcare services by integrating diverse perspectives and resources from educational institutions, healthcare providers, government agencies, community organizations, and the private sector [47].

The expanded Partnership Pentagon Plus (PPP) model addresses complex health issues by including a broader range of stakeholders, such as industry and non-profit organizations, emphasizing collaboration to address regional health disparities [48]. The PPP has been successful in addressing complex health challenges, particularly in rural and Indigenous communities, underscoring its potential for broader application in diverse healthcare settings [48]. These models enable medical schools and healthcare institutions to improve educational programs, promote health equity, and enhance overall community health outcomes.

International Federation of Medical Students' Associations (IFMSA) Students Toolkit for Social Accountability

The IFMSA Students' Toolkit for Social Accountability is designed to empower medical students to champion social accountability within their institutions [49]. This toolkit provides practical strategies and tools for assessing, advocating, and implementing social accountability principles in medical education. It emphasizes the importance of understanding social accountability, offering self-assessment tools and institutional checklists that encourage students to reflect on social accountability principles and evaluate how well their institution's curriculum, policies, and practices align with community health needs [49]. The toolkit also guides students in engaging stakeholders, executing advocacy campaigns, and promoting change through initiatives such as curriculum reforms, community-based learning, and diversity initiatives [49]. Validated in the literature [50], this toolkit equips students to actively shape their education, fostering a generation of healthcare professionals committed to equity and social justice.

National Social Accountability Frameworks

Several countries have developed national models to assess and enhance social accountability in medical education. These models provide unique perspectives and approaches, contributing significantly to the field of medical education.

Iran

Iran has implemented a national framework that emphasizes community-oriented medical education, local health needs assessment, and the integration of social accountability principles into medical school curricula [51]. This model is grounded in the local context and addresses the specific health priorities of the Iranian population. The framework involves a continuous evaluative process that ensures medical education remains aligned with public health needs, emphasizing the importance of community engagement and responsiveness to societal challenges [51].

Canada

Health Canada's pioneering national framework was the first to implement a comprehensive social accountability framework for its medical schools [52]. This framework is designed to align the activities of medical schools with the nation's health priorities, ensuring that graduates are prepared to address the diverse and evolving health needs of the Canadian population. Core components include aligning medical education with national health priorities, community engagement, the integration of social determinants of health into the curricula, and continuous evaluation and accountability [52].

Latin America

The Social Accountability Instrument for Latin American Medical Schools (SAIL) is a questionnaire developed to measure social accountability in Latin American medical schools [53]. It addresses areas not covered by traditional accreditation standards, focusing on mission alignment, public health policies, community engagement, and professional integrity. The tool was developed through a rigorous process involving focus groups, a Delphi consensus with experts, and pilot testing with 49 medical schools from 16 Latin American countries to ensure its validity and reliability [53].

Turkey

In 2020, Turkey developed a national framework to enhance the social accountability of its medical schools [54]. Created by the Association of Evaluation and Accreditation of Medical Education Programs (TEPDAD-Turkey), the framework was established through a Delphi study and a consensus workshop. The framework ensures that Turkish medical schools align their activities with local health needs, promoting public health priorities, community engagement, and continuous quality improvement [54]. The study highlights the importance of embedding these principles into accreditation standards, thereby enhancing the ability of medical schools to meet societal health needs effectively.

Korea

Researchers in Korea examined factors influencing the social accountability of medical schools. Using exploratory factor analysis and multiple regression, they identified eight key factors grouped into three broad areas: hardware (H), software (S), and partner (P), collectively referred to as the HSP model [55]. The study emphasized that strong partnerships and effective communication between stakeholders are crucial for enhancing social accountability [55]. The HSP model offers a framework tailored to the Korean context, guiding medical schools in implementing social accountability measures effectively.

Japan

A study in Japan explored how Japanese medical schools understand and implement social accountability within their educational systems [56]. Using qualitative content analysis, the study identified three main categories: societal issues, quality assurance of medical schools, and improvement of individual quality [56]. The findings reveal that while many aspects of social accountability align with global frameworks, there are unique characteristics specific to the Japanese context, such as a strong focus on disaster medicine. This study underscores the importance of adapting global concepts of social accountability to fit local contexts, ensuring that medical education remains relevant and responsive to societal needs.

Institutional-Specific Models

Institution-specific models offer medical schools unique approaches to assess and enhance their social accountability. These tools provide diverse methodologies that schools can adapt to their specific contexts, facilitating the integration of social accountability into educational practices.

CARE Model

The CARE Model was designed to foster cultural change within medical schools by enhancing social accountability through community-based learning, advocacy training, respect, and empowerment [29]. This model immerses students in local communities, providing them with practical experiences in addressing social determinants of health, particularly in underserved areas. It equips students with the skills necessary to promote health equity and social justice, integrating advocacy directly into the curriculum [29]. The model emphasizes the importance of cultural competence, addressing implicit biases, and ensuring the curriculum reflects diverse perspectives. Additionally, it encourages students to take initiative and assume leadership roles, promoting self-confidence and critical thinking.

The model has been successfully integrated into medical school curricula, particularly focusing on rural and Indigenous communities, providing evidence of its effectiveness in preparing students to address specific health challenges and drive policy changes at both local and national levels [29].

AIDER Model

The AIDER (Accountability, Interprofessional Collaboration, Diversity, Education, and Research) model provides a comprehensive framework for enhancing social accountability through continuous community engagement and integrating diverse perspectives [28]. It is structured around five key elements: assessing health concerns in underserved populations, engaging in collaborative research with community stakeholders, implementing and disseminating research outcomes to improve health outcomes, enhancing health literacy and educating healthcare providers, and continuously adapting interventions based on community feedback to ensure relevance and impact [28].

The AIDER model was successfully integrated into a Canadian medical school's curriculum, particularly through a partnership with a community serving an Indigenous population [28]. The model facilitated comprehensive assessments and tailored interventions, improving healthcare access and literacy.

DISCuSS Model

The DISCuSS (Diversity, Identify, Search, Create, Sustainability, and Social Accountability) model strengthens the connection between community needs and medical education by focusing on developing curricular content that addresses diverse healthcare needs [57]. This model incorporates diverse patient backgrounds into the curriculum, identifies and addresses gaps related to social accountability, conducts research to inform new curricular content, collaborates with community stakeholders to develop the curricula, ensures long-term integration of new modules, and continuously evaluates and updates the curriculum to meet societal needs [57].

Implemented over a five-year period at a Canadian medical school, the DISCuSS Model led to the creation of nine new curricular modules focused on health inequities. The model significantly improved students' preparedness to care for diverse populations [57].

Problem-Based Learning (PBL) Inventory

The Problem-Based Learning (PBL) Inventory integrates problem-based learning with social accountability principles in medical education by using real-world health problems to teach students about social determinants of health and community engagement [58]. It emphasizes the importance of using case scenarios directly relevant to community health needs, ensuring that students understand the impact of social determinants such as socioeconomic status and ethnicity on health outcomes, and encouraging students to engage with the community. When applied at the University of Sharjah, the PBL Inventory highlighted areas for improvement, particularly in focusing on underserved populations and cost-effective healthcare solutions [58].

REVOLUTIONS

The REVOLUTIONS framework was created to enhance social accountability in medical education by aligning schools with the health needs of underserved populations [30]. It emphasizes community-based learning, interdisciplinary collaboration, and leadership in healthcare policy, providing students with practical experiences that address social determinants of health and promote equity in marginalized communities [30].

The framework integrates community partnerships into the curriculum, preparing students to work in teams and tackle complex healthcare challenges. It also highlights the importance of faculty development to ensure educators effectively promote social accountability and cultural competence [30]. This framework supports research on health equity and encourages medical schools to influence healthcare policy, improving access to care. Through continuous evaluation, this framework has proven effective in preparing socially accountable healthcare professionals while maintaining alignment with the mission to address societal health needs.

Collaborative E2 (Evaluation & Enhancement)

The Collaborative E2 (Evaluation & Enhancement) Social Accountability Framework was designed to systematically assess and improve the alignment of medical education with community health needs [31]. The framework emphasizes collaborative evaluation between medical schools and their communities, ensuring that both stakeholders are involved in assessing the school's impact. It also focuses on enhancement, encouraging continuous improvement in curricula, research, and service activities to address social accountability goals effectively [31].

The E2 framework provides a structured approach for schools to evaluate their social accountability efforts, offering tools to measure progress and identify areas for development [31]. It highlights the importance of partnerships with local health systems and stakeholders to ensure that medical training is relevant and responsive to local health needs. The framework encourages ongoing feedback and the integration of community voices to improve medical education and foster greater social responsibility among future healthcare providers [31].

Overall, the institutional-specific models summarized above offer diverse approaches for embedding social accountability into medical education. Each model provides unique strategies to align medical school practices with community needs, ensuring that graduates are well-prepared to address health disparities and contribute meaningfully to public health. Adopting and adapting these models enables medical schools to create a more inclusive, responsive, and socially accountable educational environment.

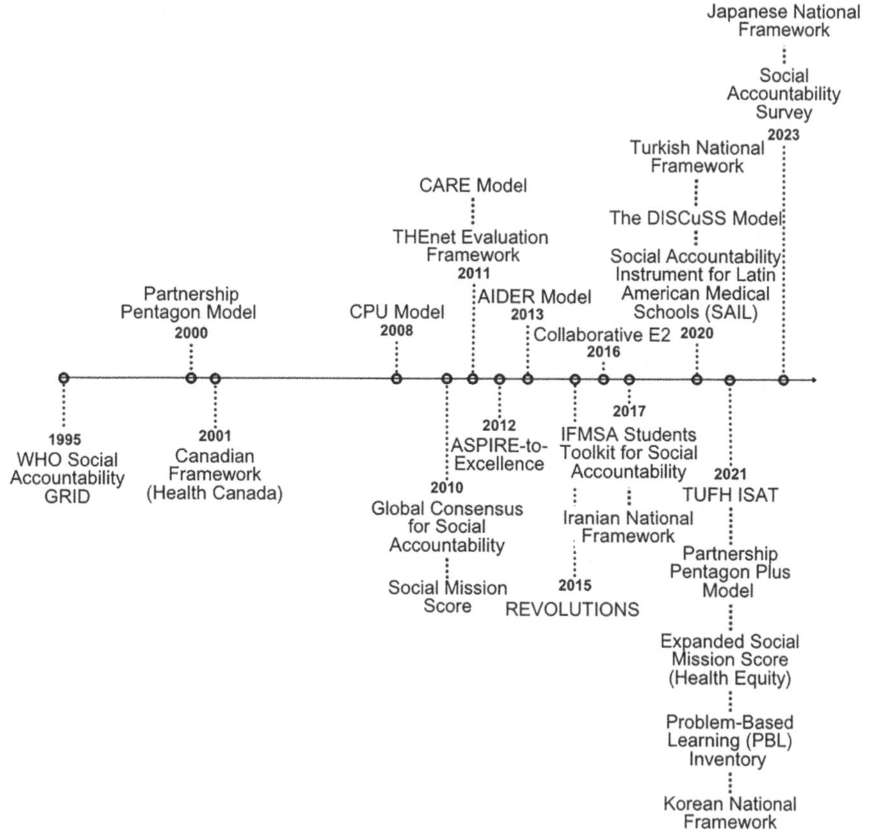

Fig. 15.1 Chronological Timeline of the Evolution of Social Accountability Tools in Medical Education (1995–2023)

Chronological Evolution of Social Accountability Tools in Medical Education

The concept of social accountability in medical education has evolved significantly over the past few decades, reflecting a growing recognition of the critical role that medical schools play in addressing societal needs. This evolution has been marked by the development of various models and frameworks, each contributing to a deeper understanding and implementation of social accountability within the field.

Figure 15.1 presents a chronological timeline of the evolution of these tools, beginning with the introduction of the WHO Social Accountability GRID in 1995 [1] and culminating in the development of the Social Accountability Survey in 2023 [42]. Each milestone on this timeline represents a significant advancement in the approach to promoting social accountability in medical schools.

The progression of these tools highlights the expanding and increasingly sophisticated understanding of social accountability in medical education. Starting with the foundational WHO GRID [1], which laid the groundwork for evaluating how well medical schools align with societal needs, the field has grown to incorporate a variety of models that offer more nuanced and comprehensive approaches. These tools emphasize the importance of aligning medical education with the health needs of the communities, promoting equity, and ensuring that medical schools have a meaningful impact on public health outcomes.

As the field continues to advance, these models serve as essential resources for institutions aiming to enhance their social accountability. They provide critical guidance for aligning educational practices with societal needs, ultimately contributing to a more equitable and responsive healthcare system. The ongoing development of these tools reflects the dynamic nature of medical education and its critical role in shaping a healthcare workforce capable of addressing the diverse challenges faced by communities worldwide.

Key Areas of Compliance Related to Social Accountability in Medical Education

The social accountability tools described above encompass policy, definition, application, and evaluation at local, national, and international levels [59]. While these tools may differ in their specific approaches, they all share common characteristics that serve as indicators for demonstrating social accountability and assessing compliance within medical education [1, 2, 8, 53].

A central theme across these tools is the emphasis on addressing local public health needs. This includes fostering collaboration with key stakeholders, increasing diversity in admissions to better reflect local demographics, producing competent medical professionals, and ensuring that the curriculum aligns with priority health needs. Despite variations in their application, these tools consistently prioritize core principles such as community engagement, alignment of curricula with health needs, and ongoing evaluation.

These tools can be used to support both formative and summative evaluation activities, aiding in strategic planning, policy development, and accreditation processes. However, it is important to recognize that while many of these tools focus on assessing school factors, they often overlook the reciprocal nature of compliance in social accountability. The relationship between the school and the community should be mutually interconnected [59].

To assist medical schools in achieving compliance with social accountability, it is essential to focus on several key areas that are consistently emphasized across the various tools described in this chapter. To facilitate this process, a comparison of these tools across key dimensions relevant to the operations of a medical school and its impacts on the community has been conducted.

Table 15.2 provides a detailed comparison of these tools, highlighting the criteria used for evaluation. This comparison is based on the interpretation of the tools by

Table 15.2 Common elements across social accountability tools in medical education by school system, programmatic, and impact compliance indicators

Tools	School system compliance			Programmatic compliance						Impact compliance			
	Governance & Leadership	Community partnerships & collaboration	Mission statement	Admission & Selection	Curricular activities	Service delivery	Interprofessional collaboration	Faculty development	Research priorities	Educational outcomes	Health policy contribution	Evaluation & Continuous Improvement	Accreditation
WHO social accountability GRID	✓	✓	✓	✓	✓			✓	✓	✓		✓	
Global consensus for social accountability (GCSA)	✓	✓	✓	✓	✓	✓	✓	✓	✓	✓	✓	✓	✓
CPU model	✓	✓	✓	✓	✓	✓	✓	✓	✓	✓	✓	✓	✓
THEnet evaluation framework	✓	✓	✓	✓	✓	✓	✓	✓	✓	✓	✓	✓	
ASPIRE-to-excellence aware	✓	✓	✓	✓	✓	✓	✓	✓	✓	✓	✓	✓	✓
ISAT	✓	✓	✓	✓	✓	✓	✓	✓	✓	✓	✓	✓	
Social accountability survey tool	✓	✓	✓	✓	✓	✓		✓	✓	✓	✓	✓	
Social Mission metrics	✓	✓	✓	✓	✓	✓			✓	✓	✓	✓	
Pentagon partnership (plus) model	✓	✓	✓		✓	✓	✓		✓		✓	✓	
IFMSA	✓	✓	✓	✓	✓	✓	✓	✓	✓	✓	✓	✓	✓
National Frameworks													
Iran	✓	✓	✓	✓	✓	✓	✓	✓	✓	✓	✓	✓	
Canada	✓	✓	✓	✓	✓	✓	✓	✓	✓	✓	✓	✓	
Latin American	✓	✓	✓	✓	✓	✓		✓	✓	✓		✓	
Turkey	✓	✓	✓	✓	✓	✓	✓	✓	✓	✓		✓	✓
Korea	✓	✓	✓		✓	✓	✓		✓	✓	✓	✓	
Japan	✓	✓	✓		✓	✓	✓		✓	✓	✓	✓	

(continued)

Table 15.2 (continued)

Tools	School system compliance			Programmatic compliance						Impact compliance			
	Governance & Leadership	Community partnerships & collaboration	Mission statement	Admission & Selection	Curricular activities	Service delivery	Interprofessional collaboration	Faculty development	Research priorities	Educational outcomes	Health policy contribution	Evaluation & Continuous Improvement	Accreditation
Institutional-specific models													
CARE model	✓	✓	✓		✓	✓	✓	✓		✓		✓	
AIDER model	✓	✓	✓		✓	✓	✓	✓	✓	✓	✓	✓	
DiSCUSS model	✓	✓			✓	✓	✓	✓	✓	✓		✓	
PBL inventory		✓			✓		✓	✓		✓		✓	
REVOLUTIONS	✓	✓	✓		✓	✓	✓	✓	✓	✓	✓	✓	
Collaborative E2	✓	✓			✓					✓		✓	

the authors of this chapter, and a thorough review of each is recommended before adoption, customization, or implementation.

In comparison, each framework is evaluated for its inclusion of indicators related to school system compliance (governance and leadership, community partnerships and collaboration, and the clarification of mission statements); programmatic compliance (admissions and selection processes, curricular activities, service delivery, interprofessional collaboration, faculty development, and research priorities); and impact compliance (educational outcomes, mechanisms for evaluation and continuous improvement, and accreditation standards).

School System Compliance

Governance and Leadership

Effective governance and leadership in medical education prioritize community health needs through strategic direction and operational oversight [8]. Twenty-one tools outline processes for integrating social accountability into strategic plans and policies, emphasizing the need for leadership to demonstrate a strong commitment by establishing governance structures that prioritize societal needs.

Community Partnerships and Collaboration

Community partnerships and collaboration are essential for medical schools to effectively address local health needs and enhance the relevance and impact of educational programs. These partnerships involve working closely with community organizations, healthcare providers, government agencies, and other stakeholders to respond to local health needs effectively [60]. Twenty-two tools emphasize the importance of creating meaningful partnerships, ensuring that medical schools remain responsive to the evolving health challenges faced by their communities.

Mission Statements

Medical schools' mission statements play a critical role in defining their commitment to social accountability, explicitly reflecting the institution's dedication to addressing community health needs and promoting health equity [1]. Nineteen tools emphasize the importance of including social accountability within a program's mission statement.

Programmatic Compliance

Admission and Selection Processes

Diversity and equity are fundamental aspects of social accountability. Admissions and selection processes should promote the inclusion of underrepresented populations and disadvantaged groups [8]. Thirteen tools highlight the need for schools to matriculate students who are reflective of the demographic composition of the local population, including race and ethnicity, Indigenous peoples, socioeconomic status, gender, and sexual orientation, and those from rural or underserved communities [1, 2, 41].

Curriculum Development

A socially accountable curriculum is designed to prepare healthcare professionals who can effectively address community health needs, incorporating topics on social determinants of health, health disparities, and community health [1]. Twenty-two tools emphasize the importance of curricular development, and community-based clinical training opportunities and experiential learning exposures.

Service Delivery

Service delivery is a critical component of social accountability, requiring medical schools to provide health services that meet the needs of local populations, especially those in underserved and marginalized communities [60]. Nineteen frameworks emphasize that schools should ensure their service delivery model prioritize equity and accessibility.

Interprofessional Collaboration

Interprofessional collaboration refers to the practice of promoting education and practice among students from various health professions to enhance communication, teamwork, and holistic care [31]. Seventeen frameworks highlight the importance of integrating interprofessional, team-based care into medical education.

Faculty Development

Faculty development programs are vital for integrating social accountability principles into medical education. Medical schools should provide ongoing professional development opportunities focused on community engagement, health equity, and interprofessional education [8]. Seventeen frameworks emphasize the need for ongoing professional development opportunities.

Research Priorities

Research priorities in medical education should align with community health needs, focusing on addressing health disparities and improving health outcomes [1]. Nineteen tools recommend engaging in community-based participatory research and collaborating with community partners to identify and address local health challenges.

Impact Compliance

Educational Outcomes

Educational outcomes measure the effectiveness of social accountability initiatives by evaluating the extent to which schools address community needs [1]. Twenty-one tools highlight the need for schools to adopt robust evaluation methods and accreditation standards. Educational outcomes should reflect the institution's commitment to producing graduates who are clinically competent and socially responsive.

Health Policy Contributions

Medical schools play a vital role in shaping health policies that promote social accountability through policy advocacy and contributions to health policy development [1, 2]. Fifteen tools emphasize the importance of leveraging institutional expertise and research findings to inform policies that address health disparities and promote health equity.

Evaluation and Continuous Improvement

Continuous evaluation and improvement are essential for maintaining social accountability. This involves the regular assessment of programs and initiatives, collecting and analyzing data on various indicators of social accountability, and using this information to inform strategic planning and policy development [60]. Twenty-two tools recommend establishing mechanisms for transparent reporting and feedback processes to ensure accountability and facilitate ongoing quality improvement.

Accreditation

Accreditation standards play a significant role in promoting social accountability in medical education [8]. Accrediting bodies should incorporate social accountability criteria into their assessment processes to ensure that medical schools meet established standards for community engagement, diversity, and health equity [8]. Five tools emphasize the importance of including social accountability in the accreditation process.

Overall, medical schools must address several key areas of compliance to be socially accountable. These areas of compliance are not prescriptive but should serve as a guide to help medical schools demonstrate social accountability. Focusing on these critical components allow medical schools to effectively address community health needs and contribute to a more equitable and responsive healthcare system.

Advantages and Limitations of Social Accountability Frameworks

This chapter provided an overview of key social accountability tools that can be used to evaluate and enhance compliance within medical education. While these tools share consistent elements, as outlined in Table 15.2, there is no universally accepted process or measure of social accountability [59]. Additionally, the empirical literature reveals marked variability in how social accountability is operationalized and measured [42]. Despite these differences, the tools discussed can be applied in various ways to establish baselines and improve the performance of health professions institutions.

These tools can be utilized formatively to identify strengths and areas for improvement, guide strategic planning, and inform policy development. Accrediting bodies can use them summatively to evaluate the social accountability of educational programs. It is essential that these tools are validated within the unique context and community in which each school operates. Moreover, policymakers and advocates can use these tools as operational guides to promote greater accountability in education. Researchers can also employ them to study the relationship between educational practices and community health outcomes, thereby building evidence on the effectiveness of socially accountable education models.

The strength of these tools lies in their comprehensive and structured approaches to integrating social accountability into medical education. They provide essential elements for planning, implementing, and evaluating activities [61], emphasize the alignment of medical education with community needs, the importance of community-participatory research, and fostering collaborations among educational institutions, healthcare providers, government agencies, and community organizations [47]. These tools are designed to develop socially accountable healthcare professionals who are prepared to address health disparities and the needs of underserved populations.

However, effective implementation of these tools requires substantial institutional commitment and resources, coordinated efforts among multiple stakeholders, and robust data collection and evaluation processes. These demands can be resource-intensive and pose challenges for institutions with limited capacities. Despite these challenges, striving towards compliance with social accountability is a goal that all schools should pursue.

Case Studies of Social Accountability Frameworks in Medical Education

To illustrate the application of social accountability frameworks, this section presents case studies from various countries, demonstrating how medical schools have implemented these principles. The examples include institutions from Sudan, Saudi Arabia, Egypt, Canada, and the Philippines, each showcasing a unique approach to integrating social accountability into medical education.

Sudan

The University of Gezira in Sudan is a prominent example of community-based medical education, closely aligning its curriculum with the health needs of the Gezira State. The institution has integrated community engagement throughout its educational programs, involving students in field training and research projects that directly address the challenges faced by underserved areas [62]. This interdisciplinary approach emphasizes primary healthcare and preventive measures, reflecting the university's deep commitment to social accountability. Focusing on local health needs, the University of Gezira prepares its students to become competent healthcare providers while also ensuring their education significantly contributes to the improvement of the community [63].

The Faculty of Medicine at the University of Gezira (FMUG) is recognized for its innovative approach to medical education, which uniquely combines social and biomedical sciences within a comprehensive curriculum [64]. Established with a mission to address the socioeconomic determinants of health, FMUG offers an immersive learning experience that actively engages students with the community to tackle priority health concerns, aligning its mission with a strong commitment to social accountability [65].

Central to FMUG's curriculum is a robust framework that integrates Community-Based Education (CBE) into all courses, ensuring students gain practical experience that directly responds to the evolving needs of the community [63]. The curriculum includes ten specialized courses, such as the Interdisciplinary Field Training Course, Research and Rural Development Programme, Primary Health Care Health Centre Practice, Family Medicine Phases I-III, Rural Residency, and Health Management and Leadership, all strategically taught in community settings. These courses provide students with in-depth exposure to community healthcare challenges and opportunities, fostering a holistic understanding of healthcare that extends beyond traditional educational boundaries [62].

The longitudinal nature of certain courses, such as Primary Health Care Centre Practice and Family Medicine Phases I-III, ensures that students gain sustained exposure to real-world scenarios, promoting a deep integration of theoretical knowledge and practical skills [66]. FMUG serves as a model of innovation in medical education, illustrating how a socially accountable curriculum can shape future healthcare professionals' skills while significantly contributing to the well-being of the community [63]. This case study highlights FMUG's commitment to holistic healthcare education, offering a blueprint for other medical institutions seeking to make a transformative impact on both their students and the communities they serve [65].

Egypt

The Faculty of Medicine at Suez Canal University (FOM/SCU) in Egypt serves as an exemplary model of integrating social accountability into medical education. Established in 1978 with a mission centered on community orientation, FOM/SCU has pioneered innovative educational strategies that emphasize addressing the social determinants of health and meeting the specific needs of the local population [39].

FOM/SCU employed the CPU model to evaluate how well its activities align with societal needs. In the *conceptualization* domain, FOM/SCU demonstrates a strong commitment to the core values of quality, equity, relevance, and effectiveness [39]. These values are deeply embedded in the institution's mission statement, strategic plan, and educational objectives, which are effectively communicated to all stakeholders. The faculty's active engagement with the community, through its involvement in the governorate and regional health council, allows FOM/SCU to identify and address the most pressing health issues in the region.

In the *production* domain, FOM/SCU excels by offering an innovative educational program that aligns with international standards, such as those set by the General Medical Council in the UK. The curriculum integrates community-based education (CBE), PBL, and early clinical exposure, ensuring that students are well-equipped to tackle the health challenges of underserved populations. The faculty, many of whom are trained in medical education, play a crucial role in maintaining the curriculum's quality and relevance [39].

However, in the *usability* domain, FOM/SCU faced certain challenges due to its reliance on the broader Egyptian health system, which is managed by the Ministry of Health (MOH). While the university hospital and affiliated primary healthcare centers enjoy some autonomy in planning activities, the school depends on the MOH for data on population health and workforce distribution. Despite these challenges, FOM/SCU has successfully implemented several impactful health programs, such as initiatives to improve maternal health services, which reflect its commitment to social accountability [39].

Overall, FOM/SCU largely meets the parameters of the CPU model, particularly in the areas of conceptualization and production. However, the institution's ability to fully realize the usability aspect is somewhat limited by external dependencies. Nevertheless, FOM/SCU's strong focus on community engagement, innovative curriculum, and faculty development positions it as a leader in socially accountable medical education [39]. Continued collaboration with the MOH and other stakeholders will be key to further advancing FOM/SCU's mission to effectively serve the health needs of the Suez Canal region.

This case study of FOM/SCU underscores the critical role that medical schools can play in improving public health through a socially accountable and community-focused curriculum. The experience of FOM/SCU offers valuable insights for other institutions seeking to enhance their impact on community health through education.

Northern Ontario School of Medicine (NOSM), Canada

The Northern Ontario School of Medicine (NOSM) stands as a pioneering institution in Canada, explicitly dedicated to social accountability in medical education. Established with a clear mandate to address the priority health concerns of Northern Ontario's diverse and often underserved populations, NOSM has developed an innovative and community-focused approach to medical education that sets it apart [67].

At the heart of NOSM's mission is its uniquely holistic curriculum, meticulously crafted through a community consultative process. This curriculum, organized around five core themes, emphasizes Distributed Community Engaged Learning (DCEL), which integrates classroom learning with clinical experiences across more than 70 communities throughout Northern Ontario [68]. This model allows students to explore medical cases from the perspective of physicians practicing in these communities, fostering a deep understanding of the region's diverse cultures and healthcare needs [69].

A standout feature of NOSM's approach is its commitment to integrated clinical learning (ICL) and interprofessional education. The school has created a dynamic environment where team teaching and learning occur across various clinical and community settings [70]. The Comprehensive Community Clerkship, a pioneering component of the MD program, immerses third-year students in family practice, offering continuity of care and exposure to community-based specialist care. This longitudinal integrated clerkship is a cornerstone of NOSM's curriculum, providing students with real-world experience in managing healthcare in rural and remote settings [69].

Early outcomes from NOSM's programs underscore the success of its social accountability mandate. Approximately 91% of NOSM's medical students come from Northern Ontario, with 61% of its graduates choosing to pursue family medicine—an area of significant need in the region. Moreover, a substantial percentage of graduates continue to practice in Northern Ontario, directly contributing to addressing local healthcare needs [70].

NOSM's impact extends beyond healthcare delivery to broader socioeconomic benefits. The school's presence has stimulated new economic activities, enhanced retention and recruitment efforts in the healthcare sector, and contributed to the development of community capacity [67]. These efforts have opened opportunities for innovation and growth within the region, further solidifying NOSM's role as a catalyst for positive change.

Through its unwavering commitment to socially accountable medical education, NOSM serves as a model for how medical schools can significantly influence the health and well-being of the communities they serve [68]. The school's focus on community-based learning, strong partnerships with local healthcare providers, and active involvement of community members in governance ensure that its educational programs remain relevant and impactful. NOSM's approach not only produces skilled healthcare providers but also cultivates advocates for community health, setting a benchmark for medical education in Canada [70].

Ateneo de Zamboanga University School of Medicine, Philippines

The Ateneo de Zamboanga University School of Medicine (ADZU-SOM) in the Philippines exemplifies a deep commitment to social accountability, particularly through its focus on community engagement, experiential learning, and addressing the priority health concerns of the Zamboanga Peninsula [71]. The school's curriculum was developed through a consultative process involving key stakeholders, ensuring that the educational content directly aligns with the most pressing regional and national health issues, such as the leading causes of morbidity and mortality in the area [72].

A cornerstone of ADZU-SOM's approach is its emphasis on community-oriented education, which seeks to transform students' attitudes toward community service and care for the underserved. The curriculum is designed to immerse students in community settings for nearly half of the four-year program [71]. This immersion goes beyond traditional classroom learning, as students actively engage with local stakeholders in joint research projects and public health activities. This hands-on approach not only enriches students' educational experience but also fosters a deep sense of responsibility towards the communities they serve [72].

ADZU-SOM's community-engaged learning program has had a profound impact on both the students and the local health services. Participating in service-learning projects and clinical rotations in rural health centers allows students to gain invaluable experience in addressing the specific health challenges of underserved populations. This experiential learning is critical in developing the skills and knowledge necessary for effective medical practice in these communities [71].

The curriculum also places strong emphasis on cultural competence. ADZU-SOM recognizes the importance of understanding and respecting the cultural beliefs and practices of the communities its graduates will serve. Incorporating cultural competence into the curriculum ensures that the school's graduates are not only medically proficient but also culturally sensitive, capable of providing compassionate and effective care in diverse settings [72].

Through these efforts, ADZU-SOM has successfully cultivated a consciousness of community service among its students and graduates, making a noticeable impact on local health services and communities. The school's approach aligns with the World Health Organization's "6 Building Blocks for Quality Health Systems" framework [73], further solidifying its vision of addressing the health workforce needs of the Zamboanga Peninsula [71].

ADZU-SOM's model of medical education, which is both cost-effective and sustainable, aims to ensure that its graduates are well-prepared to serve in rural and underserved areas upon completing their education. This commitment to social accountability is a testament to the school's mission to provide accessible and affordable medical education that directly contributes to the well-being of the communities it serves [72].

Summary

These case studies highlight the diverse approaches medical schools worldwide take to integrate social accountability into their educational, research, and service activities. Each institution demonstrates a strong commitment to addressing the health needs of its respective communities, particularly underserved and marginalized populations. Through innovative curricula, community-based training, and research focused on local health issues, these schools contribute significantly to improving public health and promoting health equity.

Best Practices and Recommendations

In the evolving landscape of medical education, it has become increasingly important to align institutional practices with social accountability principles to improve community health outcomes. Integrating these practices into their operations allows medical schools to better meet the needs of the community they serve.

Achieving compliance with social accountability is critical for ensuring that a medical school's education, research, and service activities align with the health needs of the community. Social accountability requires medical schools to produce competent healthcare professionals who are prepared to address disparities and contribute to the improvement of community health outcomes [1, 2]. This section summarizes best practices and provides recommendations for medical schools seeking to enhance their compliance with social accountability principles.

Adopting these best practices and implementing targeted recommendations significantly enhances a medical school's compliance with social accountability principles. These efforts benefit not only the institution but also have a profound impact on the communities served. Inclusive leadership, strengthened community partnerships, mission alignment, and continuous evaluation and improvement are essential for medical schools to fulfill their social responsibilities. This commitment to social accountability ultimately leads to the development of healthcare professionals equipped to address health disparities and promote equity, contributing to a more responsive and just healthcare system.

Table 15.3 presents a comprehensive overview of best practices derived from key areas of compliance in social accountability within medical education, along with specific recommendations for enhancing these practices. Implementing these

Table 15.3 Best practices and recommendations for enhancing social accountability in medical schools

Areas of compliance	Actions	Recommendations
Inclusive leadership and governance	• Establishing dedicated leadership roles focused on social accountability. • Ensuring that governance structures prioritize community health needs and support continuous improvement.	• Appoint vice-deans or senior roles specifically focused on social accountability. • Ensure these roles have the authority and resources necessary to drive significant changes.
Community Partnership & Collaboration	• Developing and maintaining strong relationships with community organizations, local health providers, and stakeholders. • Engaging in regular dialogue to align the university's objectives with local health priorities.	• Establish and maintain meaningful partnerships with community organizations, local health providers, and stakeholders. • Engage in regular dialogue to ensure the university's objectives align with community health priorities.

(continued)

Table 15.3 (continued)

Areas of compliance	Actions	Recommendations
Mission statements	• Ensuring the institution's mission statement reflects a commitment to social accountability and community health. • Reinforcing this mission across all activities, from research funding to admissions and curriculum development.	• Continuously review and update the mission statement to reflect a commitment to social accountability and community health. • Integrate this mission into all university activities.
Admissions policies	• Broadening the applicant pool to include candidates from underserved and marginalized communities. • Prioritizing admissions for those with a demonstrated commitment to serving these communities.	• Implement admissions policies that actively seek diverse candidates. • Prioritize candidates with a demonstrated commitment to serving underserved communities. • Recruit faculty dedicated to social accountability principles.
Curriculum development	• Integrating comprehensive content on social determinants of health, health equity, and community-based care into the curriculum. • Increasing practical experiences in underserved areas to provide students with hands-on learning opportunities.	• Continuously revise the curriculum to incorporate comprehensive content on social determinants of health, health equity, and community-based care. • Increase opportunities for practical experiences in underserved areas. • Collaborate with community partners to design and implement these practical experiences.
Service delivery	• Establishing student clinics supervised by faculty members in underserved areas to provide essential healthcare services and practical training for students.	• Open student clinics supervised by faculty members in underserved areas. • Ensure these clinics provide essential healthcare services and practical training for students.
Interprofessional collaboration	• Promoting collaboration between various healthcare disciplines to foster a more integrated and effective approach to patient care.	• Develop and promote programs that encourage collaboration among different healthcare disciplines. • Foster an integrated approach to patient care and community health by training students to work effectively in interprofessional teams.

(continued)

Table 15.3 (continued)

Areas of compliance	Actions	Recommendations
Faculty development	• Implementing continuous professional development programs focusing on community engagement, health equity, and interprofessional education to support faculty in their social accountability efforts.	• Provide faculty with resources, training, and incentives needed to engage in social accountability initiatives. • Implement continuous professional development programs focusing on community engagement, health equity, and interprofessional education. • Recognize and reward faculty efforts that contribute to social accountability and community health.
Research priorities	• Focusing research efforts on local and global health needs, particularly projects addressing health disparities. • Funding initial start-up grants for social accountability research to diversify the institution's research profile.	• Advocate for and allocate resources towards research that addresses health disparities and community health needs. • Provide initial grants to support faculty and student research projects focused on social accountability. • Encourage collaborations with community partners in research initiatives to ensure the research is relevant and impactful.
Needs assessments	• Use thorough needs assessments that include feedback from community stakeholders, graduates, and current students to identify gaps and align programs with community health priorities.	• Regularly perform thorough needs assessments to identify gaps in current practices. • Align programs with community health priorities based on this data.
Continuous evaluation systems	• Develop robust systems for monitoring, measuring, and evaluating social accountability initiatives. • Use data-driven approaches to assess the impact of these initiatives and inform continuous improvements. • Integrate these evaluations into the regular review processes of the institution.	• Develop systems for continuous evaluation of social accountability initiatives. • Use data-driven approaches to assess and improve the impact of these initiatives. • Integrate evaluations into regular review processes.

strategies allows medical schools to better align their activities with the health needs of their communities, fostering a more equitable and effective healthcare system.

Integrating social accountability principles into medical education represents both a strategic priority and a moral imperative. Embracing these best practices and recommendations enables medical schools to transform their educational frameworks, producing healthcare professionals who are aware of and responsive to the needs of their communities. These efforts extend beyond the academic environment, fostering healthier populations, reducing health disparities, and advancing equity in healthcare. As institutions refine their approaches to social accountability, they solidify their role as essential agents of positive change in society.

Conclusion

Sustaining and enhancing social accountability in medical education is an ongoing journey that demands regular evaluation and adaptation. Medical schools must consistently align their educational, research, and service activities with the health needs of the communities they serve. This alignment not only enhances health outcomes but also cultivates a culture of equity and social justice within the institution.

Key elements of effective social accountability include inclusive leadership, meaningful community engagement, and a strong commitment to diversity and equity in admissions and curriculum development. Establishing robust partnerships, encouraging interprofessional collaboration, and focusing on community-centered research are also critical components in this endeavor.

Ongoing monitoring, evaluation, and adaptation are essential to the success of social accountability initiatives. Utilizing data and feedback allows medical schools to make informed decisions that maximize their positive impact on community health. Ultimately, integrating social accountability principles into medical education enriches both the institution and the community, contributing to a more responsive and equitable healthcare system.

Take Home Message

- **Importance of Social Accountability:** Social accountability ensures that the missions and activities of medical schools are directly aligned with societal needs, fostering a healthcare workforce that is both competent and socially responsible.
- **Frameworks and Models:** Various frameworks offer structured approaches for evaluating and enhancing social accountability in medical education. Each provides unique perspectives and methodologies to help institutions fulfill their social obligations.
- **Integration of Best Practices:** Integrating best practices, such as inclusive leadership, community partnerships, mission alignment, and continuous evaluation, strengthens a medical school's compliance with social accountability principles.
- **Global Case Studies:** Case studies from diverse global contexts demonstrate how different institutions have successfully implemented social accountability frameworks to improve public health outcomes and promote equity.

- **Ongoing Commitment:** Sustaining social accountability in medical education requires a commitment to regular evaluation, adaptation, and continuous alignment of educational practices with community health priorities.

Incorporating these principles into their operations allows medical schools to enhance their educational programs while playing a pivotal role in improving public health, reducing health disparities, and advancing equity in healthcare on a broader scale. This chapter serves as a guide for institutions seeking to make meaningful contributions to the communities they serve and to develop healthcare professionals who are deeply committed to social justice.

References

1. Boelen C, Heck JE. Defining and measuring the social accountability of medical schools. Geneva: World Health Organization; 1995.
2. Global Consensus for Social Accountability of Medical Schools. Global consensus for social accountability of medical schools. 2010. http://healthsocialaccountability.org.
3. Barber C. Aligning education to societal needs: evaluating social accountability in health professions education [Doctoral Thesis, Maastricht University]. Maastricht University; 2023. https://doi.org/10.26481/dis.20231220cb.
4. Cruess RL, Cruess SR. Expectations and obligations: professionalism and medicine's social contract with society. Perspect Biol Med. 2008;51:579–98.
5. Cruess R, Cruess S. Updating the Hippocratic oath to include medicine's social contract. Med Educ. 2014;48:95–100.
6. Parboosingh J, Campbell C, Silver I, Horsley T, Richardson D, Dath D, et al. Pursuing excellence in practice: a CanMEDS scholar program on lifelong learning. Ottawa: The Royal College of Physicians and Surgeons of Canada; 2008.
7. Barber C, van der Vleuten C, Leppink J, Chahine S. Social accountability frameworks and their implications for medical education and program evaluation: a narrative review. Acad Med. 2020;95(12):1945–54.
8. Boelen C, Woollard B. Social accountability and accreditation: a new frontier for educational institutions. Med Educ. 2009;43:887–94.
9. Woollard RF. Caring for a common future: medical schools' social accountability. Med Educ. 2006;40(4):301–13.
10. Walling E, Lachance E, Yeo L, Koepke K, Wasik A, Woollard R. Key drivers of social accountability in nine Canadian medical schools. Med Teach. 2021;43(2):182–8.
11. Flexner A. Medical education in the United States and Canada: a report to the Carnegie Foundation for the advancement of teaching. New York, NY: Carnegie Foundation; 1910.
12. Ployhart RE, Holtz BC. The diversity–validity dilemma: strategies for reducing racioethnic and sex subgroup differences and adverse impact in selection. Pers Psychol. 2008;61:153–72.
13. Kravitz DA. The diversity-validity dilemma: beyond selection—the role of affirmative action. Pers Psychol. 2008;61:173–93.
14. Larkins S, Michielsen K, Iputo J, et al. Impact of selection strategies on representation of underserved populations and intention to practise: international findings. Med Educ. 2015;49:60–72.
15. Young ME, Razack S, Hanson MD, et al. Calling for a broader conceptualization of diversity: surface and deep diversity in four Canadian medical schools. Acad Med. 2012;87:1501–10.
16. Girotti JA, Park YS, Tekian A. Ensuring a fair and equitable selection of students to serve society's health care needs. Med Educ. 2015;49:84–92.

17. Patterson F, Roberts C, Hanson MD, et al. 2018 Ottawa consensus statement: selection and recruitment to the healthcare professions. Med Teach. 2018;40:1091–101.
18. Allan J, Barwick TA, Cashman S, et al. Clinical prevention and population health: curriculum framework for health professions. Am J Prev Med. 2004;27:471–6.
19. Dharamsi S, Ho A, Spadafora SM, Woollard R. The physician as health advocate: translating the quest for social responsibility into medical education and practice. Acad Med. 2011;86:1108–13.
20. Kaprielian VS, Silberberg M, McDonald MA, et al. Teaching population health: a competency map approach to education. Acad Med. 2013;88:626–37.
21. Maeshiro R, Johnson I, Koo D, et al. Medical education for a healthier population: reflections on the Flexner report from a public health perspective. Acad Med. 2010;85:211–9.
22. Strasser RP. Community engagement: a key to successful rural clinical education. Rural Remote Health. 2010;10:1543.
23. Strasser R, Hogenbirk JC, Minore B, et al. Transforming health professional education through social accountability: Canada's Northern Ontario School of Medicine. Med Teach. 2013;35:490–6.
24. Worley P, Prideaux D, Strasser R, Magarey A, March R. Empirical evidence for symbiotic medical education: a comparative analysis of community and tertiary-based programmes. Med Educ. 2006;40:109–16.
25. Worley P, Silagy C, Prideaux D, Newble D, Jones A. The parallel rural community curriculum: an integrated clinical curriculum based in rural general practice. Med Educ. 2000;34:558–65.
26. Cruess RL, Cruess SR, Johnston S. Professionalism: an ideal to be sustained. Lancet. 2000;356(9224):156–9.
27. Buchman S, Woollard R, Meili R, Goel R. Practising social accountability: from theory to action. Can Fam Physician. 2016;62(1):15–8.
28. Sandhu G, Garcha I, Sleeth J, Yeates K, Walker GR. AIDER: a model for social accountability in medical education and practice. Med Teach. 2013;35(8):e1403–8.
29. Meili R, Ganem-Cuenca A, Leung JW, Zaleschuk D. The CARE model of social accountability: promoting cultural change. Acad Med. 2011;86(9):1114–9.
30. Ventres W, Dharamsi S. Socially accountable medical education—the REVOLUTIONS framework. Acad Med. 2015;90:1728.
31. Kirby J, O'Hearn S, Latham L, Harris B, Davis-Murdoch S, Paul K. Introducing a collaborative E2 (Evaluation & Enhancement) social accountability framework for medical schools. Int J High Educ. 2016;5:216–21.
32. Elsanousi S, Elsanousi M, Khalafallah O, Habour A. Assessment of the social accountability of the Faculty of Medicine at University of Gezira, Sudan. East Mediterr Health J. 2016;22(4):258–66. https://doi.org/10.26719/2016.22.4.258.
33. Alrebish SA, Taha MH, Ahmed MH, Abdalla ME. Commitment towards a better future for medical education in Saudi Arabia: the efforts of the College of Medicine at Qassim University to become socially accountable. Med Educ. 2020;25(1):1710328. https://doi.org/10.1080/10872981.2019.1710328.
34. Drees S, Peters H. ASPIRE-to-excellence academy. Educ Med. 2016;17(3):115–8.
35. ASPIRE-to-Excellence Academy. ASPIRE recognition of excellence in social accountability of a medical school: criteria - Version 2.0. Dundee, UK: AMEE; 2023. https://amee.org/wp-content/uploads/2023/10/Social-Accountability-Criteria.pdf
36. Rourke J. Social accountability: a framework for medical schools to improve the health of the populations they serve. Acad Med. 2018;93(8):1120–4.
37. AMEE. ASPIRE academy award winners 2013–2023 [internet]. Dundee, UK: AMEE; 2023. https://amee.org/wp-content/uploads/2023/10/ASPIRE-Academy-Award-Winners-2013-2023.pdf
38. Towards Unity for Health (TUFH). International Social Accountability Toolkit (ISAT) implementation guide. 2021. https://socialaccountabilityhealth.org/wp-content/uploads/2021/04/ISAT-Implementation-Guide.pdf.

39. Hosny S, Ghaly M, Boelen C. Is our medical school socially accountable? The case of Faculty of Medicine, Suez Canal University. Med Teach. 2015;37(Suppl 1):S47–55.
40. Larkins S, Michielsen K, Iputo J, et al. Measuring social accountability in health professional education: development and international pilot testing of an evaluation framework. Med Teach. 2013;35(1):32–45.
41. Ross SJ, Preston R, Lindemann IC, Matte MC, Samson R, Tandinco FD, et al. The training for health equity network evaluation framework: a pilot study at five health professional schools. Educ Health. 2014;27(2):116–26.
42. Barber C, Chahine S, Leppink J, van der Vleuten C. Global perceptions on social accountability and outcomes: a survey of medical schools. Teach Learn Med. 2023;35(5):527–36.
43. Mullan F, Chen C, Petterson S, Kolsky G, Spagnola M. The social mission of medical education: ranking the schools. Ann Intern Med. 2010;152:804–11.
44. Mullan F, Fair M, Meiri A, et al. Beyond Flexner: a novel framework to implement the social mission of medical education. Educ Health Prof. 2021;4(2):50–7. https://doi.org/10.4103/EHP.EHP_6_21.
45. Batra S, Orban J, Zhang H, et al. Analysis of social mission commitment at dental, medical, and nursing schools in the US. JAMA Netw Open. 2022;5(5):e2210900.
46. Batra S, Orban J, Guterbock TM, Butler LA, Mullan F. Social mission metrics: developing a survey to guide health professions schools. Acad Med. 2020;95(12):1811–6.
47. Boelen C. The partnership pentagon: working together for health. Geneva: World Health Organization; 2000.
48. Markham R, Hunt M, Woollard R, et al. Addressing rural and indigenous health inequities in Canada through socially accountable health partnerships. BMJ Open. 2021;11(11):e048053.
49. World Federation for Medical Education. Basic medical education: WFME global standards for quality improvement. Copenhagen, Denmark: WFME; 2015. https://wfme.org/standards/bme
50. Coşkun Ö, Timurçin U, Kıyak YS, et al. Validation of IFMSA social accountability assessment tool: exploratory and confirmatory factor analysis. BMC Med Educ. 2023;23:138.
51. Abdolmaleki M, Yazdani S, Momeni S, Momtazmanesh N. A social accountable model for medical education system in Iran: a grounded-theory. J Med Educ. 2017;16(2)
52. Health Canada. Social accountability: a vision for Canadian medical schools. Ottawa: Health Canada; 2001. https://www.afmc.ca/future-of-medical-education-in-canada/medical-doctor-project/pdf/sa_vision_canadian_medical_schools_en.pdf
53. Püschel K, Riquelme A, Moore P, et al. What makes a medical school socially accountable in Latin America? A report from a Latin American panel based on a qualitative approach. Med Teach. 2017;39(4):415–21.
54. Sayek I, Turan S, Batı AH, Demirören M, Baykan Z. Social accountability: a national framework for Turkish medical schools. Med Teach. 2020;43(2):223–31.
55. Lee ST, Yang EB. Factors affecting social accountability of medical schools in the Korean context: exploratory factor and multiple regression analyses. Med Educ Online. 2022;27(1):2054049.
56. Mori H, Izumiya M, Hayashi M, Eto M. Current perception of social accountability of medical schools in Japan: a qualitative content analysis. Med Teach. 2023;45(5):524–31. https://doi.org/10.1080/0142159X.2022.2140033.
57. Goez H, Lai H, Rodger J, Brett-MacLean P, Hillier T. The DISCuSS model: creating connections between community and curriculum–a new lens for curricular development in support of social accountability. Med Teach. 2020;42(9):1058–64.
58. Abdalla ME, Dash N, Shorbagi S, Taha MH. Development and validation of inventory tool to evaluate social accountability principles in case scenarios used in problem-based curriculum (social accountability inventory for PBL). Med Educ Online. 2021;26(1):1847243. https://doi.org/10.1080/10872981.2020.1847243.
59. Reddy AT, Lazreg SA, Phillips RL Jr, Bazemore AW, Lucan SC. Toward defining and measuring social accountability in graduate medical education: a stakeholder study. J Grad Med Educ. 2013;5(3):439–45.

60. Boelen C, Dharamsi S, Gibbs T. The social accountability of medical schools and its indicators. Educ Health. 2012;25(3):180–94.
61. Gibbs T. Sexy words but impotent curricula: can social accountability be the change agent of the future? Med Teach. 2011;33:605–7.
62. Ahmed KA, Alneel SM. The role of Gezira University's medical education in community health improvement. J Community Med. 2017;35(2):101–10.
63. Elamin AM, Ahmed KA, Hamad B. Community-based education: the foundation of Gezira University's curriculum. J Med Educ Pract. 2018;9(1):15–22.
64. Abdalla ME, Ahmed KA, Alneel SM. Integrating community-based education in medical curriculum: a case study of Gezira University's Faculty of Medicine. Med Educ Online. 2022;25(1):1710328.
65. Elsanousi S, Hamad B, Ahmed KA. Social accountability in medical education: the case of Gezira University. J Glob Health. 2016;6(2):020406.
66. Hamad B. The genesis of community-based medical education in Gezira. Med Educ J. 1985;19(4):305–8.
67. Strasser R, Peltier R. The Northern Ontario School of Medicine: a long-term strategy to create quality doctors for rural and northern Ontario communities. Healthc Manag Forum. 2014;27(3):67–70.
68. Ross S, Cervin C. Distributed community engaged learning: a novel approach to medical education. J Med Educ. 2020;45(2):123–30.
69. Zhang J, Mitra G, Strasser R. Comprehensive community clerkship: preparing medical students for rural and underserved practice. Can Med Educ J. 2019;10(3):91–8.
70. Mitra G, Zhang J, Strasser R. Social accountability in action: NOSM's success in addressing rural healthcare needs. Can Fam Physician. 2018;64(7):508–12.
71. Guignona J, Woolley T, Ross S. Community engagement and experiential learning in the curriculum of Ateneo de Zamboanga University School of Medicine. J Med Educ. 2021;46(3):225–34.
72. Punzalan RC, de Vera J, Ross S. The impact of community-engaged learning on medical education at Ateneo de Zamboanga University School of Medicine. Med Teach. 2023;45(1):85–92.
73. World Health Organization. Monitoring the building blocks of health systems: a handbook of indicators and their measurement strategies. Geneva: World Health Organization; 2010.

Further Reading

Abdalla ME, Ahmed KA, Alneel SM. Integrating community-based education in medical curriculum: a case study of Gezira University's Faculty of Medicine. Med Educ Online. 2022;25(1):1710328. This article examines the integration of community-based education at Gezira University, demonstrating how medical schools can align educational programs with local health priorities.

Barber C, Chahine S, Leppink J, van der Vleuten C. Global perceptions on social accountability and outcomes: a survey of medical schools. Teach Learn Med. 2023;35(5):527–36. This survey explores global perceptions of social accountability in medical education, offering insights into how schools align their activities with community health outcomes.

Boelen C, Heck JE. Defining and measuring the social accountability of medical schools. Geneva: World Health Organization; 1995. This seminal report by the WHO introduces the concept of social accountability in medical education, laying the foundation for subsequent frameworks such as the WHO Social Accountability GRID.

Boelen C, Woollard R. Social accountability and accreditation: a new frontier for educational institutions. Med Educ. 2009;43:887–94. This paper explores the intersection of social accountability and accreditation in medical education, proposing that accreditation bodies adopt social accountability as a core standard.

Global Consensus for Social Accountability (GCSA) of Medical Schools. Global Consensus for Social Accountability of Medical Schools. 2010. http://healthsocialaccountability.org. This GCSA outlines key principles and measures for achieving social accountability in medical schools, providing an international perspective on aligning education with societal needs.

Larkins S, Michielsen K, Iputo J, et al. Measuring social accountability in health professional education: development and international pilot testing of an evaluation framework. Med Teach. 2013;35(1):32–45. This article presents the THEnet Evaluation Framework, designed to assess social accountability in health professional education, with an emphasis on underserved populations and community engagement

Mullan F, Chen C, Petterson S, et al. The social mission of medical education: ranking the schools. Ann Intern Med. 2010;152:804–11. A landmark study that ranks U.S. medical schools based on their social mission, particularly focusing on the production of primary care physicians and service to underserved areas.

Rourke J. Social accountability: a framework for medical schools to improve the health of the populations they serve. Acad Med. 2018;93(8):1120–4. Rourke's article emphasizes the importance of medical schools adopting social accountability as a framework to produce health professionals equipped to serve diverse populations.

Strasser R, Hogenbirk J, Minore B, et al. Transforming health professional education through social accountability: Canada's Northern Ontario School of Medicine. Med Teach. 2013;35:490–6. This case study on the Northern Ontario School of Medicine illustrates how a medical school can successfully implement a socially accountable curriculum that addresses the needs of rural and underserved communities.

Toward Unity for Health (TUFH). International Social Accountability Toolkit (ISAT) Implementation Guide. 2021. https://socialaccountabilityhealth.org/wp-content/uploads/2021/04/ISAT-Implementation-Guide.pdf. The ISAT provides a comprehensive toolkit for evaluating and improving social accountability in medical schools, emphasizing the importance of community engagement and institutional governance.

Chapter 16
Social Accountability and Accreditation of Medical Schools

Somaya Hosny and Mona Ghaly

Learning Outcomes

1. Explain how accreditation standards can be used as a tool to integrate and promote social accountability in medical education.
2. Evaluate the strengths and limitations of current accreditation systems in fostering socially accountable medical schools.
3. Compare how different global accreditation bodies incorporate social accountability principles.
4. Recognize the importance of aligning accreditation standards with community health needs.

Introduction

The landscape of medical education is undergoing a crucial shift, driven by the pressing need to equip future physicians with a deeper understanding of their social responsibility. Thus, the focus is no longer on only equipping future doctors with clinical knowledge and skills. Traditionally, medical schools have focused on disease management and preparing doctors for a specialist-driven healthcare system. This approach, however, is evolving. Today's focus is shifting towards a more community-oriented approach to equip graduates for addressing the health needs of the population [1, 2]. Despite the increasing specialization and advances in medical technology, disparities and inequalities persist. Additionally, an important challenge is to bridge the gap in essential healthcare services for all with properly qualified medical graduates [3].

S. Hosny (✉) · M. Ghaly
Faculty of Medicine, Suez Canal University, Ismailia, Egypt

M. E. Abdalla et al. (eds.), *Social Accountability of Medical Schools*,
https://doi.org/10.1007/978-3-031-94435-2_16

The disparities and inequalities in health, paired with the burden of chronic diseases, highlighted the critical need of medical schools to be socially accountable [4]. A socially accountable school anticipates the community's health needs through its impact on society. This anticipation should be reflected in all functions and stages of the medical education programme [5]. Accordingly, the socially accountable medical schools' graduates will serve the healthcare requirements of their communities and contribute to a more equitable and sustainable system.

Socially accountable medical schools are not only accountable for what is under the control of the governance of the school, but also should try to influence matters, that currently are beyond the ability of the school and determined by political or financial priorities. This demands a transformation not only in educational philosophies but also in the mechanisms that regulate and assess medical education [6]. Thus, accreditation bodies of medical schools have an important role in this regard.

Accreditation bodies, tasked with ensuring the compliance of the medical programmes with quality and integrity standards, possess the power to incorporate social accountability into their standards and evaluation process. In this way, accreditation bodies can be powerful driver of change that help medical schools to provide, not only competent graduates but also socially responsive to the evolving needs of their communities.

This chapter delves into the intricate and crucial interplay between social accountability and accreditation in medical education. Through a critical analysis of current practices and a proposal for future advancements, it seeks to illuminate the path toward a more socially accountable medical education system through well-defined accreditation standards, ultimately contributing to a healthier and more equitable future for all.

The Role of Accreditation Bodies in Promoting Social Accountability

- **The global perspective of accreditation in medical education**

Accreditation in medical education is defined as "a voluntary peer review process designed to test the educational quality of the new and established medical programmes" [7].

Medical education accreditation was first developed 60 years ago. In 1980 there were only eight accreditation Bodies, in 2021 there were 71 accreditation agencies. Nowadays, The Council for Higher Education Accreditation (CHEA) International Directory lists over 550 quality assurance bodies, accreditation agencies, and Ministries of Education in 175 countries [8] . Despite the fact that the use of medical education accreditation and standards is increasing, it is not universal. Although most countries have some undergraduate accreditation systems in place, the majority of these do not use standards that are specific to medical education, especially in the Sub-Saharan African region [9].

There are currently over 3000 medical schools providing education and training to aspiring physicians around the world [9]. The variability in educational models, combined with the rapid increases in the number of medical schools worldwide [10] and the increasing international movement for education and employment [11] need oversight of quality assurance, and formal accreditation systems, to ensure medical educational institutions function properly [12]. The landscape of medical education accreditation spans international margins, involving a diverse range of bodies implementing varied standards and procedures.

Many countries have developed their standards and processes for accreditation. The Liaison Committee on Medical Education (LCME) is responsible for the accreditation of medical schools in the United States and Canada. The Committee issued "Functions and Structure of a Medical School" [13, 14], uses standards for the accreditation of medical education programmes leading to the M.D. degree. The Australian Medical Council (AMC) is the responsible body for the accreditation of medical schools in both Australia and New Zealand [13, 15–17].

Regional cooperation and international agencies seem to be a growing trend. These international agencies have recognized multinational programmes and supported physician migration and mutual degree recognition [9]. Recently, the development of WFME recognition in collaboration with the World Health Organization (WHO) indicates the spread of globalization in this area. This effort aims to provide a general quality assurance instrument for medical education to be used worldwide voluntarily [18]. This work has resulted in the publication of "Basic Medical Education: WFME Global Standards for Quality Improvement" [19]. These standards are proposed to be used mainly as a tool for the development of medical programmes and to enable international accreditation and recognition of medical schools [20] while tackling the issue of addressing national problems and challenges [21]. The standards are now widely used by many countries worldwide and WFME has recognized more than 100 Accrediting agencies. WFME recognition has many benefits as the existence of an accreditation system that has not been recognized does not guarantee the quality of programmes, Thus, it protects students against education in sub-standard medical schools, and for accrediting agencies, it represents an indicator of international best practice [22].

- **Strengths and weaknesses of the accreditation process in addressing social Accountability**

Accreditation standards play a significant role in driving change within medical schools. As indicated in the Global Consensus for the Social Accountability of Medical Schools [23], accreditation standards are considered one of the most important factors in promoting social accountability in medical schools. The social accountability of medical education must be included in all accreditation processes at all levels [24]. Including social accountability within accreditation process strengthens medical education's commitment to social justice, health equity, and community engagement, ultimately fostering a more sustainable and equitable healthcare system [25].

Accreditation standards can be generally classified into three types: input standards, process standards, and outcome standards. Input standards focus on the resources and infrastructure required, such as staff qualifications, equipment availability, and physical facilities. Process standards emphasize the activities and procedures used to deliver services or products. Outcome standards assess the actual results or impacts achieved, such as the quality of care, patient satisfaction, or environmental effects [26].

The current predominant method used for accrediting medical education is the process standards [27, 28]. These standards typically guarantee that organizations follow established protocols, procedures, and guidelines. While process standards can help maintain quality and consistency, they may not adequately address the social accountability of organizations as it may not capture the extent to which an organization is addressing social determinants of health, promoting equity, or collaborating with community stakeholders [29]. Thus, to better address social accountability, a shift towards outcome-based accreditation standards may be more appropriate as it would assess the actual impact of an organization's activities on the well-being of the community, rather than just the adherence to predetermined processes. This would encourage organizations to be more responsive to the communities' needs and demonstrate their commitment to social responsibility [29, 30] .

Many examples can be included in outcome-based accreditation standards to address social accountability. Medical institutions could be assessed on their ability to improve the overall health and well-being of the communities they serve, such as measures of health equity, access to healthcare, and community-level health indicators [30]. For educational institutions, standards could include measures of Graduates' ability to contribute to the social and economic development of their communities [29]. Moreover, institutions could be evaluated on their ability to minimize the environmental impact and contribute to the sustainability of the communities they serve, such as waste management and ecosystem preservation [30]. Outcome standards could also assess the level of satisfaction and engagement of various stakeholders, including community members, policymakers, and industry partners, with the institution's activities and their perceived impact on the community [31].

Despite the fact that including social accountability concepts in accreditation processes for medical education has many benefits for the programme and the graduates, it also has some limitations. Here's a breakdown of both:

- **Strengths**

  When social accountability concepts are inculcated into the accreditation standards, this will ensure graduates have the necessary skills to serve their communities [25]. Beyond clinical expertise, these skills include effective communication abilities, and cultural competency, both are crucial for addressing community health needs [24] . Moreover, this will encourage the medical schools to include in their curricula, important topics such as population health, social medicine, health promotion as well as risk and disease prevention, among other topics which will prepare future doctors to understand the broader social determinants of health and health disparities [25]. By considering local health workforce needs in accreditation standards, this can encourage medical schools to graduate doctors who are well-prepared to work in underserved areas and address local health challenges [32]. Finally, Accreditation serves as a framework for medical schools to continually improve their educational programmes and this can lead to better alignment with community needs over time [33].

- **Weaknesses**

  Overall, accreditation can be a tool to promote social accountability in medical education, but it has limitations [32]. Accreditation might prioritize individual graduate competency, measured through exams, which may not necessarily directly translate to improved population health outcomes. Accreditation standards may lack emphasis on practical experience in underserved communities. Experience in working with real populations can be crucial for social accountability [33]. Also, standards may not be specific enough to address the social determinants of health, like poverty or lack of sanitation which are factors that greatly impact population health but might not be well-addressed in curriculum [25]. Finally, the rigor of accreditation processes can vary across regions which can lead to uneven social impact, with some graduates better prepared to address population health needs than others [34]. Addressing these weaknesses through stronger outcome standards, community engagement requirements, and a focus on population health outcomes can make accreditation a more effective driver of social responsibility in future doctors.

- **Initiatives of some accrediting bodies in incorporating the concepts of social accountability in their accreditation standards**

  The WFME, LCME, and AMC are used as the basis for the development of accreditation systems in many countries around the world [13, 35, 36]. These bodies have started promoting social accountability through incorporating social accountability standards into their frameworks [37].

  The concept of social accountability is embedded in many parts of the WFME standards documents [38]. The WFME standards stimulate medical schools to encompass social accountability when developing their mission and objectives, where area 1, Mission and values, states that medical schools must respond to the health needs of society [36] and one of the key questions concerning the mission is "How does mission statement address the role of the medical school in the community?". In Area 2 "curriculum" some key question are also related to the society "How do they relate to the intended career roles of graduates in society?", "What makes the chosen outcomes appropriate to the social context of the school?", "What elements of behavioral and social sciences are included in the curriculum? How are the choices made and time allocated for these elements?" Thus Area 2 considered societal needs as one of the basis for curricular developments, and programme evaluation, the behavioral and social sciences and medical ethics [38, 39].

  The LCME Document [14] proposed 12 standards, in which some criteria of social accountability are included into these standards. Under Standard 6 "competencies, curricular objectives and curricular design" they stated that "The faculty of a medical school ensure that the medical education programme provides sufficient opportunities for, encourages, and supports medical student participation in service-learning and/or community service activities". Standard 7, "Curriculum content," 7.1 requires students to apply updated scientific knowledge to act on individual and population health and recognize possible impacts of socio-economic and cultural factors on patients' health [30] and 7.2 "Societal problems" were also indicated as an important component of curricular contents which was defined in the standards as "The faculty of a medical school ensure that the medical curriculum includes instruction in the diagnosis, prevention, appropriate reporting, and treatment of the medical consequences of common societal problems. Finally, 7.3 "structural competence, cultural competence, and health inequities" were defined also as important component of curricular contents emphasizing the importance of health care disparities and health inequities, and the impact of disparities in health care on all populations and approaches to reducing health care inequities [14].

The AMC standards, under Standard 1 "Purpose, context and accountability" there is encouragement for the medical schools to incorporate social accountability when making their purpose include learning, teaching, research, and social and community responsibilities. The same standard also mentions partnerships with communities and engagement with stakeholders including community groups who experience health inequities that should participate in defining the medical programme outcomes, designing and implementing the curriculum and assessment system, and evaluating the medical programme and its outcomes. Some concepts of social accountability are also embedded on standard 5 "learning environment" 5.2.5: staff resources where it states that "The medical education provider recruits, supports and trains patients and community members who are formally engaged in planned learning and teaching activities. The provider has processes that are inclusive and appropriately resourced for recruiting patients and community members, ensuring the engagement of community groups who experience health inequities and Aboriginal and/or Torres Strait Islander and Māori communities" [15].

Moreover, other committees such as the Accreditation Commission on Colleges for Medicine (ACCM) which is a medical accreditation body whose members (Commissioners) are senior medical educators, together with a lay member representing the public, serve countries that may not have a medical accreditation body of their own. The Commission is independent of the countries it serves and of the schools it inspects and evaluates. The ACCM standards of accreditation for schools of medicine also have considered some concepts related to social accountability, particularly in standard 5 "curricular content" where they included criteria related to "service to society and the community" and "cultural competence and health care disparities". The standard states that "The curriculum provides opportunities for, and encourages, medical student participation in, service-learning and/or community service activities." Furthermore, this standard encourages medical curricula to include an appreciation of basic principles of culturally competent health care, the impact of disparities in health care on medically underserved populations and the potential solutions to eliminate these disparities [40].

The Committee on Accreditation of Canadian Medical Schools (CACMS) also shares the same 12 standards as the LCME but has added an accreditation element under Standard 1. Element 1.1.1 explicitly addresses the social accountability mandate of medical schools and states that "A medical school is committed to address the priority health concerns of the populations it has a responsibility to serve". Hence, CACMS considered the medical school's social accountability is fulfilled in its educational programme through admissions, curricular content, and types and locations of educational experiences; evidenced by specific outcome measures." [37, 41].

All the previous accreditation bodies set of standards have sincere efforts to include some dimensions of Social accountability, however, innovative evaluation methods measuring all aspects of social accountability should be explicit in those standards to ensure that medical schools are obliged to apply these aspects.

Incorporating Social Accountability in Accreditation Standards for Greater Accountability

The accreditation system can be a strong drive for change [29] and can consider the effect of educational programmes rather than the process of delivering these programmes [42]. Previous studies have shown that social aspects are considered in evaluations of medical schools if they receive funds and support from society and their graduates should be evaluated for their responsibilities toward their communities [43]. Thus, it would be essential to include assessment of social accountability as a major component of accreditation standards and processes [36, 44].

Definitions of standards to address social accountability should consider three principles. First, the current social goals, necessities and difficulties should be defined through community discussion [5, 25]. Second, the goals should be specific. Third, the standards should be based on evidence that links them to the community objectives [43].

For strengthening social accountability within accreditation standards, accreditation bodies should focus on many points. Measurable outcomes should be available where institutions would report on key performance indicators (KPIs) disaggregated by race, ethnicity, socioeconomic status, gender, and other relevant demographics. This allows for the identification of areas where certain groups are not being well-served [45]. Standards could mandate surveys or focus groups to assess the community's perception of the institution's responsiveness to their needs [24]. Representatives from the community could be included on accreditation review teams. This will ensure a broader perspective is incorporated into the evaluation process [46]. Moreover, institutions should be mandated to openly report on their social accountability efforts, including initiatives undertaken and progress made towards stated goals.

Certainly, Social accountability in the context of institutions extends beyond the educational or service delivery functions. It also encompasses the research and service activities of these institutions. Social accountability requires institutions to ensure that their research agenda and outputs are aligned with the needs and priorities of the communities they serve [29]. This means that institutions should also engage with stakeholders, including community members, policymakers, and practitioners, to identify research topics that are relevant and impactful for addressing societal challenges [30]. Additionally, institutions should strive to disseminate their research findings in accessible and actionable ways to facilitate the translation of knowledge into practice [47].

Furthermore, the service function of institutions, such as providing technical assistance, consulting, or community outreach, should also be guided by principles of social accountability [29]. Institutions should actively seek to collaborate with community partners, understand their needs, and tailor their service offerings to address local priorities and challenges. Institutions should establish mechanisms to continuously evaluate the impact of their research and service activities on the communities they serve and use this feedback to refine their approaches and priorities [29].

Thus, by integrating the evaluation of institutional research and service activities in accreditation KPIs, accreditation standards will ensure institutional commitment to addressing the broader societal impact of their work and contribute to the well-being of the communities they serve [30].

Other points that may help accrediting bodies to consider institutions accountable to the communities they serve may include the presence of standards for measuring the following:

- Graduate preparedness to serve diverse populations effectively, through integrating social justice issues and culturally responsive pedagogy into the curriculum [38] .
- Institutions regular assessments of the community's health needs and tailoring their services accordingly [48].
- Publicly reporting on healthcare disparities in the community served [49]
- Institutional tracking and reporting on patients' outcomes to demonstrate the effectiveness of services in meeting community needs [50].
- Degree of involvement of the different stakeholders [29].

The Implementation of the previous items requires resources for data collection, training, community engagement, and potentially enforcement mechanisms. While the implementation holds promise for strengthening social accountability, several challenges can hinder it. These challenges may be related to institutions, accreditation bodies, or communities.

Challenges for institutions include the following:

- Disaggregated data collection can be resource-intensive, require new reporting systems and analyzing this data and translating it into actionable insights can also be demanding [49].
- Fears of external influence on decision-making could arise when including community representatives in the accreditation team.

- Some transparency concerns may arouse as publicly reporting on shortcomings or negative outcomes can damage an institution's reputation.
- There might be resistance to disclose disaggregated data if it reveals inequalities.

Accreditation Bodies challenges may be summarized as following:

- Difficulty in standardization, where developing a fair and effective way to assess social accountability initiatives across diverse institutions can be difficult.
- Metrics need to be adaptable to different contexts.
- Some Accreditation bodies might lack the resources to train reviewers on social accountability frameworks and conduct in-depth community engagement.

Communities' challenges may include the following:

- Community members might lack the knowledge, skills, or resources needed to effectively participate in accreditation processes.
- Marginalized communities might be hesitant to participate with powerful institutions due to historical distrust or fear of retribution.
- Encouraging consistent community participation requires ongoing outreach and education efforts [50].

All the previous challenges should not deter efforts to strengthen social accountability in accreditation standards. By acknowledging these difficulties, institutions, accreditation bodies, and communities can work together to develop feasible strategies that lead to positive change.

Take Home Message

- Social accountability is an ongoing process, not a one-time fix. Sustaining efforts over time requires commitment from all stakeholders.
- Medical graduates should be well trained to address the health needs of the communities they serve.
- Accreditation standards can play a pivotal role in driving social accountability.
- Focusing on measurable outcomes, broadening stakeholder representation, and fostering transparency are essential criteria in accreditation process
- While incorporating social accountability into accreditation standards presents challenges for institutions, accreditation bodies and communities, efforts should be pursued by all three parties
- Institutions must embrace transparency and invest in data collection and community engagement. Accreditation bodies need to develop robust and adaptable frameworks for assessing social accountability. Finally, communities must be empowered to actively participate in shaping the education of future healthcare providers.

References

1. Murray RB, Larkins S, Russell H, Ewen S, Prideaux D. Medical schools as agents of change: socially accountable medical education. Med J Aust. 2012;196(10):653.
2. Greer PJ, Brown DR, Brewster LG, Lage OG, Esposito KF, Whisenant EB, et al. Socially accountable medical education: an innovative approach at Florida International University Herbert Wertheim College of Medicine. Acad Med. 2018;93(1):60–5.
3. Boelen C. Coordinating medical education and health care systems: the power of the social accountability approach. Med Educ. 2018;52(1):96–102.
4. Boelen C, Pearson D, Kaufman A, Rourke J, Woollard R, Marsh DC, et al. Producing a socially accountable medical school: AMEE Guide No. 109. Med Teach. 2016;38(11):1078–91.
5. Boelen C, Woollard R. Social accountability: the extra leap to excellence for educational institutions. Med Teach. 2011;33(8):614–9.
6. Boelen C, Dharamsi S, Gibbs T. The social accountability of medical schools and its indicators. Educ Health. 2012;25(3):180–94.
7. World Health Organization. Accreditation of Hospitals and Medical Education Institutes, challenges and future directions. Cairo: WHO, EMRO; 2005.
8. https://www.chea.org/
9. Bedoll D, van Zanten M, McKinley D. Global trends in medical education accreditation. Hum Resour Health. 2021;19:70. https://doi.org/10.1186/s12960-021-00588-x.
10. Duvivier RJ, Boulet JR, Opalek A, van Zanten M, Norcini J. Overview of the world's medical schools: an update. Med Educ. 2014;48(9):860–9. https://doi.org/10.1111/medu.12499.
11. Forcier MB, Simoens S, Giufrida A. Impact, regulation and health policy implications of physician migration in OECD countries. Hum Resour Health. 2004; https://doi.org/10.1186/1478-4491-2-12.
12. Boulet J, van Zanten M. Ensuring high-quality patient care: the role of accreditation, licensure, specialty certification and revalidation in medicine. Med Educ. 2014; https://doi.org/10.1111/medu.12286.
13. Van Zanten M, Boulet JR, Greaves I, Rothman A. Overview of accreditation of undergraduate medical education programmes worldwide. Med Educ. 2008;42(9):930–7.
14. LCME. Functions and structure of a Medical School, standards for accreditation of Medical Education Programmes leading to M.D. Degree March 2024. www.lcme.org
15. AMC. Assessment and Accreditation of Medical Schools: standards for assessment and accreditation of primary medical programmes July 2023. www.amc.org
16. Hamilton J. Medical Schools Accreditation: the Australian Experience. Commun Oriented Educ. 1993;6:231–42.
17. Hamilton J. Establishing standards and measurement methods for medical education. Acad Med 1995.
18. WHO. WHO guidelines for quality assurance of basic medical education in the Western Pacific Region. Manila: WHO, Regional Office for the Western Pacific; 2001.
19. WFME. Basic medical education WFME global standards for quality improvement. World Federation for Medical Education; 2003. www.wfme.org
20. Karle H. International recognition of basic medical education programmes. Med Educ. 2008;42(1):12–7.
21. Karle H. European specifications for global standards in medical education. Med Educ. 2007;41(10):924–5.
22. https://wfme.org/recognition/accrediting-agencies-status
23. GCSA. Global consensus for social accountability of medical schools. 2010. http://healthsocialaccountability.sites.olt.ubc.ca/files/2011/01/GCSA-Consensus-Document-English.pdf
24. Lindgren S, Karle H. Social accountability of medical education: aspects on global accreditation. Med Teach. 2011;33(8):667–72. https://doi.org/10.3109/0142159X.2011.590246.
25. IFMSA. IFMSA policy document social accountability of medical schools. 2024. https://ifmsa.org/social-accountability/

26. Donabedian A. The quality of care: how can it be assessed? JAMA. 1988;260(12):1743–8. https://doi.org/10.1001/jama.1988.03410120089033.
27. Accreditation Council for Graduate Medical Education. ACGME Common Programme Requirements 2022. 2022. https://www.acgme.org/what-we-o/accreditation/common-programme-requirements/
28. Council for the Accreditation of Educator Preparation. CAEP Standards 2022. 2022. https://caepnet.org/standards/introduction
29. Boelen C, Woollard B. Social accountability and accreditation: a new frontier for educational institutions. Med Educ. 2009;43(9):887–94. https://doi.org/10.1111/j.1365-2923.2009.03413.x.
30. Frenk J, Chen L, Bhutta ZA, Cohen J, Crisp N, Evans T, et al. Health professionals for a new century: transforming education to strengthen health systems in an interdependent world. Lancet. 2010;376(9756):1923–58. https://doi.org/10.1016/S0140-6736(10)61854-5.
31. Wallerstein NB, Duran B. Community-based participatory research contributions to intervention research: the intersection of science and practice to improve health equity. Am J Public Health. 2010;100(S1):S40–6. https://doi.org/10.2105/AJPH.2009.184036.
32. Frenk J, Chen L, Green AR, et al. The future of medical education: strengthening its social accountability. Med Teach. 1995;17(6):417–22.
33. World Health Organization (WHO). Guidance on social accountability in medical education. 2013. https://www.who.int/publications/i/item/defining-and-measuring-the-social-accountability-of-medical-schools
34. World Federation for Medical Education (WFME). Global standards for quality improvement for medical education programmes. n.d. https://www.wma.net/what-we-do/education/the-world-federation-for-medical-education/
35. Lilley PM, Harden RM. Standards and medical education. Med Teach. 2003;25(4):349–51.
36. WFME. WFME global standards for quality improvement in medical education, European specifications. Denmark: Quality Assurance Taskforce, WFME Office, University of Copenhagen; 2007. www.wfme.org
37. Boelen C, Blouin D, Gibbs T, Woollard R. Accrediting excellence for a medical school's impact on population health. Educ Health. 2019;32:41–8.
38. World Federation for Medical Education. WFME global standards for quality improvement in medical education. Copenhagen: WFME; 2020. https://wfme.org/standards/bme/
39. Abdalla ME. Social accountability of medical schools: do accreditation standards help promote the concept? J Case Stud Accredit Assess. 2014:3.
40. ACCM. Standards for Accreditation for Schools of medicine, 2021. https://accredmed.org/wp-content/uploads/2021/03/STANDARDS-OF-ACCREDITATION-FOR-SCHOOLS-OF-MEDICINE-March-2021.pdf
41. Committee on Accreditation of Canadian Medical Schools. CACMS Accreditation Standards; 2017. https://cacms-cafmc.ca/sites/default/fles/documents/CACMS_Standards_and_Elements_-_AY_2019-2020.pdf
42. Boelen C. Adapting the health care institutions and medical schools to societies needs. Acad Med. 1999;74(8 Supplement):S11–20.
43. Peabody JW. Measuring the social responsiveness of medical schools: setting the standards. Acad Med. 1999;74(8 Supplement):S59–68.
44. Boelen C, Boyer MH. A view of the world's medical schools: defining new roles. 2001. http://www.iaomc.org/WHOReptMedSchools.pdf
45. Association of American Medical Colleges (AAMC). Core Entrustable Professional Activities for Entering Residency. 2021, October. https://www.aamc.org/media/20211/download
46. Lindgren S, Karle H. Social accountability of medical education: aspects on global accreditation. Med Teach. 2011;33(8):667–72.
47. Kraft JM, Paina L, Boydell V, Elnakib S, Sihotang A, Bailey A, Tolmie C. Social Accountability Reporting for Research (SAR4Research): checklist to strengthen reporting on studies on social accountability in the literature. Int J Equity Health. 2022;21(Suppl 1):121. https://doi.org/10.1186/s12939-022-01716-2.

48. Hosny S, Ghaly M, Boelen C. Is our medical school socially accountable? The case of Faculty of Medicine, Suez Canal University. Med Teach. 2015;37(S1):S47–55. https://doi.org/10.3109/0142159X.2015.1006600.
49. Barber C, van der Vleuten C, Leppink J, Chahine S. Social accountability frameworks and their implications for medical education and programme evaluation: a narrative review. Acad Med. 2020;95(12):1945–54. https://doi.org/10.1097/ACM.0000000000003731.
50. Accreditation Council for Graduate Medical Education (ACGME). Common programme requirements. 2023. https://www.acgme.org/programmes-and-institutions/programmes/common-programme-requirements/

The manufacturer's authorised representative in the EU is Springer Nature Customer Service Centre GmbH, Europaplatz 3, 69115 Heidelberg, Germany. If you have any concerns regarding our products, please contact ProductSafety@springernature.com

Printed and bound by CPI Group (UK) Ltd, Croydon, CR0 4YY
01/10/2026
02225971-0013